# HEALTH AND HEALTHCARE IN INDIAN SUBCONTINENT

## By the Same Author

- Education in North East India: Experience & Challenge (Jointly Edited with Biloris Lyndem)
- Resource and Development in India: Special Focus on Tourism, Entrepreneurship and Natural Resources of North East.

---

## About the Editors

**Utpal Kumar De** is currently a Professor of Economics at the North Eastern Hill University, Shillong, Meghalaya, India. Prof. De has been teaching at post-graduate level since 1994. His research interests include agricultural economics and rural development, issues on environmental and natural resources, climate change adaptation, and empowerment of women. Prof. De has visited Europe and Asia in connection with research and delivered keynote and invited lectures at a number of conferences. Besides presenting over 60 research papers in various international and national conferences he has published 85 research articles in reputed national and international journals. His recent publications include *Inequality, Poverty and Development in India: Focus on the North-Eastern Region, Issues on Health and Healthcare in India: Focus on the North-Eastern Region*, both from Springer Nature Singapore Pvt. Ltd. and *Deprivation, Development and Empowerment of Women in India: North-East Perspectives,* from Bookwell, New Delhi.

**Premananda Bharati** is Professor (Retired) of the Biological Anthropology Unit, Indian Statistical Institute (ISI), Kolkata. His research interests include human biology, physical anthropology, growth, nutrition, poverty, gender issues, and demography. He has also taught at the Centre of Statistics, Human Sciences Research Council, Pretoria, South Africa. Professor Bharati was awarded the International Man of the Year (1993/94) by the International Biographical Centre, Cambridge, England; and Man of the Year 1994 by the American Biographical Institute, North Carolina, USA. He is a fellow of the Human Biology Association, Michigan, USA. He has published more than 100 research papers in journals of national and international repute and completed a number of research projects. He has visited America, Europe, and Asia extensively in connection with short-term courses and has delivered invited lectures and presented papers at various conferences.

# Health and Healthcare in Indian Subcontinent

## Special Focus on North East India

*Edited by*

Utpal Kumar De
Premananda Bharati

CONCEPT PUBLISHING COMPANY PVT. LTD.
NEW DELHI-110059

**ISBN-13: 978-93-86682-84-0**

First Published 2019

*Published and Printed by:*

Concept
Since 1974

**Concept Publishing Company Pvt. Ltd.**
A/15-16, Commercial Block, Mohan Garden,
New Delhi-110059 (INDIA)
*T* : +91 11 25351460, +91 11 25351794
*E* : publishing@conceptpub.com, *W* : www.conceptpub.com

**Cataloging in Publication Data**--Courtesy: D.K. Agencies (P) Ltd. <docinfo@dkagencies.com>

**National Seminar on "Poverty, Inequality and Health in India with Special Reference to North East India" (2015 : Shillong, India)**

Health and healthcare in Indian Subcontinent : special focus of North East India / edited by Utpal Kumar De, Premananda Bharati.

pages cm

"The volume is basically an outcome of the selected research papers presented in the National Seminar on "Poverty, Inequality and Health in India with Special Reference to North East India" held at North Eastern Hill University, Shillong, Meghalaya during 8-10 October, 2015 ..."--Acknowledgements.

Includes bibliographical references and index.

ISBN 9789386682840

1. Public health--India, Northeastern--Congresses. 2. Public health--Bangladesh--Congresses. 3. Medical care--India, Northeastern--Congresses. 4. Medical care--Bangladesh--Congresses. I. De, Utpal Kumar, 1968- editor. II. Bharati, Premananda, editor. III. North Eastern Hill University, host institution. IV. Title.

LCC RA530.N67N38 2015 | DDC 362.109541 23

# Preface

Health and healthcare are very important for the generation of human resource and thus occupied an important place in the UN Millennium Development Goals, which later on replaced with Sustainable Development Goals. This book is a comprehensive document on health and healthcare in Indian Subcontinent with a special focus on North East India. It covers a wide range of broad issues related to dimensions of health and healthcare in the subcontinent, connections of various socio-economic factors leading to health related issues, institutional mechanism and healthcare and role of education and pattern of nutritional intake on healthcare status as well. In depth statistical analyses of health and healthcare dynamics and its regional pattern are provided with empirical observations for the occurrence of drug resistant Tuberculosis, attitude of people towards the same and behaviours of HIV/AIDS among Female Sex Workers in Bangladesh.

Changing healthcare expenditure in India, its relation to economic reform and growth, along with the understanding of maternal and child healthcare and solutions to healthcare needs are some important aspects that have been addressed in this volume. Further, an innovative contingency theory of management of public health and government healthcare organisations are included in a separate section.

Also, multidisciplinary dimension of healthcare like deprivation across societies or social groups, and institutional arrangements are analysed in some chapters, which are crucial for addressing various healthcare issues in appropriate manner. The text also includes case studies substantiating theoretical models that would be helpful for the readers to cross-refer and understand others' perspectives.

Nutritional intake, which is directly related to the economic status and socio-economic relationship matters for the human development and performance of the workers in various sectors and that in turn affect nutritional intake through income. In many societies nutritional intake of women and girl children is comparatively poorer than that of men or boys. Also, it reflects an aspect of deprivation of women in the society. Education helps in removing such bottleneck significantly through changing human attitude and behaviour of several matters of health and hygiene. This volume also addressed some of these issues in a separate section.

Therefore, this book addressed a number of health and healthcare related issues with appropriate interactive analyses of healthcare and various socio-economic and institutional dimensions. Perspective on varied socio-cultural North East India also added a newer dimension of the analyses. This compilation would thus be of interest to students, researchers, professionals and policy-makers.

**Utpal Kumar De**
**Premananda Bharati**

# Acknowledgements

This volume *Health and Healthcare in Indian Subcontinent: Special Focus on North East India* is concentrated in some important aspects of health and healthcare in Indian sub-continent. Special attention is given to North East India. Moreover, the book addresses a number of healthcare issues in Bangladesh, in the pre- and post-reform period in India and of spatio-temporal pattern of healthcare in Orissa. Health care issues in Bangladesh are discussed in a number of chapters, e.g., the emergence of Multi-Drug Resistant (MDR) TB cases in Bangladesh, prevalence of HIV-AIDS among the female sex workers and their clients in Bangladesh and factors associated with cesarean delivery among women in Rajshahi city of Bangladesh.

The volume is basically an outcome of the selected research papers presented in the national seminar on "Poverty, Inequality and Health in India with special reference to North East India" held at North Eastern Hill University, Shillong, Meghalaya during 8-10 October, 2015, where over 200 researchers, academicians and practitioners presented their research outputs and expressed their views. Though it was a national level seminar, there were participants from many other countries like Bangladesh, Nepal, Australia, USA etc. Here selected papers after proper review and corrections have been included in this volume. We express our sincere thanks to all the scholars who presented their research outputs relevant to MDGs, particularly various aspects of healthcare.

Indian Statistical Institute, Kolkata and NABARD, Mumbai were the important parts of the programme. We sincerely acknowledge the contributions of these institutions for academic achievements. Prof. Manoranjan Pal of Economic Research Unit, Indian Statistical Institute, Kolkata took special initiative with other scholars for completing the review process and providing useful comments for the improvements of research papers presented in the conference. We offer our special gratitude from our side to him and his team for all sorts of cooperation.

Various socio-economic challenges related to health and healthcare which are given much stress in the Millennium Development Goals (MDGs) and studies on measures for solving health and healthcare as well as their statistical analyses are also incorporated in this volume.

Finally, we are thankful to Concept Publishing Company (P.) Ltd., New Delhi for taking necessary steps to publish this volume.

**Utpal Kumar De**
**Premananda Bharati**

# Contents

## PART 2
## SOCIO-ECONOMIC FACTORS AND HEALTH ISSUES



## PART 3
## INSTITUTION AND HEALTHCARE

## PART 4
## EDUCATION, NUTRITION AND HEALTH

## List of Contributors

**A.E. Cantanhêde,** Student in Business Administration at the Foundation Federal University of Rondônia, Brazil.
**E-mail:** *du-dek@hotmail.com*

**Atanu Sengupta,** Professor, Economics Department, Burdwan University, Burdwan-713104, West Bengal.
**E-mail:** *sengupta_atanu@yahoo.com*

**B.T. Langstieh,** Research Scholar, Department of Anthropology, NEHU, Shillong, Meghalaya. **E-mail:** *lagstieh.banrida@gmail.com*

**Dr. Bisworanjan Behuria,** Department of Geography, North Eastern Hill University, Shillong-793022, Meghalaya, India.
**E-mail:** *biswobehuria90@gmail.com*

**F. de São P. Filho,** Professor and Researcher at the Foundation Federal University of Rondônia, Brazil. **E-mail:** *flavio1954@gmail.com*

**Dr. Farhana Hasan,** Associate Professor, Department of Statistics, University of Rajshahi, Rajshahi-6205, Bangladesh.
**E-mail:** *fswatee07@yahoo.com*

**Ganesh Naskar,** Research Scholar, Department of Economics, University of Burdwan, Burdwan-713104, West Bengal.

**Gyan Chandra Kashyap,** Research Scholar, International Institute for Population Sciences, Govandi Station Road, Donor, Mumbai-400088, India. **E-mail:** *statskashyap@gmail.com*

**Himangshu Karmaker,** Regional Coordinator, TB CARE II Project, Rajshahi Division, Bangladesh. **E-mail:** *hossain95@yahoo.com*

**Hoineilam Kipgen,** Research Scholar, Department of Anthropology, NEHU, Shillong, Meghalaya. **E-mail:** *hoineilamkips@gmail.com*

**Ismail Hossain,** Department of Statistics, University of Rajshahi, Rajshahi-6205, Bangladesh. **E-mail:** *ismail_gm@ru.ac.bd*

**J.D.M. dos Santos,** Student in Business Administration at the Foundation Federal University of Rondônia, Brazil.
**E-mail:** *jose.moura.sd@hotmail.com*

**Jayashree Patil-Dake,** Faculty in Economics, KPB Hinduja College of Commerce, Mumbai-04, Maharashtra.
**E-mail:** *js_patil2001@rediffmail.com, jayashree.patil@gmail.com*

**Kakoli Choudhury,** Ph.D. scholar, Department of Sociology, Assam University, Silchar-788011, Assam. **E-mail:** *kakoli3001@gmail.com*

**Kh. Jitenkumar Singh,** Scientist-C, National Institute of Medical Statistics, ICMR, I-242, Ansari Nagar, AIIMS Campus, R.K. Puram, New Delhi-110029, New Delhi. **E-mail:** *jitensinghkh@gmail.*

**Laiamonriti P. Soh,** Research Scholar, Department of Commerce, North-Eastern Hill University, Shillong, Meghalaya.
**E-mail:** *laiamonriti4@gmail.com*

**Dr. Mauli Sanyal,** Assistant Professor, New Alipore College, 0/5, Durgapur Colony, Block L, New Alipore, Kolkata-700053, West Bengal. **E-mail:** *mauli_sanyal@yahoo.co.in*

**Dr. Md. Golam Hossain,** Professor of Health Research Group, Department of Statistics, University of Rajshahi, Rajshahi-6205, Bangladesh. **E-mail:** *hossain95@yahoo.com*

**Md. Masud Rana,** Department of Population Science & HR Development, University of Rajshahi, Rajshahi-6205, Bangladesh.
**E-mail:** *masud7648@gmail.com*

**Md. Rafiqul Islam,** Department of Population Science & HR Development, University of Rajshahi, Rajshahi-6205, Bangladesh.
**E-mail:** *skmri@yahoo.com*

**Dr. Md. Sabiruzzaman,** Associate Professor, Department of Statistics, University of Rajshahi, Rajshahi- 6205, Bangladesh.
**E-mail:** szsuza@ru.ac.bd

**N. Talita A. Nascimento,** Student in Business Administration at the Foundation Federal University of Rondônia, Brazil.
**E-mail:** *natalia.kimpos163@hotmail.com*

**Nayanakhee Sarma,** Department of Humanities and Social Science, Indian Institute of Technology, Guwahati-781039, Assam.
**E-mail:** *nayanakheesarma@gmail.com*

**Prahlad Kumar,** Professor, Department of Economics, University of Allahabad, Senate House, University Road, Old Katra, Allahabad-211002, Uttar Pradesh.
**E-mail:** *prahladkumar20_3@rediffmail.com*

**Rajiya Shahani,** Assistant Professor, Department of Sociology, Assam University, Silchar-788011, Assam.
**E-mail:** *rajiyasoc@yahoo.com*

**Sheikh Moin Uddin**, Population Services and Training Center (PSTC), 30, Shahid Shangbadik Selina Parveen Sarok (Old-103, New Circular Road), Dhaka-1217, Bangladesh. **Email:** moin.lipu@gmail.com

**Shri Kant Singh**, Professor, Department of Mathematical Demography & Statistics, International Institute for Population Sciences, Mumbai, Maharashtra. **E-mail:** *sksingh1992@yahoo.co.in*

**Dr. Sidhartha Sankar Laha,** Assistant Professor of Economics, Tufanganj Mahavidyalaya, Tufanganj, Suknirpar Dham, Andaran Phulbari, West Bengal-736159. **E-mail:** *sidharthasankar09@gmail.com*

**Sonam Gupta,** Research Scholar, Department of Economics, University of Allahabad, Senate House, University Road, Old Katra, Allahabad-211002, Uttar Pradesh.
**E-mail:** *guptasonam_31@rediffmail.com*

**Utpal Kumar De,** Professor, Department of Economics, North Eastern Hill University, Shillong-793022, Mehalaya.
**E-mail:** *utpalkde@gmail.com*

# Introduction

Apart from reduction in Poverty, inequality, promoting gender equality and empowerment of women, ensuring environmental sustainability some health related issues like reducing child mortality, improving maternal health and halting the spread of HIV/AIDS were very important UN Millennium Development Goals (MDGs) that were targeted to be achieved by 2015.

In this volume, we concentrate on various aspects of health and healthcare, which are given much stress in the MDGs. We selected the papers specific to health and health care and included on the basis of the quality and relevance to the present day situation.

Despite progress in several dimensions hunger, malnutrition and starvation deaths are common in many parts of the world, particularly in a number of countries in Asia and Sub-Saharan Africa. Health still remains a critical issue and without proper health human resource development remain incomplete, which is crucial for the overall progress of any country. Proportion of underweight children in India has come down from 43 per cent in 1998-99 to only 40 per cent in 2005-06. This proportion, for the children below 3 years, was expected to reach about 33 per cent by 2015. In this respect, discrimination between men and women is also prevalent in India. Moreover, there is also spatial variation in the achievement of nutritional intake. Some states have prevalence of underweight children above the national average. These states are namely Madhya Pradesh (57.9%), Bihar (54.9%), Jharkhand (54.6%), Chhattisgarh (47.8%), Meghalaya (42.9%), Uttar Pradesh (41.6%) and Gujarat (41.1%). Thus, it remains a challenge to achieve the target. The trend shows that MMR may come down to 140 per lakh population, which was above 31 points of the targeted figure of 2015. Also, in terms of infant mortality rate, India may be behind the target by 27 points in 2015. Several cases of malaria, incidences of malnutrition and work related hazards have been observed all over the country and that is also prevalent in North East India.

Nutritional intake, which is directly related to the economic status and socio-economic relationship matters for the human development and performance of the workers and that in turn affect nutritional intake through income. In many societies nutritional intake of women and girl children is comparatively poorer than that of men or boys. Also, it reflects an aspect of deprivation of women in the society.

From the above discussion it is clear that we could not achieve the MDGs in all targets and there are also significant spatial variations in healthcare, nutritional intake, healthcare infrastructure etc. Thus, it is high time we review our achievements and lapses incurred in comparison with the targets of the MDGs.

We hope that the readers of the volume will be highly benefited and be encouraged to do further studies to meet up the gaps which still remain. The research outputs presented here will also help the planners, politicians and the social workers.

We have divided the volume into four parts: 1. Health and Healthcare in Indian Subcontinent, 2. Socio-Economic Factors and Health Issues, 3. Institution and Healthcare, 4. Education, Nutrition and Health.

In Chapter 1, **Himangshu Karmaker** and **Golam Hossain** estimate the emergent issue of Multi-Drug Resistant (MDR) TB cases in Bangladesh. They observe prevalence of MDR TB mostly among males in the age group of 16-45 years. MDR or Non-MDR TB cases have a little role in developing MDR TB. The study would assist government to take different activities to save lives from MDR TB at most productive age and thus prevent economic loss.

In Chapter 2, "Healthcare Spending in India: Pre- and Post-Reforms Perspectives" have been examined by **Sidhartha Sankar Laha** using the Indian national data. India as a nation has been growing economically at a rapid pace particularly after the adoption of New Economic Policy. Rapid economic growth has not been accompanied by social development particularly health sector development. Health sector has been accorded very low priority in terms of allocation of resources. Public expenditure on health is less than one per cent of GDP in India. Growth rate during different macro-economic changes vary considerably across the states. There also exists a high inter-state variation in per capita health expenditure. The paper suggests for significant increase in healthcare expenditure across the states.

**Sheikh Moin Uddin** *et al.* tried to establish the relationship between Female sex workers (FSWs) and their clients are the major sources of spread of HIV/AIDS in Bangladesh. The purpose of the study is to find the high risk factors and testing behaviour of HIV among FSWs in urban area of Bangladesh. The age range of FSWs has been 16 to 41 years. More than 88 per cent of FSWs reported to have practicing unprotected sex because of client's insistence. FSWs that traded sex at residence, already tested for STI, were in the age group 21-30 years, and were found to be secondary and higher educated, came from rich family and mostly used condom and asked new clients for HIV testing. They also mention that authorities of the country should focus their HIV/AIDS prevention efforts on illiterate, married and poor FSWs. Consequently, FSWs are considered as a vulnerable group for spreading HIV/AIDS, authority should take steps to promote HIV testing for FSWs in Bangladesh.

Chapter 4 examines the temporal and spatial patterns of fertility in Odisha, a socio-economically lagging state of India. It also aims at finding the socio-economic factors affecting district level differentials in fertility in the state. Two indicators of fertility namely Crude Birth Rate (CBR) and Total Fertility Rate (TFR) have been used in this chapter. Besides, several district level socio-economic indicators such as female literacy rate, female work participation rate, percentage of non-agricultural worker, sex-ratio, level of urbanization, proportion of Scheduled Tribe and Scheduled Caste population, contraceptive prevalence rate and Infant Mortality Rate have been used to examine the association of fertility with socio-economic development. Findings show a declining trend of Crude Birth Rate and Total Fertility Rate in Odisha. The rate of decline was more consistent in 1990s and in the first decade of twenty first century as contrast to 1970s and 1980s. Regional divide in fertility rate is persistent in Odisha. It is observed that the degree of regional differences in CBR and TFR has increased over time. District-level analyses reveal that the women's agency (female literacy and female work participation) has significant negative effect on fertility. Economic prosperity and use of modern contraceptives have also some role in influencing fertility in the state.

In the fifth chapter, **Farhana Hasan** *et al.* aim to determine the prevalence and factor associated with cesarean delivery among women in Rajshahi city, Bangladesh. Considering drastic prevalence of caesarean delivery, this study demonstrates that the roles of selected risk factors are not the main source of influence on the rate of caesarean delivery. The c-section delivery is more costly than vaginal deliveries, and there are many risks for cesarean deliveries. Consequently, health authorities improve policy to make awareness among the women in Bangladesh for vaginal deliveries.

Chapter 6 attempts to understand the various determinants of utilisation of maternal and child health care services among the Thadou-Kuki of Manipur. An anthropological fieldwork has been conducted among 560 ever married women aged between 15 and 49 years. The findings of the study reveals that majority of deliveries happen to be at home and less in hospital.

**Gyan Chandra Kashyap** and **Shri Kant Singh** in chapter 7 evaluate the pattern and correlates of tobacco use and quitting tobacco among smokers as well as users of smokeless tobacco. This study finds that the trend of use of tobacco in upward direction, whereas the probability of quitting is very low in Northeast. Reduction in tobacco consumption is advised for avoiding the health risks and ban on smoking in public places and workplaces, comprehensive bans on advertising and promotion of such products are prescribed.

The chapter 8 by **Laiamonriti P. Soh** examines the challenges faced by India to meet the increasing patient population needs and how innovative solutions help in addressing such challenges. The buzz around innovation in health care and its services has been steadily increasing over the past few years. Innovation in healthcare today is no longer a luxury but a necessity. Indian healthcare industry has a huge scope for investing in new specialty/ multi-specialty hospitals or expansion of existing facilities in recent years and installation of advanced equipments and technology up gradation. These factors would enable healthcare players to serve the increasing patient population to access qualitative diagnosis and treatment at adorable price models. Private healthcare is coming forth as one of the fastest growing sectors in India, with chain hospital explorations into various cities. Further, various states have launched innovative initiatives to attract Public Private Partnership (PPP) investments into healthcare. These PPP initiatives may help in improving the infrastructure and healthcare provisions in the country and at the same time introduce various healthcare innovations.

**Natália Talita Araújo Nascimento** *et al.* in chapter 9 examines the causal relationship between the confrontation between an environment and an individual that is defended by Contingency Theory of Management in the Public Health Government (hospital) services organizations. The study is done through the qualitative analysis, by questionnaires from stakeholders in the location of investigations and by support from the focus group. The results of individual behaviour are described after investigation in the context of the processes of the service delivery. The participation of social actors in the interaction with the public body in order to infer in the quality of service delivery is analysed. Following the scientific recommendations, the citizen participation in the projects can improve this process. This research activity contributes as an academic tool for improvement of the service delivery quality offered by public institutions. The findings and suggestions developed from the analysis of data obtained from employees delivering services and the service users would be used to diagnose the necessities and opportunities aiming the elaboration of government policies for the process of community development.

**Atanu Sengupta** and **Ganesh Naskar** (chapter 10) capture three dimensions of the inequity apparatus—social, economic and residential (Rural and Urban) and observe that deprivation in the North East India was manifold and often cumulative. Inequity in one dimension enhances inequity of other dimension. For example rural poor *Dalit* family is worse off than the richer, upper caste urban households in North East India. It appears that a prolong attack across the dimensions is necessary to fight this evil. For our analysis we have used the household level data pertaining to the NSSO 60th Round (January-June 2004) survey. Their analysis revealed that across the states of North East India, socially and economically deprived classes are always in a disadvantageous position in regards to health infrastructure provision. However, inequity has been much less in developed states in comparison to the relatively backward regions of North East India.

In chapter 11, **Sonam Gupta** and **P. Kumar** examines budget allocation and expenditure, the utilization and per capita investment etc. for health and family welfare in India as a whole and for states separately. They also propose to analyse the comparative status of North-Eastern states (Arunachal Pradesh, Assam, Manipur, Meghalaya, Mizoram, Nagaland and Tripura) *vis-à-vis* rest of the states in respect of the above variables.

**Nayanakhee Sarma** (chapter-12) however tries to see if there is difference in effective functioning of ICDS in selected rural and urban areas of Assam and how community participation and involvement of women in ICDS increase its effectiveness. The study is based on both secondary and primary data. The analysis of the primary data collected from the Anganwadi Workers and mothers whose children attend Anganwadi centre. The second part of the analysis is devoted to comparing difference between the effectiveness of rural and urban and to know if the differences are statistically significant Mann Whitney U test has been used since the data collected were categorical in nature. Today ICDS has spread to every block in Assam but still gap exist in terms of available infrastructure, coverage by health personnel, regularity of supplementary nutrition etc. There is also significant presence of underweight children under the Anganwadi centres.

*Masud Rana et al.*, in chapter 13 tries to assess the knowledge about TB among Rajshahi University students in Bangladesh. The study finds the lack of basic knowledge about TB among the university students. Consequently, health education programme is needed to improve the knowledge among university students regarding TB. Government should take initiative to form a medical team to sensitize the non-medical university students.

**Rajiya Shahani** and **Kakoli Choudhury** on the other hand, in their study examine the impact of education on hygiene and sanitation practices among Scheduled Caste People. It also explores the effect of other socio-economic indicators on health condition of the Scheduled Caste People. The study has been conducted in Silchar town of Cachar District in Assam. Poverty and education are found to be principle reasons for choosing traditional sanitation practices in the area.

**Kh. Jitenkumar Singh** in chapter 15 assesses the prevalence of EBF and associated factors among mothers having children age 0-6 months in North East India. The study concludes that prevalence of EBF was low in the region. The length of median duration of EBF is 2 month. Strengthening health education programmes such as infant feeding advice/counselling both at the community and institutional levels targeting to mother who are residing in urban areas, more educated and are from wealthier households may be necessary.

In the last chapter on non-communicable disease (NCD) epidemic, **Mauli Sanyal** suggests that the poor are equally affected by NCDs. Considering the formidable costs of treatment for NCDs and lack of adequate financial coverage by the state, out-of-pocket expenditure emerges as the principle mode of health care financing. This leads to impoverishment and financial catastrophe for the poor. The chapter identifies a vicious cycle involving incidence of diseases, health care utilization in terms of hospitalization and financial impoverishment. Again the inter-state variation involving these parameters is noteworthy. A short study of the situation prevailing in the North-Eastern states of India has been attempted for in this regard. The analysis is crucial because in the presence of any anomaly between the development programmes and the target group, the victim will be none other than the economically weak and the deprived.

The book, therefore, captures some important aspects of health and healthcare in Indian sub-continent and North East India occupied a special space in this volume. I am sure that the interactive analyses of healthcare with various socio-economic and institutional aspects presented in this book will benefit the students, researchers, academicians and policy-makers as well.

The book, therefore, addresses a wide range of issues including tourism and hospitality aspects of development, entrepreneurship and socio-economic development interface, which are crucial for understanding overall progress of a region. Also, it provides the guidelines for the future actions by the policy-makers and further studies to unearth other related socio-economic issues concerning welfare. The volume, therefore, will surely attract the researchers, academicians and policy-makers and benefit all sections of readers.

**Utpal Kumar De**
**Premananda Bharati**

# PART 1

# Health and Healthcare in Indian Subcontinent

# 1
# Pattern of Drug Resistant Tuberculosis at Northern Part of Bangladesh and Associated Risk Factors

*Himangshu Karmaker* and *Md. Golam Hossain*

## Introduction

Tuberculosis (TB) is a major Public health problem in Bangladesh since long. The history of Tuberculosis in Bangladesh has different stages. In 1965, tuberculosis services were mainly curative and based in TB clinics and TB hospitals. TB services were expanded to 124 Upazila Health Complexes (UHCs) during the 2nd Health and Population Plan (1980-86), and were operationally integrated to Leprosy during the 3rd Health Population Plan (1986-91) under the Mycobacterium Disease Control (MBDC) unit of the Directorate General of Health Service (DGHS). The National TB Control Programme (NTP) adopted the revised DOTS strategy during the 4th Population and Health plan (1992-98) under the project "Further Development of TB and Leprosy Control Services". The NTP started its field implementation in November 1993 in four Thanas (Upazilas) and progressively expanded to cover all Upazilas by mid 1998. The NTP was integrated into the Communicable Disease Control component of the Essential Service Packages under the Health and Population Sector Programme (HPSP). In 2003, HPSP was renamed as Health Nutrition and Population Sector Programme (HNPSP) (2003-2011). Now, Ministry of Health and Family Welfare (MOHFW) has been implementing the Health Population and Nutrition Sector Development Programme (HPNSDP) for a period of five years from July 2011 to June 2016. In all the sector programmes tuberculosis control programme has been recognized as one of the priority programme (National Guidelines and Operational Manual for Tuberculosis Control 5th Edition, 2014). The programme is maintaining the high treatment success rates from the beginning and met the target of 85 per cent treatment success since 2003. The programme has been maintaining the treatment success rate of new smear positive cases over 90 per cent since 2006. Regarding case notification of NSP cases, the programme made slow and steady progress till 2003. Since then due to multi–sectoral approach and support from development partners the notification rate increased from 40 in 2003 to 61 in 2005 and 73 in 2006. Afterwards, the case notification rate remain static till 2008, and in 2009 it increased slightly to reach the peak of 74/1,00,000 population. Since 2010 the notification rate is showing a decreasing trend with 70.5 and 65 per 1,00,000 populations in 2010 and 2011 respectively. During 2012 finally, it was 70 and in 2013 it became 68/1,00,000 Population.

*Global Situation:* Tuberculosis (TB) remains one of the world's deadliest communicable diseases. In 2013, an estimated 9.0 million people developed TB and 1.5 million died from the disease, 3,60,000 of whom were HIV-positive. Worldwide, the proportion of new cases with multidrug-resistant TB (MDR-TB) was 3.5 per cent in 2013 and has not changed compared with recent years. Of the estimated 9 million people who developed TB in 2013, more than half (56%) were in the South-East Asia and Western Pacific Regions. India and China alone accounted for 24 per cent and 11 per cent of total cases, respectively. Globally, the TB mortality rate fell by an estimated 45 per cent between 1990 and 2013 and the TB prevalence rate fell by 41 per cent during the same period. Progress needs to accelerate to reach the Stop TB Partnership targets of a 50 per cent reduction by 2015 (Global TB Report, WHO, 2014).

*Global MDR-TB situation:* Globally, 3.5 per cent of new and 20.5 per cent of previously treated TB cases was estimated to have had MDR-TB in 2013. This translates into an estimated 4,80,000 people having developed MDR-TB in 2013. On average, an estimated 9.0 per cent of patients with MDR, TB had extensively drug resistant TB (XDR-TB). In 2013, 1,36,000 MDR Cases were diagnosed and notified. A total of 97,000 patients were started on MDR-TB treatment in 2013, a three-fold increase compared with 2009. The most recent treatment outcome data are for patients started on MDR-TB treatment in 2011. Globally the success rate was 48 per cent. Five of the 27 high MDR-TB burden countries achieved a treatment success rate of 70 per cent (Global TB Report, WHO, 2014).

*MDR situation at Bangladesh:* At present, MDR-TB cases in Bangladesh are relatively low and a few XDR-TB Cases exist. Along with the present MDT-TB Case load, Bangladesh falls into the category of High MDR-TB Burden Country and ranks 11th among 27 such High MDR TB Burden Countries. The NTP has carried out its first nation-wide Drug Resistance Survey in Tuberculosis Patients in collaboration with WHO and SNRL, ANTWERP, Belgium in 2010-2011. The result shows the overall number of MDR-TB cases is low, 1.4 per cent among new cases and 28.5 per cent among retreatment cases. Although, the rates of MDR TB in Bangladesh do not appear to be high, the absolute number of MDR-TB Cases is higher considering the overall high TB burden. MDT-TB prevalence of 1.4 per cent in new cases and 28.5 per cent in Retreatment cases translate approximately an estimate of 4,496 MDR-TB cases among notified TB cases in 2013 (National Guidelines and Operational Manual for Programmatic Management of Drug Resistant TB - PMDT). In August 2008 NIDCH started enrollment of MDR-TB patients with GLC approved 24 months regimen and supported by the Global Fund. By the end of December 2013 a total of 1301 confirmed MDR-TB patients including 330 in 2013 have been enrolled. As a part of Programmatic Management of Drug Resistance TB (PMDT) plan NTP established one Regional TB Reference Laboratory (NTRL) at Chest Disease Hospital (CDH) of Chittagong in 2011 and also managing MDR-TB patients from that year. In 2013 NTP has also started managing MDR-TB in CDH Pabna and Khulna. The MDR-TB patients are also managed in the CDH of Rajshahi division and in three other hospitals of Damien Foundation at Jalchatra under Tangail Hospital, Anantapur under Netrakona District and Shambhuganj under Mymensingh district with shorter regimen of 9 months and supported by Damien Foundation, Bangladesh under operational Research. Since May 2005 those centres have been managing MDR-TB patients, and by end of December 2013 a total of 1161 patients including 189 in 2013 have been enrolled (National Guidelines and Operational Manual for Programmatic Management of Drug Resistant TB - PMDT).

From the above discussion, we can have a clear picture of the problem of MDR-TB case diagnosis and management situation in Bangladesh. In comparison with the yearly estimation, the diagnosis is very low. In 2011, 2012 and 2013 we could diagnose only 10 per cent, 12 per cent and 15 per cent of the estimated cases. From this point of view this research has been designed and aimed to know the real situation that can make us think in new way.

## Study Objectives

*General Objective:* To collect information and data from diagnosed DR TB patients to know the DR TB pattern and assess the risk factors associated for developing DR TB.

*Specific Objectives*

- To list diagnosed DR TB cases from functioning diagnostic and treatment facilities of Rajshahi and Rangpur Division.
- To Interview each patient.
- To Review available documents.
- To find out the patterns of DR TB and risk factors behind developing DR TB.
- To know the socio-economic and demographic characteristics of DR TB Patients.

## Literature Review

To conduct a survey or study, it is very important to review related books, documents, abstracts, articles etc. Accordingly, I have to searched and gone through different literature.

The most important book that I found is the Global TB report 2014 by WHO. This was published in September 2014 and it contains the latest Global situation of all aspects of TB and this data are used by all as reference. TB is present in all regions of the world and the Global Tuberculosis Report 2014 includes data compiled from 202 countries and territories (Global TB Report, WHO, 2014).

Several studies were reviewed on risk factors of MDR-TB on Bangladesh and other country perspective. On Bangladesh perspective, the study conducted by Dr. Mahfuza Rifat *et al.* is mentionable. The title of the study was mentioned as "Development of multidrug resistant tuberculosis in Bangladesh: a case-control study on risk factors". The objective of the study was to determine the risk factors for developing multidrug resistant tuberculosis in Bangladesh.

Another study was reviewed namely "Risk factors of multidrug resistant tuberculosis in central Nepal: a pilot study." This study was conducted by Marahatta, S.B., Kaewkungwal, J., Ramasoota, P., Singhasivanon, P. They mentioned in their study that Tuberculosis is the most widespread infectious disease in Nepal and poses a serious threat to the health and development of the country. Incidences of drug resistant tuberculosis in Nepal are increasing and this tuberculosis a major threat to successfully controlling tuberculosis. The general objective of the study was to assess the risk factors of multi-drug resistant tuberculosis among the patients attending the National Tuberculosis Centre, Bhaktpur Nepal.

A literature was found in an Indian Health journal named "Operational Research for Healthcare". In its Volume 1, Issues 2–3, June–September 2012, Pages 45–53, there was a study on "Drug-resistant tuberculosis in Mumbai, India: An agenda for operations research". This study describes the status of MDR-TB at Mumbai City, associated risk factors and need for operational research in the field. The research say that Multidrug-resistant TB is a significant problem in Mumbai, India's most populous city, and there have been recent reports of totally resistant TB. The study attempts to summarize the major challenges to TB control in Mumbai, with an emphasis on drug resistance.

There was a study which was conducted in Nepal and published in the official website of Health Research and Social Development Forum Thapathali, Kathmandu, Nepal under completed research category by name "Risk factors of MDR-TB: a case control study in selective DOTS Plus Clinics in Nepal". The study was conducted to identify the risk factors for MDR-TB among people with MDR-TB registered in National TB control programme at selected DOTS plus clinics in Nepal. The findings of the study say that more than a quarter of the respondents were engaged in job or private business (28.1% and 27.6% respectively in cases and controls). Likewise, almost similar proportion was daily wage labourer and students. Nearly, half of the cases (48.2%)

worked more than eight hours a day as compared to 34.2 per cent among the controls (http://www.herd.org.np/resources/research-survey/risk-factors-mdr-tb-case-control-study-selective-dots-plus-clinics-nepal).

I reviewed a study published in the Indian journal of tuberculosis on 28-12-2011 namely "An epidemiological study of multi-drug resistance tuberculosis cases registered under revised National Tuberculosis control programme of Ahemadabad City". The study was conducted by Geneyaa Bhatt, Sheetal Vyas and Kartik Trivedi. The study was initiated to study socio-demographic profile, housing environment, health-seeking behaviour, present and past-history regarding the treatment of tuberculosis, drug resistance patterns and the preventive practice adopted by the patients (Bhatt, 2011).

## Research Materials and Methodology

It was a Cross-sectional Descriptive study.

*Study Area:* Eight districts under Rajshahi division and 8 districts under Rangpur division. They are: Bogra, Joypurhat, Natore, Naogaon, Nawabgonj, Pabna, Rajshahi, Sirajgonj, Dinajpur, Gaibanda, Kurigram, Lalmonirhat, Nilphamary, Panchagar, Rangpur, Thakurgaon.

*Study Period:* The period of the study was May 2014 to December 2014.

*Study Population:* The target population included all enrolled MDR-TB patients at Rajshahi Chest Disease Hospital and Pabna Chest Disease Hospital. Also some MDR patients of selected study area who were diagnosed and registered at NIDCH, but taking treatment at selected study area are also included.

*Sampling Technique:* Non-random purposive sampling technique is used for selecting the sample. All registered patients during 2013 and 2014 at Pabna and Rajshah CDH are taken into consideration. Finally, 164 respondents are included to avoid dropout and to confirm the size. As the number of patients of Pabna hospital are less, maximum of them are included. For Rajshahi, maximum are taken from 2014 and rest to meet target, taken from 2013. By doing this, 15 districts out of 16 are covered and no sample could be found from Panchagar district.

*Inclusion criteria:* All registered and treatment started MDR patients from defined divisions are included.

*Exclusion criteria:* Registered at Rajshahi and Pabna CDH but resident of out of the study area are excluded from the study to make it confined within Rajshahi and Rangpur divisions.

*Data Collection Method:* To collect the data, available registers, treatment cards of individual patients maintained and preserved at Rajshahi and Pabna CDH are reviewed. Secondary data are collected from those cards and registers. Afterwards, direct interview method with respondents is used to collect primary data in this study. Data are collected following pre-designed and approved questionnaire by study supervisor.

*Data Management:* The completed questionnaire was collected and checked for the completeness and clarity of the information to exclude missing or inconsistent data and then compiled together. Data was edited properly before analysis. A Excel Spreadsheet as master document was prepared first. Data analysis was done through SPSS 16.0.

*Data Analysis:* Final analysis of the data was carried out using percentage, absolute numbers for categorical variables in IBM SPSS 16.0. For some purpose Excel programme was also used.

## Results

The study has been conducted in 16 districts of Rajshahi and Rangpur Division. From the MDR register of Pabna and Rajshahi CDH, all patients registered during 2013 and 2014 were listed and selected for interviewed. 164 patients were enrolled from total registration. Seven patients, who were registered at NIDCH, but taken treatment at study area under supervision of Pabna CDH, were included. Finally, 106 respondents from Rajshahi CDH, 51 patients from Pabna and 7 from NIDCH make 164 all together.

**Table 1.1:** Distribution of Respondents by Sex

| *Sex* | *Respondents* | |
|---|---|---|
| | *No.* | *(%)* |
| Male | 113 | 68.9 |
| Female | 51 | 31.1 |
| **Total** | **164** | **100** |

*Source:* Data collected from Rangpur division, Bangladesh.

**Table 1.2:** Distribution of Respondents by Age

| *Age group (in years)* | *Respondents* | | | | | |
|---|---|---|---|---|---|---|
| | *Male* | | *Female* | | *Total* | |
| | *No.* | *(%)* | *No.* | *(%)* | *No.* | *(%)* |
| 6 – 15 | 2 | 40 | 3 | 60 | 5 | 3 |
| 16 – 25 | 31 | 57 | 23 | 43 | 54 | 33 |
| 26 – 35 | 32 | 67 | 16 | 33 | 48 | 29 |
| 36 – 45 | 21 | 78 | 6 | 22 | 27 | 16 |
| 46 – 55 | 10 | 77 | 3 | 23 | 13 | 8 |
| 56 – 65 | 11 | 100 | 0 | 0 | 11 | 7 |
| 66 – 75 | 4 | 100 | 0 | 0 | 4 | 2 |
| 75+ | 2 | 100 | 0 | 0 | 2 | 1 |
| **Total** | **113** | **69** | **51** | **31** | **164** | **100** |

*Source:* Data collected from Rangpur division, Bangladesh.

From Table 1.2 the most vulnerable age for MDR-TB can be marked as 16 to 45. In this group total number of respondents is 129 which is 79 per cent of total respondents. This is the most productive age group for human life while this group is mostly vulnerable for MDR TB as well as non-MDR TB. If we check it in more specific, we can see that the highest number is from 16 – 25 (33%) age group, second highest is from 26 – 35 (29%) age group and third one id from 36 – 45 (16%) age group. The result is quite significant and interesting.

## Geographical Distribution of Respondents

Table 1.3, shows the division and district-wise distribution of 164 respondents. 72.6 per cent respondents are from Rajshahi division and only 27.4 per cent respondents are from Rangpur division. It is clear that most MDR cases are detected at Rajshahi division. There may be a gap of surveillance at Rangpur division or there may have other reason which could be explored by further study.

Huge variety of occupation was noted and those occupations are finally grouped in to 9. Male has more variety in occupation than female. The data shows that among female most are housewife and they are 18 per cent among total. For male, most are Farmer and they are 21 per cent among total. There is a good number of Students among male and female. Student occupies 14 per cent

**Table 1.3:** Division and District-wise Distribution of Respondents

| Sl. No. | Districts | Respondents | | | | | |
|---|---|---|---|---|---|---|---|
| | | Male | | Female | | Total | |
| | | No. | (%) | No. | (%) | No. | (%) |
| 1. | Bogra | 9 | 56 | 7 | 44 | 16 | 10 |
| 2. | Joypurhat | 3 | 60 | 2 | 40 | 5 | 3 |
| 3. | Naogaon | 11 | 85 | 2 | 15 | 13 | 8 |
| 4. | Natore | 4 | 100 | 0 | 0 | 4 | 2 |
| 5. | Nawabgonj | 3 | 75 | 1 | 25 | 4 | 2 |
| 6. | Pabna | 16 | 59 | 11 | 41 | 27 | 16 |
| 7. | Rajshahi | 17 | 81 | 4 | 19 | 21 | 13 |
| 8. | Sirajgonj | 20 | 69 | 9 | 31 | 29 | 18 |
| **Total** | Rajshahi Division | 83 | 70 | 36 | 30 | 119 | 73 |
| 9. | Dinajpur | 1 | 100 | 0 | 0 | 1 | 1 |
| 10. | Gaibanda | 9 | 64 | 5 | 36 | 14 | 9 |
| 11. | Kurigram | 3 | 38 | 5 | 63 | 8 | 5 |
| 12. | Lalminirhat | 1 | 50 | 1 | 50 | 2 | 1 |
| 13. | Nilphamari | 5 | 83 | 1 | 17 | 6 | 4 |
| 14. | Panchagar | 0 | 0 | 0 | 0 | 0 | 0 |
| 15. | Rangpur | 8 | 67 | 4 | 33 | 12 | 7 |
| 16. | Thakurgaon | 2 | 100 | 0 | 0 | 2 | 1 |
| **Total** | Rangpur Division | 29 | 64 | 16 | 36 | 45 | 27 |
| | **Grand Total** | **112** | **68** | **52** | **32** | **164** | **100** |

*Source:* Data collected from Rangpur division, Bangladesh.

**Table 1.4:** Occupation-wise Distribution of Respondents

| Sl. No. | Occupation | Respondents | | | | | |
|---|---|---|---|---|---|---|---|
| | | Male | | Female | | Total | |
| | | No. | (%) | No. | (%) | No. | (%) |
| 1. | Farmer | 35 | 100 | 0 | 0 | 35 | 21 |
| 2. | House wife | 0 | 0 | 29 | 100 | 29 | 18 |
| 3. | Student | 12 | 52 | 11 | 48 | 23 | 14 |
| 4. | Garments Worker | 6 | 43 | 8 | 57 | 14 | 9 |
| 5. | Service | 6 | 86 | 1 | 14 | 7 | 4 |
| 6. | Business | 10 | 100 | 0 | 0 | 10 | 6 |
| 7. | Day Labour | 13 | 87 | 2 | 13 | 15 | 9 |
| 8. | Transport worker | 6 | 100 | 0 | 0 | 6 | 4 |
| 9. | Other | 24 | 96 | 1 | 4 | 25 | 15 |
| | **Total** | **113** | **68** | **51** | **32** | **164** | **100** |

*Source:* Data collected from Rangpur division, Bangladesh.

among total respondents. Garment Sector is the high risk place for TB incidence. It is also displayed in Table 1.4, that nine per cent of the total respondents are in this occupation. Several other occupation of male consist a good percentage of MDR TB. Besides, all sorts of day labour accounts for 9 per cent, different service occupy 4 per cent and business occupies 6 per cent among the respondents.

**Table 1.5:** Educational level of Respondents

| *Education level* | *Respondents* | | | | | |
|---|---|---|---|---|---|---|
| | *Male* | | *Female* | | *Total* | |
| | *No.* | *(%)* | *No.* | *(%)* | *No.* | *(%)* |
| No Education | 39 | 73 | 14 | 27 | 53 | 32 |
| Class 1 -- 5 | 30 | 67 | 15 | 33 | 45 | 28 |
| Class 6 – <SSC | 24 | 69 | 11 | 31 | 35 | 21 |
| SSC + HSC | 15 | 60 | 10 | 40 | 25 | 15 |
| Graduate + | 5 | 80 | 1 | 20 | 6 | 3 |
| **Total** | **113** | **69** | **51** | **31** | **164** | **100** |

*Source:* Data collected from Rangpur division, Bangladesh.

Table 1.5 shows that a high number of respondents have no education. The percentage of no education is 32 per cent. Twenty eight per cent of respondent has an educational level from class 1 – class 5 which is very preliminary level.

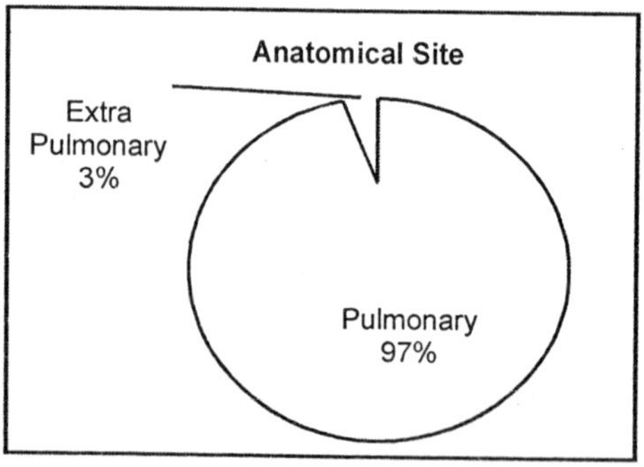


**Fig. 1.1:** Anatomical site of TB among Respondents

*Source:* Data collected from Rangpur division Bangladesh.

Figure 1.1, we can see that most of the MDR cases have pulmonary TB (97%). Only 3 per cent have Extra Pulmonary MDR-TB.

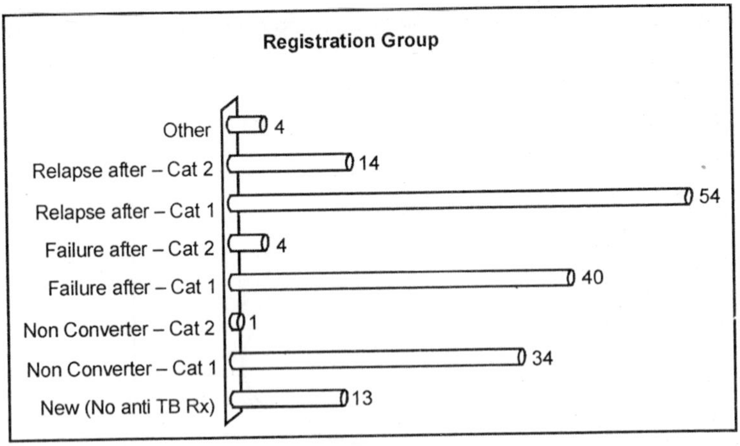


**Fig. 1.2:** Registration Group of the Respondents
*Source:* Data collected from Rangpur division, Bangladesh.

Registration group are determined based on previous treatment history of MDR cases. Here, in this figure, it shows that most of the MDR-TB cases fall in the group of Relapse after receiving Category 1 treatment. It consist 33 per cent among total. Next high group is Failure after Receiving Category 1 treatment and it is 24 per cent among total. Non-Converter after category 1 treatment also has high number which is 21 per cent. One interesting finding is that MDR patients who never took any anti-TB treatment consist 8 per cent among total. If we make a total, we can see that 88 per cent of the respondents are from new or first time treatment group and 12 per cent from re treatment group.

**Table 1.6:** Monthly Family Income of the Respondents

| *Family Income (BDT/Month)* | *No. of Respondent* | *%* |
|---|---|---|
| ≤ 10000 | 105 | 64 |
| 10001 - 20000 | 49 | 30 |
| ≥ 20001 | 10 | 6 |
| **Total** | **164** | **100** |

*Source:* Data collected from Rangpur division, Bangladesh.

During the interview it was difficult to translate monthly income of respondents in to *taka*. Finally, a figure could be worked out asking probing questions. It is observed from the table that most of the respondents fall under group of BDT =10,000. It consist 64 per cent among the total. In 2nd group there are 49 respondents which consist of 30 per cent among total. Another 6 per cent comes from the group of ≥20,001, which is very few in number among total respondents. In general we can say that most of the MDR-TB patients are from very low income group.

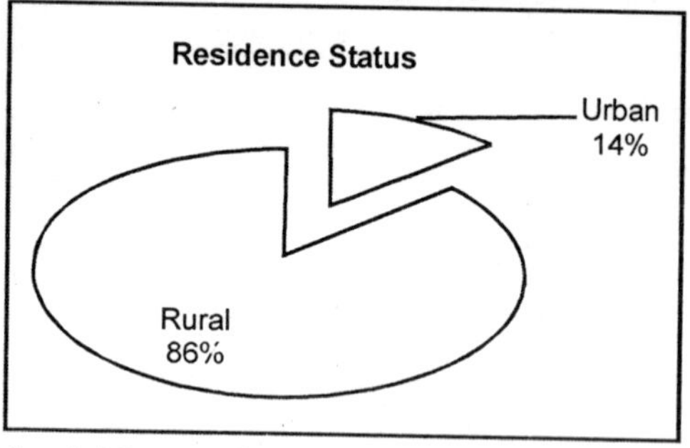


**Fig. 1.3:** Residential Status of Respondents

*Source:* Data collected from Rangpur division, Bangladesh.

Figure 1.3, we can see that most respondents are from rural area (86%) and only 14 per cent are from urban area.

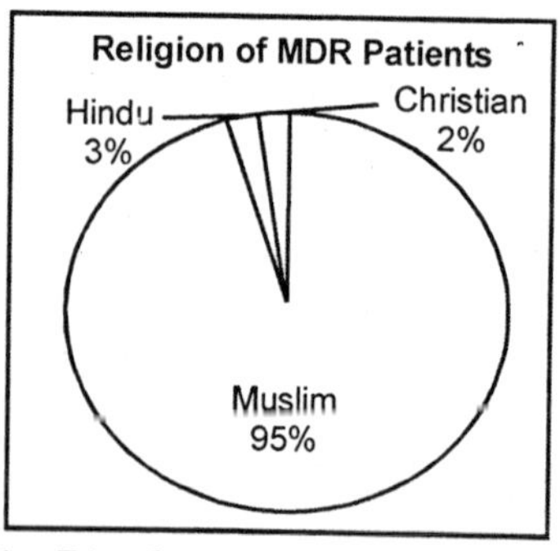


**Fig. 1.4:** Religion wise Distribution of Respondents

*Source:* Data collected from Rangpur division, Bangladesh.

Figure 1.4 shows that among 164 respondents, 95% are Muslim, 3 per cent Hindu and 2 per cent Christian.

**Table 1.7:** History of Previous Anti-TB Treatment among Respondents

| *Previous $R_x$* | *No. of Respondents* | *Regularity Maintained No. (%)* | *DOT maintained No. (%)* |
|---|---|---|---|
| Episode – 1 | 150 | 139 (93) | 126 (84) |
| Episode – 2 | 20 | 15 (75) | 15 (75) |
| Episode – 3 | 1 | 1 (100) | 1 (100) |

*Source:* Data collected from Rangpur division, Bangladesh.

After compiling and analysing the response, Table 1.7 shows that 150 respondents have received one episode of anti-TB treatment of any duration among 164. Among those 150, 139 took the treatment regularly (93%) and 126 took the treatment under DOT (84%). Table 1.7, we can find that 20 respondents among 164 received 2 episodes of treatment. Among those 20, 15 (75%) took the treatment regularly and 15 (75%) took the treatment under DOT. Only one respondent found among 164, who received 3rd episode which is actually treatment of MDR-TB. That was 9 month regimen and he failed that treatment.

History of contact with known TB cases, DR or Non DR TB, was checked during interview with respondent. Table 1.8, we can see that only 44 MDR-TB case has a history of contact with known TB cases (27%). Among 44 cases, 20 (45%) have a history of contact with known DR TB patients and 24 have history of contact with non-DR TB patients. The contact cases are also divided in to 2 groups – family members and non-family members. It is found Table 1.8, that 27 (61%) MDR cases among 44, have contact TB patients within their family members and 17 (39%) have contact with known TB cases who are not their family member.

**Table 1.8:** History of having Contact with Known TB cases by Respondents

| *Contact History* | *No. of Respondents* | *% of Yes and No* | *Contact with DR TB* | *Contact with Non DR TB* | *Contact is Family Member* | *Contact is Non-Family member* |
|---|---|---|---|---|---|---|
| Yes | 44 | 27 | 20 | 24 | 27 | 17 |
| No | 119 | 73 | | | | |
| **Total** | **163** | **100** | **45%** | **55%** | **61%** | **39%** |

*Source:* Data collected from Rangpur division, Bangladesh.

**Table 1.9:** Respondents Having Other Chronic Disease besides MDR-TB

| *Having Other Chronic Disease* | *No. of Respondents* | *(%)* |
|---|---|---|
| Yes | 34 | 21 |
| No | 129 | 79 |
| **Total** | **163** | **100** |

*Source:* Data collected from Rangpur division, Bangladesh.

**Table 1.10:** Respondents having other Chronic Disease with MDR-TB

| *Disease Name* | *No. of Respondents* | *(%)* |
|---|---|---|
| Asthma | 15 | 43 |
| Diabetics | 12 | 34 |
| Other | 8 | 23 |
| **Total** | **35** | **100** |

*Source:* Data collected from Rangpur division, Bangladesh.

From Table 1.9, we can see that only 34 (21%) respondents were suffering with other chronic diseases beside MDR-TB. Those chronic diseases are mainly Asthma and Diabetics. Among 35 MDR patients having other chronic diseases, 15 (43%) have Asthma and 12 (34%) have Diabetics (Table 1.10). Rest of 35 has other diseases like HTN, Eye problem, Hypothyroidism etc. During interview, most of the respondents told that they have General weakness. But, it is not considered as disease as it is an unstable physical condition due to many reasons.

**Table 1.11:** Respondents having any Addiction and its Nature

| *Addiction Status* | *Respondents – No. and %* | | | | | |
|---|---|---|---|---|---|---|
| | *Male* | *%* | *Female* | *%* | *Total* | *%* |
| Having No addiction | 42 | 48 | 45 | 52 | 87 | 53 |
| Having any Addiction | 70 | 92 | 6 | 8 | 76 | 47 |
| **Total** | **112** | **69** | **51** | **31** | **163** | **100** |

*Source:* Data collected from Rangpur division, Bangladesh.

From Table 1.11, we can see that among 112 male respondents, 70 have any addiction which is 92 per cent among respondents having any addiction. Only 6 female (8%) have addiction. At the same time, 45 female and 42 male do not have any addiction. In total, 76 respondents have any addiction among 163 respondents which is 47 per cent. 53 per cent have no addiction.

**Table 1.12:** Type of Addiction among Respondents

| | *Type of Addiction* | *No.* | *%* |
|---|---|---|---|
| Among Female | Tobacco (*Jarda*) | 6 | 8 |
| | Smoking | 51 | 67 |
| | Smoking + *Ganja* | 7 | 9 |
| Among Male | Smoking + Alcohol | 6 | 8 |
| | Tobacco (*Jarda*/Powder) | 3 | 4 |
| | Other | 3 | 4 |
| | **Total** | **76** | **100** |

*Source:* Data collected from Rangpur division, Bangladesh.

Table 1.12, explains the types of addiction. Among 6 female, all are addicted with tobacco (*jarda*). Among 70 male, most are addicted with smoking of biri or cigarette. It is found from Table 1.12 that 7 respondents smoke *Ganja* along with cigarette or *biri*, 6 used to drink alcohol with smoking. One respondent confesses that he used to take all sorts of addiction materials like Heroin, Fensidril, *Ganja*, Alcohol etc.

From the slide culture result I came to know that only 16 patients out of 105 have additional drug resistance beside Rifampicine (by slide culture). They are displayed in Table 1.13. Most important finding from the table is that one Patient was identified as **XDR TB**. The XDR case is a female of 40 years of age and Failure of Category 1.

**Table 1.13:** Respondents having other Drug Resistance *Rifampicine*

| *Resistance drugs* | *No. of respondents* |
|---|---|
| R + Z | 11 |
| R + Z + O | 3 |
| R + Z + K | 1 |
| R + Z + O + K + C + S | 1 |
| **Total** | **16** |

*Note:* *R* = Rifampicine, *Z* = Pyrazinamide, *O* = Ofloxacine, *K* = Kenamycine, C = Clofazimine, *S* = Streptomycine.

*Source:* Data collected from Rangpur division, Bangladesh.

## Discussions

This study has intended to identify the risk factors more in specific as well as explore the practical situation of MDR-TB at Rajshahi and Rangpur division. The results from the study are discussed below in brief.

*Age and Sex:* Male are more prevalent and the age group from 16-45 are mostly vulnerable. In late age, women are less likely to develop MDR-TB, but there are evidences of male having TB in the age of 80 or more. A study was conducted by Geneyeea Bhatt *et al.* at Ahemedabad of India on the age and sex distribution of MDR-TB. That tells almost same finding in this regard. The study reports 2/3rd Male and highest age group is 1645 (Bhatt, 2011).

*Region:* More MDR-TB is diagnosed at Rajshahi division and less in Rangpur division. It is a very important finding from the point of geographical distribution of MDR-TB in Bangladesh. It needs further research to explore of facts and under lying causes.

*Education:* Most of the MDR patients have no education or low education. So, awareness level, motivation, understanding of risks may be low due to education. There is no study found on educational impact of MDR-TB. It also found in the study performed by Geneyaa Bhatt *et al.*, in 2010 where the educational levels of the MDR cases were found primary level. Further, study may help to conclude the findings (Bhat, 2011).

*Registration Group:* Most MDR Cases are diagnosed from Category 1 or having no treatment. They are about 80 per cent. From Re-treatment MDR cases are 20 per cent of Total. Primary MDR may be more emerging. It needs to conduct an analytical study only on this topic (DRS, 2012).

*Monthly family Income:* In general, it is said that TB is a disease of poverty. MDR is prevalent to low socio-economic group of people. Due to low income, their life style may be affected positively to develop MDR-TB. This was also established by several other studies (Rifat, 2012).

*Residential status and ethnicity:* In general, rural people are mostly affected by MDR-TB and there is no ethnic sensitivity. MDR-TB developed from different religion group. This study is not suitable to make any comment on whether any religion is more vulnerable for TB or not.

*Occupation:* A number of occupations have been identified

among the respondents. This study does not shows that Farmers for Male and House wife for Female are predominating. At the same time Garments worker, students, private business and day labour are common.

*Previous history:* Previous history is important for developing MDT-TB. Most of the MDR cases have previous anti TB drug history (Rifat, 2012), (Marahatta, 2010).

*Contact history:* It is an important risk factor. Contact with MDR-TB is most likely to produce MDR-TB. MDR-TB cases may have contact with Non-MDR-TB, but there may not have association to be transmitted from each other. Both may have different source of infection (Rifat, 2012).

*Other disease:* No comments can be made on the findings except one and that is Diabetics. DM patients are most vulnerable to develop MDR-TB. Also Asthma is a remarkable chronic disease among MDR-TB. Diabetics are also considered a risk factor in the study (Bhatt, 2011).

*Addiction:* Addiction may influence MDT-TB. Numbers of MDR patients have different addiction. Among them smoking is dominant. Addictions with multiple items are also vulnerable for developing MDR-TB. Several other studies proved it (Marahatta, 2010).

*Existence of XDR case:* By performing slide culture for 2nd line drugs, one XDR cases have been diagnosed.

This study gives us a clear view of socio-economic demographic status of registered MDR-TB cases at Rajshahi and Rangpur divisions over the years 2013 and 2014. From the analysis, risk factors associated with MDR-TB can be identified. It is shown in the part of literature review that several other studies were performed with same objective and results are almost similar.

## Conclusion

The study concluded that among the respondents majority were productive age group age group (16–45). Surveillance programme need to conduct at Rangpur division to explain low MDR case detection in spite of high notification rate. No highly remarkable risk factors are found from the study. But some indicative risk factors are identified such as education, low income, previous history etc. This study opens several scopes of further study and research on multiple issues. In this case, this study has successfully sketched the pattern of the MDR situation at Rajshahi and Rangpur division.

## List of Abbreviations

CDH: Chest Disease Hospital, DF: Damien Foundation, DGHS: Directorate General of Health Services, DOT: Directly Observed Treatment, DST: Drug Susceptibility Test, GLC: Green Light Committee, HPSP: Health and Population Sector Programme, HPNSDP: Health Population and Nutrition Sector Development Programme, MDR: Multi-Drug Resistance, MBDC: Mycobacterium Disease Control, MOHFW: Ministry of Health and Family Welfare, NSP: New Smear Positive, NTP: National TB Control Programme, NIDCH: National Institute of Diseases of Chest and Hospital, NTRL: National TB Reference Laboratory, PMDT: Programmatic Management of Drug Resistance TB, PPM: Public Private Mix, RTRL: Regional TB reference Laboratory, SNRL: Supranational Reference Laboratory, UHC: Upazila Health Complex, WHO: World Health Organization, XDR: Extensively Drug Resistance.

## Acknowledgements

I would like to extend my sincere gratitude to the authority of Rajshahi Chest Disease Hospital, Pabna Chest Disease Hospital and implementing partners of NTP at Rajshahi and Rangpur divisions for permitting me to conduct the study. I would also like to convey my gratefulness to all field staff members of partner organizations for their warm support to accomplish the study. I would also like to express my eternal thanks and appreciation to the respondents who were the source of information without which this research would not been possible.

## References

Barroso, E.C., Motà, R.M.S., Santos, R.O., Sausa, A. L. O., Barroso, J. B., Rodrigues, L. N. (2003). Risk factors for acquired multidrug-resistant tuberculosis. *Journal de pneumologia, 29*(2): 89-97.

Bhatt, G.; Vyas, S.; Trivedi, K. (2012). An Epidemiological study of Multi Drug Resistant Tuberculosis cases registered under Revised National

Tuberculosis Programme of Ahemadabad City. *Indian Journal of Tuberculosis, 59*(1): 18-27.

Blackman, C., Browning, R., Kogut, D., Young H. (n.d.). Multiple Drug-Resistant Tuberculosis-MDR-TB and XDR-TB. Retrieved from Boston University web site: http://sphweb.bumc.bu.edu/otlt/MPH-Modules/PH/MDR-TB/MDR-TB_print.html

Faustini, A.; Hall, A. and Perucci, C. (2006). Risk factors for multidrug resistant tuberculosis in Europe: a systematic review. *Thorax 61*(2): 158–163.

Jose, A.C. (Ed.). (2013). *Guidelines for Clinical and Operational Management of Drug-Resistant Tuberculosis.*. 68 boulevard St. Michel, 75006 Paris, France. International Union Against Tuberculosis and Lung Diseases (The Union). Available at http://www.theunion.org/what-we-do/publications/technical/english/mdr-tbguide_6-19-13_web.pdf.

Kamal, S.M., Hossain, A., Sultana, S., Begum, V., Haque, N., Ahmed, J., Rahman, T. M., Hyder, K. A., Hossain, S., Rahman, M., Chowdhury, R. A., Aung, K. J., Islam, A., Hasan, R., Van Deun, A. (2015). Anti-tuberculosis drug resistance in Bangladesh: reflections from the first nationwide survey. *International Journal of Tuberculosis and Lung Disease, 19*(5): 622.

Marahatta, S.B., Kaewkungwal, J., Ramasoota, P., Singhasivanon, P. (2010). Risk factors of multi-drug resistant tuberculosis in central Nepal – a pilot study. *Kathmandu University Medical Journal (KUMJ), 8*(32): 3927.

Mistry, N., Tolani, M., Osrin, D. (2012). Drug-resistant tuberculosis in Mumbai, India: An agenda for operations research. *Operations Research for Health Care, 1*(2–3): 45–53.

*Tuberculosis Control in Bangladesh, Annual Report* (2014). National Tuberculosis Control Programme: DGHS, Dhaka, pp. 17-23.

*National Guidelines and Operational Manual for Programmatic Management of Drug Resistance TB (PMDT).* (2013). 2nd Edition. National TB Control Programme, DGHS, Dhaka and WHO, pp. 45-50.

*National Guidelines and Operational Manual for Tuberculosis Control* (2014). 5th edition. National TB Control Programme: DGHS, Dhaka and WHO, pp. 50-54.

Peter, D.O. *Multi-Drug Resistant Tuberculosis.* (2009). Director of the Tuberculosis Research Unit, Cardiothoracic Centre, Thomas Drive, Liverpool. Retrieved from: http://www.priory.com/cmol/TBMultid.html

Rifat, M., Milton, A.H., Hall, J., Oldmeadow, C., Islam, M.A., Husain, A., Akhanda, M.W., Siddiquea, B. N. (2014). *Development of multidrug resistant tuberculosis in Bangladesh: a case-control study on risk factor,* 19; 9(8):e105214. doi: 10.1371/journal.pone.0105214.

WHO (2015). *Tuberculosis (TB).* Own website of WHO. http://www.who.int/tb/challenges/mdr

USAID, TB CARE II. (October 2011). *Community – Based care for Drug-Resistance Tuberculosis: A guide for implementers.* 1st Edition. Available at: https://drtbnetwork.org/community-based-care-drug-resistant-tuberculosis-guide-implementers

WHO and TB CARE II Bangladesh. (2013). Standard Operating Procedure (SOP) – Community based Programmatic Management of Drug Resistance TB. 1st edition (Chapters 1 and 2).

WHO. (2013). *Global Tuberculosis Report*. Available at: http://www.health-e.org.za/2013/10/23/global-tuberculosis-report-2013/

WHO. (2014). *Global Tuberculosis Report-2014*. Available at: http://www.who.int/tb/publications/global_report/en/

# 2
# Health Care Spending in India
## Pre- and Post-Reforms Perspective

*Sidhartha Sankar Laha*

### Introduction

Health is one of the vital indicators reflecting the quality of life and, therefore, it has been rightly said, "Health is wealth". Though preservation and promotion of health is one of the most basic human rights, India is still lagging behind in realizing this distant dream. Public health is concerned with the health of the community as a whole. Its key goal is to reduce population's exposure to disease. It has been said that: "Health care is vital to all of us some of the time, but public health is vital to all of us all of the time".

For several decades, public sector reforms have been premised on the assumption that improving the ability of the government to manage its business will lead to improved social and economic position of the country. The Indian economy grew at a comparatively low rate of growth of 3.5 per cent from 1950 to 1980. The plethora of procedures, permits, bureaucratic controls and protectionist policies created under import substitution strategy (ISS) along with other factors landed us into economic crisis of 1991, which was reflected in macro-economic mismanagement of the economy judged from parameters such as high fiscal deficit, high balance of payment deficit, double digit inflation, low forex reserves etc. An attempt was made to resolve this crisis through the introduction of stabilization and structural adjustment programme (SAP)/economic reforms. One of the important planks of the stabilization measures is the compression of public expenditure and that of SAP is raising efficiency and international comparative no.ce

It is apprehended that any economic reform package that relates to compression in public expenditure will adversely affect the vulnerable sections of the society as this will lead to reduction in social sector spending. The experience of many developing countries which have embarked upon a process of macroeconomic reforms during the last 20 years shows that the accentuation of reforms lead to reduction in public spending on basic services and programmes directly related to social sector development or human resource development (Gupta and Sarkar, 1994). Even the European countries which have experienced reforms have had diverse experiences with respect to the social impact of reforms (Panchamukhi, 2000). It is from this angle a study of impact of economic reforms on public health expenditure which is a component of social sector expenditure in India becomes important. During the 1970's "growth with social justice" was the popular slogan. But from 1980's onwards that is from the onset of reforms the slogan of "equity with stabilization and SAP" appears to be more relevant.

But SAPs have been evaluated as having a negative impact on social sector expenditure (Cornia, Jolly and Steward, 1987; Tusjita, 2005; Dev and Mooji, 2002). The reduction of fiscal deficits is normally included in the conditionality of SAPs and consequently government expenditures have to be cut in order to meet the targets for reducing fiscal deficits. There are a number of studies which have pointed out the declining trend in social sector expenditures. UNICEF's Adjustment with a Human Face (Cornia, Jolly and Steward, 1987) was the first major criticism of SAPs and if pointed out the negative impact on the vulnerable. In the present study public expenditure on health sector has been considered for the impact of economic reform. As already mentioned there are handful studies which have found the negative impact of economic reform on health expenditure. At the same time the time frame considered by these studies is very limited. Furthermore, most studies were restricted to only revenue expenditure. Expenditure by combined (Centre and States), centres, all states and individual states are very few. An attempt has been made here to fill this research gap. The chapter aimed at firstly to examine the growth of public health expenditure of India and to measure its trends over-time period, secondly to measure the nature and level of inter-state disparities in health status in India, thirdly to examine the public health system and health related policies over time in India and lastly to identify and policy implications to improve health status in India.

## Data and Methodology

The study is largely based on secondary data. The required data sources namely, Indian Public Finance Statistics, RBI Bulletin, National Human Development Reports, Central Statistics Office, Economic Survey of India, Finance Account of the State Governments, Ministry of Health and Family Welfare and National Rural Health Mission are utilized. Fifteen major Indian states have been selected for the analysis as they covered around ninety per cent of the Indian population. The states covered in the study include, Andhra Pradesh, Assam, Bihar, Gujarat, Haryana, Karnataka, Kerala, Madhya Pradesh, Maharashtra, Orissa, Punjab, Rajasthan, Tamil Nadu, Uttar Pradesh and West Bengal. Public Health expenditure includes expenditure on (a) medical and public health, water supply and sanitation and (b) family welfare. The time period considered for analysis of trends of public expenditure on health sector is from 1976-77 to 2005-2006 (15 years of pre-reform period) [from 1976-77 to 1990-91] and 15 years of post-reform period [from 1991-92 to 2005-06]. The first reason for selecting this period is that – two appropriate divisions can be done for pre- and post-economic reform, and second is that before 1975-76, in budgetary classification the head health was not defined properly.

In order to remove the impact of price rise, the growth and composition of public health expenditure has been considered at constant prices with 1999-2000 as the base year. By using the GDP deflator method, the current expenditure items were converted into constant prices (1993-94). The GDP deflator is the ratio of nominal GDP to real GDP. In other words, it is equal to nominal GDP divided by real GDP. To get a value at constant prices we need to divide the value of current prices with GDP Deflator, in case of individual states Gross State Domestic Product (GSDP) deflators have been used. To analyse the pattern of public expenditure on health, the present study has included plan and non-plan expenditure of revenue and capital accounts; loans and advances have been excluded. The study does not analyse government programmes or schemes relating cost to health sector development. Also the allocations of Central Government expenditure to individual states have been excluded from the scope of this study.

## Origin of Reforms in India

Health Sector reforms in India were a direct outcome of economic reforms post-1991. Before this, the Indian economy was committed to socialism with slack foreign exchange flow. India followed planned economic development with a strong import substitute orientation. There was no balance of payment crisis till 1980s owing to the gulf boom and large worker remittances. With the oil crisis and an import dependent growth strategy there was a balance of payment crisis post-gulf war in 1991. During this period, the social indicators too were poor. India had to go for loan under the Structural Adjustment Programme (SAP) of the World Bank (Narayana, 2008). The period also coincided with many other developing countries going for the World Bank loan. In the mean time there were two significant documents which later became the basis for reforms in many developing countries. One such document was "Financing Health Services in Developing Countries" in 1987 by the World Bank. This document was a paradigm shift with respect to the role of government in health care provision. It called for introduction of user fee, insurance or other risk coverage, effective use of non-governmental resources and decentralization. The World Development Report in 1993, 'Investing in Health' advocated the development of ideal environment for health, increased government spending and promoting diversity and promotion (Health Sector Reforms in India). With the fiscal deficit, the centre had to cut its total expenditure, which fell more on the capital disbursement and the revenue expenditure remained unaltered. This led to a decrease in the capital expenditure and decrease in the loans given to the States and the Union Territories (Narayana, 2008). In the meantime, there were policy shifts in the Five Year Plans. The Eighth Five Year Plan proposed revoking of free medical care and encouraged initiatives by private sector. The Ninth Five Year Plan emphasized the need to increase the involvement of voluntary, private organizations and the self-help groups and ensure intersectoral coordination. It also placed the need to enable Panchayati Raj

Institutions (PRIs) in planning and monitoring of health programmes. The Tenth Five Year Plan, in addition to the above points, recognized the need to address the issue of equity and the need to devise a targeting mechanism by which the population living below the poverty line will have access to subsidized health care (Health Sector Reforms in India). Despite the cut in central total expenditure in the form of capital expenditure, health sector remained relatively protected. There was increase in absolute spending on health post-economic reforms, though the central health spending as a percent of GDP remained stagnant. The cut fell more on the service sector. As 50 per cent of the States' debt is to the Centre, total expenditure remained stagnant post-1991. The Interest of payment rose (as a % of GDP); there was a decrease in discretionary spending. Spending on public health and water, sanitation decreased post-economic reforms. Hence, the states had to go for loans form World Bank under the Structural Adjustment Programme. Seven states went for the Health System Development Project (HSDP) as a part of the structural adjustment between 1994-97. Though the health system development project recognizes the need to increase the public spending on health, the public spending as a share of total spending decreased. The decline in spending on public health water and sanitation was milder in the reforming states. Fifteen per cent of the cost of health system development project had to be borne by the states, which already had scarce resources. The loan came with a pre-condition that 65 per cent of loan had to be used for strengthening of hospitals, institutions and purchasing equipment. Hence, the states could not use this money exclusively to improve primary health care. Despite health being a state subject, tax resources are largely controlled by the centre. The planning commission and finance commission give money to the states, but there is no mention in the constitution on the fixed proportional spending on health. The states with decreased central grant, submitted the most promising budget with the assurance of increasing health sector spending, privatization, introduction of user fee and decentralization. The HSDP was used by reforming states as a tool for leveraging external financing (Narayana, 2008). Structural adjustment pushed the states to cut health sector investments, opening up of medical care to private sector, introduction of user fee and private investments in public hospitals (Qadeer, 2000), therefore revoking free and affordable healthcare. Health sector spending remained stagnant with increase in health inequity. Economic reforms sought to achieve rapid economic development, overall increase in productivity with free access to market, to eliminate poverty and finally leading to improved standard of living (Health Sector Reforms in India). It was thought that this effect would trickle down to health sector, which did not happen (Qadeer, 2000). Even though evidence was available that market based health sector reforms were not able to achieve equity, it was pursued (Bennett *et al.*, 1994). These changes in health financing only or donor driven changes that were non-purposive are not health sector reforms in true sense.

## Pre- and Post-Health Reforms in India

Before going to the analysis of trends and pattern of public health expenditure a quick review of private and public expenditure on health sector in different states gives us the proportion spent by public as against private, and it also shows the position of different states in both sectors. Table 2.1 shows the per capita public and private expenditure on health by Indian states during 2001-2002. Per capita public health expenditure is Rs. 207 in India while it is Rs. 790 from private sector. Public sector spends only 20 per cent of the total health expenditure. One can easily argue that private expenditure is very important, but the thing is not so uncomplicated, people who are rich can spend on health, although health expenditure has not been considered as luxurious expenditure, for poor people health spending is the territory expenditure after food and cloth. In case of health expenditure considerable inter-state disparity can be observed from the table, while private expenditure (Coefficient of Variation 28.21%) has less disparity than that of public expenditure (CV 46.23%). At the same time we can observe that there is no significant relationship between public and private expenditures. Kerala, Punjab, Haryana, Uttar Pradesh are the highest spending states in private as well as total health expenditure with the amount of more than Rs. 1100 per person, per year. While in case of public expenditure of Punjab, Kerala, Tamil Nadu, and Karnataka are the highest spending states with the amount more than Rs. 220 per person, per year. If we see the relationship with poverty of these expenditure-public expenditure turns a negative significant relationship with poverty

**Table 2.1:** Per Capita Public Private Expenditure on Health in Indian States, 2001-02

| *States/Rank* | *Public Exp.* | *Private Exp.* | *Total Exp.* | *% of Public Exp. to Total Exp.* |
|---|---|---|---|---|
| Andhra Pradesh | 182 (6) | 858 (5) | 1039 (5) | 17.5 (9) |
| Assam | 1766 (9) | 393 (15) | 569 (15) | 30.9 (1) |
| Bihar | 92 (14) | 687 (8) | 779 (10) | 11.8 (13) |
| Gujarat | 147 (11) | 670 (9) | 816 (9) | 18.0 (8) |
| Haryana | 163 (10) | 1408 (2) | 1570 (2) | 10.4 14) |
| Karnataka | 206 (3) | 506 (12) | 712 (12) | 28.9 (3) |
| Kerala | 240 (2) | 1618 (1) | 1858 (1) | 12.9 (12) |
| Madhya Pradesh | 132 (13) | 733 (7) | 864 (7) | 15.2 (11) |
| Maharashtra | 196 (5) | 815 (6) | 1011 (6) | 19.4 (7) |
| Orissa | 134 (12) | 449 (13) | 582 (14) | 23.0 (6) |
| Punjab | 258 (1) | 1273 (3) | 1530 (3) | 16.8 (10) |
| Rajasthan | 182 (7) | 415 (14) | 597 (13) | 30.4 (2) |
| Tamil Nadu | 202 (4) | 644 (10) | 846 (8) | 23.9 (4) |
| Uttar Pradesh | 84 (15) | 1040 (4) | 1124 (4) | 7.5 (15) |
| West Bengal | 181 (8) | 593 (11) | 775 (11) | 23.5 (5) |
| All India # | 207 | 790 | 997 | 20.8 |
| CV (%) | 28.21 | 46.23 | 39.91 | 37.74 |

*Note:* # All India public expenditure including expenditure by the Ministry of Health and Family Welfare, Central Ministries and local bodies, while private expenditure includes health expenditure by NGO, firms and household.

Figures in parenthesis indicate rank computed on the basis of data.

*Source:* Economic Survey of India, 2005-2006.

(correlation coefficient –0.673), whereas it not so in case of private expenditure. Thus, it is clear that public health expenditure is mainly for the poorer and private health expenditure comes from the rich.

However, present study has the intension to analyse the impact of economic reform on public health expenditure and not to trace out the relationships and behaviours of public and private expenditure, which is important theme of the study. India has a federal government. Indian Constitution prescribes different areas in three lists, i.e. State list, Central list and Concurrent list. Health comes under the state list. But Centre has a strong influence on State Government expenditure *via* its fiscal transfers. We have tried to analyse public health expenditure at four levels: combined Centre and States, Centre, all States and each of the fifteen major States. While most of the studies use only revenue expenditure, in this study we include both revenue and capital accounts of plan and non-plan expenditure.

### Public Health Expenditure of Centre and States Combined

India's finest dedication or commitments to the public health expenditure can be seen in Centre and States combined expenditure. Table 2.2 shows the combined health expenditure from 1976-77 to 2005-06. In the absolute term expenditure increased significantly about 50 times from Rs. 978 crores to Rs. 47,220 crores. This impressive growth is offset by escalation of price and rapid growth in population. After converting these figures into constant prices of 1999-2000, the increase is less than 6 times. If we view this growth in per capita terms at 1999-2000 prices, the picture does not look so impressive. In per capita terms, expenditure increased only 3 times. In sum, increase of public health expenditure is only three times from 1976-77 to 2005-06 (over 30 years). Measuring Health expenditure as a share of total budgetary expenditure is another way to understand the commitment of budget to health sector. The share was less than 4 per cent until 1981-82, 1982 onwards it increased and reached 4.68 per cent in 1984-85. Thereafter, the share has started declining except for some years, like 1993-94 which has second highest share (4.63%) during the study period. Measuring health expenditure as a share of GDP is also considered as an important way especially when comparing with other nations. Health expenditure as a percentage of GDP was between 1.08 per cent and 1.83 per cent in the period under reference.

The share rose from 1.08 per cent in 1977-78 to 1.83 per cent in 1987-88, but later on declined significantly. The share is 1.44 in 2006-07, which is more than 6 per cent in developed countries. Public expenditure on health in per capita term, as a share to total expenditure and percentage of GDP is less in India. In Organisation for Economic Co-operation and Development (OECD) countries public health expenditure as a share of GDP is more than 6 per cent. In France it is 10 per cent and in Germany it is more than 11 per cent (Lalitha and Guennif, 2007). Moreover, the share has shown declining trend during the period of economic reforms. Growth rates of public health expenditure in different terms in pre-reform period are high as compared that of post-reform period, which can be seen in the last columns of Table 2.1.

**Table 2.2:** Combined (Centre and State Governments) Expenditure on Health

| *Years* | *Current Prices* | *Constant Prices* | *Per-Capita Exp.* | *As a share to Total Budget* | *As a Percentage of GDP* |
|---|---|---|---|---|---|
| 1976-77 | 978 | 6579 | 102 | 3.84 | 1.18 |
| 1977-78 | 1024 | 6486 | 98 | 3.56 | 1.08 |
| 1978-79 | 1195 | 7430 | 109 | 3.47 | 1.18 |
| 1979-80 | 1420 | 7670 | 111 | 3.85 | 1.28 |
| 1980-81 | 1724 | 8351 | 118 | 3.79 | 1.30 |
| 1981-82 | 2087 | 9120 | 126 | 4.14 | 1.35 |
| 1982-83 | 2497 | 10053 | 136 | 4.19 | 1.44 |
| 1983-84 | 3034 | 11263 | 149 | 4.39 | 1.50 |
| 1984-85 | 3909 | 13434 | 174 | 4.68 | 1.72 |
| 1985-86 | 4486 | 14371 | 182 | 4.60 | 1.76 |
| 1986-87 | 5132 | 15381 | 191 | 4.47 | 1.81 |
| 1987-88 | 5876 | 16084 | 196 | 4.59 | 1.83 |
| 1988-89 | 6492 | 16403 | 196 | 4.44 | 1.69 |
| 1989-90 | 6990 | 16271 | 190 | 4.12 | 1.58 |
| 1990-91 | 8088 | 17016 | 195 | 4.12 | 1.57 |
| 1991-92 | 9056 | 16751 | 188 | 4.13 | 1.52 |
| 1992-93 | 10291 | 17486 | 192 | 4.25 | 1.51 |
| 1993-94 | 12794 | 19766 | 213 | 4.63 | 1.62 |
| 1994-95 | 13999 | 19701 | 208 | 4.34 | 1.51 |
| 1995-96 | 15426 | 19893 | 206 | 4.33 | 1.42 |
| 1996-97 | 17322 | 20725 | 211 | 4.29 | 1.37 |
| 1997-98 | 20138 | 22599 | 226 | 4.38 | 1.44 |
| 1998-99 | 24214 | 25148 | 247 | 4.44 | 1.50 |
| 1999-00 | 27306 | 27306 | 263 | 4.46 | 1.53 |
| 2000-01 | 29963 | 29018 | 275 | 4.45 | 1.56 |
| 2001-02 | 30869 | 29028 | 271 | 4.47 | 1.47 |
| 2002-03 | 35551 | 32200 | 295 | 4.15 | 1.57 |
| 2003-04 | 35209 | 30834 | 262 | 4.15 | 1.39 |
| 2004-05 | 42191 | 35017 | 291 | 4.17 | 1.47 |
| 2005-06 | 47220 | 37665 | 313 | 4.18 | 1.44 |
| **Pre-reform period** | **17.73** | **8.22** | **5.95** | **1.48** | **3.35** |
| **Post-reform period** | **12.23** | **5.89** | **3.63** | **0.27** | **–0.27** |
| **Total period** | **14.57** | **5.90** | **3.71** | **0.49** | **0.45** |

*Note:* Total expenditure is Rs. in Crores and per capita expenditure in Rupees.

*Source:* Computed from the Budgetary Documents of India, Indian Public Finance Statistics and RBI Bulletin (Various Issues).

## Central Government Expenditure

As it is already mentioned health is a state subject in India. This means that the primary responsibility of financing and providing health care rests with the State Governments. The Central Government's role has been to fund centrally sponsored schemes, to develop policies and guidelines and provide statutory grants or general transfers to the states (Bajpai and Goyal, 2005). In this connection, analysing the role of Central Government on health spending before and after economic reform becomes imperative. There are a number of studies who have indicated the increasing public spending of Central Government notably Dev and Mooij (2002), Prabhu, (1994), Panchamukhi (2002), Joshi (2005). In the present section we analyse the same with broadening of the time period and we look how much increase/decrease has taken place over time on various counts. Table 2.3 gives us the growth of Central Government expenditure on health from 1976-77 to 2005-06. As we have seen in the above section expenditure at current prices is very impressive and not so in constant prices and in per capita constant prices. One thing here to be noted is that in per capita constant prices the increase is around 5 times from Rs. 20 in 1976-77 to Rs. 97 in 2005-06, while it is only 3 times in combined (Centre and State) expenditure. Moreover, public expenditure on health of combined in the reform period is less as compared with that of pre-reform period. In case of central expenditure the growth rates are high in reform period in all type of measurements; growth rate in per capita expenditure was 5.3 per cent per annum, which increased to 8.6 per cent per annum in the post-reform period. Health expenditure as a share of total expenditure and as a percentage of GDP has increased around 2 times in the study period from 1.41 per cent to 2.84 per cent and from 0.23 per cent to 0.45 per cent respectively from 1976-77 to 2005-06. This increase is mainly due to implementation of many centrally sponsored health and development programmes like Rajiv Gandhi National Drinking Water Mission, National Rural Health Mission, and Jawaharlal National Urban Renewal Mission (JNURM), others.

## Expenditure on Health of All States

From the above analysis we found that combined (Centre and

**Table 2.3:** Central Government Expenditure on Health in India

| *Years* | *Current Prices* | *Constant Prices* | *Per-Capita Exp.* | *As a share to Total Budget* | *As a Percentage of GDP* |
|---|---|---|---|---|---|
| 1976-77 | 192 | 1291 | 20 | 1.41 | 0.23 |
| 1977-78 | 194 | 1229 | 19 | 1.25 | 0.21 |
| 1978-79 | 187 | 1163 | 17 | 1.00 | 0.18 |
| 1979-80 | 197 | 1064 | 15 | 1.04 | 0.18 |
| 1980-81 | 238 | 1153 | 16 | 1.05 | 0.18 |
| 1981-82 | 290 | 1267 | 18 | 1.15 | 0.19 |
| 1982-83 | 386 | 1554 | 21 | 1.25 | 0.22 |
| 1983-84 | 447 | 1659 | 22 | 1.26 | 0.22 |
| 1984-85 | 611 | 2100 | 27 | 1.40 | 0.27 |
| 1985-86 | 685 | 2194 | 28 | 1.30 | 0.27 |
| 1986-87 | 754 | 2260 | 28 | 1.20 | 0.27 |
| 1987-88 | 887 | 2428 | 30 | 1.30 | 0.28 |
| 1988-89 | 1062 | 2683 | 32 | 1.34 | 0.28 |
| 1989-90 | 1110 | 2584 | 30 | 1.19 | 0.25 |
| 1990-91 | 1271 | 2674 | 31 | 1.21 | 0.25 |
| 1991-92 | 1374 | 2542 | 28 | 1.2 | 0.23 |
| 1992-93 | 1630 | 2770 | 30 | 1.33 | 0.24 |
| 1993-94 | 2182 | 3371 | 36 | 1.54 | 0.28 |
| 1994-95 | 2490 | 3504 | 37 | 1.55 | 0.27 |
| 1995-96 | 2974 | 3435 | 40 | 1.67 | 0.27 |
| 1996-97 | 3084 | 3690 | 38 | 1.53 | 0.24 |
| 1997-98 | 3575 | 4012 | 40 | 1.54 | 0.26 |
| 1998-99 | 4477 | 4650 | 46 | 1.60 | 0.28 |
| 1999-00 | 6004 | 6004 | 58 | 2.01 | 0.34 |
| 2000-01 | 6303 | 6104 | 58 | 1.94 | 0.33 |
| 2001-02 | 8837 | 8310 | 77 | 2.44 | 0.42 |
| 2002-03 | 7736 | 7007 | 64 | 1.87 | 0.34 |
| 2003-04 | 9263 | 8112 | 69 | 1.97 | 0.36 |
| 2004-05 | 11891 | 9869 | 82 | 2.35 | 0.41 |
| 2005-06 | 14631 | 11670 | 97 | 2.84 | 0.45 |
| **Pre-reform period** | **17.03** | **7.58** | **5.32** | **0.65** | **2.73** |
| **Post-reform period** | **17.63** | **10.99** | **8.62** | **4.80** | **4.53** |
| **Total period** | **16.81** | **7.97** | **5.74** | **2.61** | **2.41** |

*Note:* Total expenditure is Rs. in Crores and per capita expenditure in Rupees.

*Source:* Computed from the Budgetary Documents of India, Indian Public Finance Statistics and RBI Bulletin (Various Issues).

States) expenditure on health decreased after economic reforms while it increased in Central Government. States have the lions' share in health spending as these spend around 80 per cent of the total spending. Comparatively changes of states spending affect a lot on the population of the country. Table 2.4 depicts the public health expenditure of all states from 1976-77 to 2005-06. In the current prices public health expenditure increased around 42 times from Rs. 897 crore in 1976-77 to Rs. 37,523 crore 2005-05. It is not necessary to mention that the picture is not so impressive in constant and per capita terms. In per capita constant term is less the 3 times, which is less than Centre and combined expenditures. Furthermore, growth rates are very low in the post-reform period and in case of as a share of total budget and as a share of GDP growth rates turned to negative in the post-reform period.

**Health Expenditure of Major States**

Now, we discuss the main and crucial issues about the trends and. pattern of public health expenditure of 15 major states. State-wise analysis of trends of public expenditure becomes critical when the states are reorganised or divided. So, the economists normally analyse trends and pattern of public expenditure in per capita terms, as a share of GSDP or National State Domestic Product (NSDP), or as a share of total expenditure. In the present study selecting of 30 years of long period is not exception for the same (*see* Table 2.4).

During this long period of time many states were newly restructured (e.g.: Chhattisgarh was carved out from Madhya Pradesh, Uttarakhand from Uttar Pradesh, Jharkhand from Bihar). Consequently, the trends and pattern of public expenditure on health is examined in per capita current and constant prices, as a share of total expenditure and also as a share of NSDP. Public health expenditure as a share of total budget in all states is around 7 per cent in the study period. It gets around 25 per cent of the social services expenditures it is most important component after education, which occupies 55 per cent in social services expenditure. Average of per capita public expenditure on health of major 15 states increased from Rs. 114 in 1976-77 to Rs. 285 in 2005-06. The increase is not same in all states there is huge inter-state disparity exists. Coefficient of variation was 30.75 per cent in 1976-77 which hovered between 25 per cent and 35 per cent during the study period and reached at 35.49 per cent in 2005-06.

**Table 2.4:** Public Expenditure on Health of All States in India

| Years | Current Prices | Constant Prices | Per-Capita Exp. | As a share to Total Budget | As a Percentage of GDP |
|---|---|---|---|---|---|
| 1976-77 | 897 | 6031 | 93 | 7.57 | 1.08 |
| 1977-78 | 937 | 5937 | 89 | 7.07 | 0.99 |
| 1978-79 | 1104 | 6866 | 101 | 7.04 | 1.09 |
| 1979-80 | 1338 | 7226 | 104 | 7.46 | 1.21 |
| 1980-81 | 1608 | 7790 | 110 | 7.10 | 1.21 |
| 1981-82 | 1949 | 8518 | 118 | 7.74 | 1.26 |
| 1982-83 | 2329 | 9377 | 127 | 8.10 | 1.34 |
| 1983-84 | 2843 | 10555 | 140 | 8.48 | 1.40 |
| 1984-85 | 3181 | 10931 | 142 | 7.98 | 1.40 |
| 1985-86 | 3679 | 11785 | 150 | 8.20 | 1.45 |
| 1986-87 | 4259 | 12765 | 159 | 8.22 | 1.50 |
| 1987-88 | 4963 | 13586 | 165 | 8.29 | 1.54 |
| 1988-89 | 5480 | 13846 | 165 | 8.17 | 1.43 |
| 1989-90 | 5962 | 13878 | 162 | 7.77 | 1.35 |
| 1990-91 | 6815 | 14338 | 164 | 7.48 | 1.32 |
| 1991-92 | 7674 | 14195 | 159 | 7.11 | 1.29 |
| 1992-93 | 8569 | 14560 | 160 | 7.18 | 1.26 |
| 1993-94 | 10646 | 16447 | 177 | 7.91 | 1.34 |
| 1994-95 | 11586 | 16305 | 172 | 7.17 | 1.25 |
| 1995-96 | 12884 | 16614 | 172 | 7.26 | 1.19 |
| 1996-97 | 14522 | 17375 | 177 | 7.16 | 1.15 |
| 1997-98 | 16964 | 19037 | 190 | 7.44 | 1.21 |
| 1998-99 | 20221 | 21001 | 206 | 7.59 | 1.25 |
| 1999-00 | 22294 | 22294 | 215 | 7.10 | 1.25 |
| 2000-01 | 24672 | 23893 | 226 | 7.11 | 1.28 |
| 2001-02 | .24892 | 23408 | 218 | 6.60 | 1.19 |
| 2002-03 | 29030 | 26294 | 241 | 6.56 | 1.28 |
| 2003-04 | 28353 | 24830 | 211 | 6.59 | 1.12 |
| 2004-05 | 34291 | 28460 | 236 | 6.90 | 1.19 |
| 2005-06 | 37523 | 29930 | 248 | 7.06 | 1.15 |
| **Pre-reform period** | **16.62** | **7.20** | **4.95** | **0.78** | **2.37** |
| **Post-reform period** | **11.83** | **5.52** | **3.26** | **–0.68** | **–0.62** |
| **Total period** | **13.98** | **5.36** | **3.18** | **–0.43** | **–0.06** |

*Note:* Total expenditure is Rs. in Cores and per capita expenditure in Rupees.

*Source:* Computed from the Budgetary Documents of India, Indian Public Finance Statistics and RBI Bulletin Various Issues.

Looking at the averages from pre (1975-76 to 1990-91) to post-reform (1991-92 to 2005-06) periods it increased from 27.64 per cent to 31.91 per cent respectively. Going by the respective position of states, Bihar, Orissa, Uttar Pradesh and West Bengal are the lowest spending states, while Kerala, Haryana, Rajasthan and Punjab are the highest spending states in most of the selected years. Assam was in the 3rd position in 1976-77, which heightened its position to 2nd during 1987-88, but failed to maintain and fell to 10th position in 2004-05. Gujarat's position hovered between 6 and 9, but with an interesting exception of 1st position in 1999-00 and 2000-01.

Average per capita expenditure of all states increased between 1.2 times (lowest in Assam) and 1.9 times (highest in Karnataka) from pre-reform period to post-reform period. In case of growth rates of per capita health expenditure 7 out or 15 states show an increase in the reform period. Significant growth rate can be observed in Andhra Pradesh, Haryana, Kerala and West Bengal during reform period. Going by health expenditure as a share to NSDP, 7 out of 15 states' average health spending is high in post-reform period, while growth rate has fell down in all states in post-reform period. Moreover, except Haryana, Maharashtra, Punjab and Rajasthan remaining 11 states experienced a negative growth rate in this respect.

Another important way of analysis of public health expenditure is that of as a share of total expenditure. Seeing by average shares of total expenditure, only 4 out of 15 states shown the improved shares, whereas, Gujarat and Haryana are the two states who improved in growth rates; and notably no state experienced a positive growth rate. Totally, 8 states have negative impact of economic reform on health spending as a share of total expenditures. A simple cross comparison across states in terms of their base level per capita expenditure on health and growth rates in it in the subsequent period would give us a clear indication of the nature of disparities and would help us in grouping the states as well. While there has been no change in the absolute number of states with higher than the mean level of per capita expenditure on social services or higher than the mean growth of it, the relative positions have changed overtime. Punjab, Gujarat, Maharashtra and Rajasthan have performed consistently by performing well above mean rate of growth.

On the other hand, Orissa and Bihar have continued to remain in the lower rungs of health sector spending. In the pre-reform period, Kerala and Haryana recorded lower rates of growth despite having higher than mean per capita expenditure on health; in the post-reform period they joined the group of high growth rate and high per capita expenditure. Andhra Pradesh and West Bengal improved their position from low expenditure and low growth rate in pre-reform period to low expenditure and high growth rate in post-reform period. Assam, Madhya Pradesh and Uttar Pradesh have not shown high growth rate in post-reform period, hence moved to the low expenditure and low growth rate group. Karnataka moved from high growth rate and low spending group to high spending and high growth rate group during the same period.

| *States Public Health Expenditure ranking in Pre- and Post-Reform Regime* | | | |
|---|---|---|---|
| Description | | States with higher and lower mean growth in Per capita Expenditure on Health in Pre-Reform period | |
| | | High (9) | Low (6) |
| **States with higher and lower than average in per capita Health Expenditure in Pre-Reform Period (Average 1976-77 to 1990-91)** | High (8) | Punjab, Rajasthan, Maharashtra, Assam, Gujarat, Tamil Nadu | Kerala, Haryana |
| | Low (7) | Karnataka, Madhya Pradesh, Uttar Pradesh | West Bengal, Bihar, Orissa, Andhra Pradesh |
| | | States with higher and lower mean growth in Per capita Expenditure on Health in Post-Reform period | |
| | | High (9) | Low (6) |
| **States with higher and lower than average in per capita Health Expenditure in Post-Reform Period (Average 1991-92 to 2005-06)** | High (8) | Rajasthan, Haryana, Punjab, Kerala, Gujarat, Maharashtra, Karnataka | Tamil Nadu |
| | Low (7) | Andhra Pradesh, West Bengal | Assam, Orissa, Madhya Pradesh, Uttar Pradesh, Bihar |

*Source:* (1) Ministry of Health and Family Welfare, Government of India.
(2) National Rural Health Mission, Government of India.

## Inter-State Variation in Per Capita Public Expenditure

The health expenditure in real per capita terms shows high inter-state variation. This inter-state variation in health expenditure is increasing over the period. The value of coefficient of variation was recorded around 0.55 in the period 1987 to 1992 and increased to 0.64 in the period 2005 to 2011 (Table 2.5). The per capita spending in most of low income states is recorded lower than the high income states. Interestingly, in some of the high income states (like Gujarat and Maharashtra) the per capita expenditure is recorded lower than the average spending of all states. The variations in health expenditure themselves is not a matter for concern if it is due to the exercising of preferences by individual states on the basis of prevailing disease or mortality rate in the state. But, it became problematic when states with high prevalence of disease and/or mortality rates and states with high level of income allocate little/low funds in health sector. This may mean that either these states are shying away from fulfilling its constitutional commitment of 'Right to Health' for its citizens or

**Table 2.5:** Inter-State Variation in Per Capita Public Expenditure on Health

| *States* | *1987-1992* | *1993-1998* | *1999-2004* | *2005-2011* |
|---|---|---|---|---|
| Andhra Pradesh | 113 | 176 | 198 | 195 |
| Assam | 139 | 106 | 124 | 250 |
| Bihar | 69 | 80 | 94 | 108 |
| Gujarat | 164 | 170 | 223 | 211 |
| Haryana | 146 | 184 | 221 | 336 |
| Karnataka | 130 | 142 | 183 | 205 |
| Kerala | 146 | 135 | 164 | 236 |
| Madhya Pradesh | 120 | 149 | 180 | 175 |
| Maharashtra | 131 | 141 | 178 | 195 |
| Orissa | 102 | 110 | 128 | 169 |
| Punjab | 151 | 148 | 199 | 243 |
| Rajasthan | 200 | 227 | 252 | 267 |
| Tamil Nadu | 198 | 204 | 247 | 243 |
| Uttar Pradesh | 86 | 79 | 83 | 149 |
| West Bengal | 88 | 95 | 129 | 135 |
| Mean | 150 | 163 | 200 | 245 |
| STDEV | 82.3 | 90.0 | 118.6 | 157.5 |
| CV | 0.55 | 0.55 | 0.59 | 0.64 |

*Source:* Finance Account of States and RBI-State Finances: A Study of Budget.

consider health as low priorities sector. It has been observed from the discussion that the differences in health expenditure across states probably arise either because of preference or income of the state. The differences may also arise because of fiscal disabilities of the states arising from unequal capacities in raising revenues or due to varying cost of providing health services. The regional diversity and socio-economic conditions of a particular state however can also be the cause of inter-state variation in health expenditure. In order to fully evaluate the reason behind the differences in health expenditure, one needs to identify the degree to which the discrepancy in health expenditure is explained by the differences in states income, fiscal capacity, priority of State Governments or by other demographic factors. This however does not come under the preview of this study but can be the part of future research.

**Summary and Conclusion**

It is well known fact that improved education and health positively affect economic growth. Although private expenditure is 80 per cent of the total health expenditure, government spending is necessary in a developing country like India due to poor financial position of the majority of the population. Especially in the rural area, accounting around 72 per cent of the total population in the country, expenditure on health is the territory expenditure. Cutting down of the health services affects a lot for rural people. India accepted "Structural Adjustment Programme" in its new economic reforms, which suggests fewer government interventions in the economy including basic social services. In this paper an attempt has been made to analyse the trends and pattern of public health expenditure pre- and post-economic reform periods. Public health expenditure of combined Centre and States increased impressively in current prices about 50 times from Rs. 978 crores in 1976-77 tc Rs. 47,220 crores in 2005-06. This impressive growth has been eaten into escalation of price and rapid growth in population. In the per capita constant prices (1999-00) expenditure increased only 3 times. Compared to 1980s public health expenditure as a share of total budget as a percentage to GDP are less in 1990s and 2000s. Moreover, growth rate is also less in post-reform period. On the other hand centre has increased its spending after economic reforms not only in per capita term, but also in case of as a share of total expenditure and percentage to GDP. In case of All States, economic reform affected negatively, spending as a share of total expenditure and as a percentage of GDP decreased after reforms, further the growth rate is also less. Whereas analysis of 15 major states reveals that with having the continuation of increased inter-state disparity economic reforms affected differently on health sector for different states. Bihar, Orissa, Uttar Pradesh and West Bengal are the lowest spending states, while Kerala, Haryana, Rajasthan and Punjab are the highest spending states in most of the selected years. In case of growth rates of per capita health expenditure in 7 out or 15 states show an increase in the reform period. Significant growth rate can be observed in Andhra Pradesh, Haryana, Kerala and West Bengal during reform period. This means more than 50 per cent of the selected states affected negatively by economic reform. In case of health expenditure as a share of total budget it is less in 11 out of 15 states compared spending of 1980s.

The overall explanation reveals that public health expenditure decreased in India after economic reforms. Seeing of the lagging behind in Human Development Index, India needs to improve its education and health condition of the people. Huge investment is necessary to improve. In case of education Sarva Shiksha Abhiyan is the Central Government ambitious scheme to attain the goal of universalisation of primary education by 2007 and the universalisation elementary education by 2010. Three donors have assured for $ 1 billion in the estimated $ 3.5 billion. Similarly, as Bajapai and Goyal suggested a Health for All programme (Sarva Svasthya Abhiyan) is to be launched in India to improve the health from the ground level. Not only increasing of funds by the government is important, but the efficient use of the fund is also important. Along with this encouraging of the private and public partnership also appreciated. Last, but not least awareness improvement of the people is very important.

The impact of different macro-economic conditions shows that health expenditure is highly and negatively affected under adverse macro-economic conditions. Analysis at the state level shows that growth rate in per capita health expenditure in some of the low income states is recorded negative and significant. Interestingly, some of the high income states found unable to maintain significant positive growth rate in health expenditure. The co-efficients of growth rate during different macro-economic changes vary considerably across states. There also exists a high inter-state variation in per capita health expenditure in India.

The whole analysis confirms that India and its states are shying away from fulfilling its constitutional commitment of 'Right to Health' for its citizens. We have observed that public health sector have never been given change to perform well in India. Given the low level, declining and fluctuating behaviour of health expenditure over the last twenty five years, it is not surprising that the health sector performance in improving the health outcomes is not satisfactory. The failing nature of better health outcomes however can easily be reverse with the high level of public funds allocation in this sector. Specifically, India needs to double or triple its health spending from its existing level. Along with the commitments of health spending, it became important to ensure that the allocated additional public funds get spend effectively across its constituent states, which have shown low absorptive capacity to utilize the fund properly/effectively.

## References

Cornia, Giovanni A., Richard Jolly and Frances Stewort (1990). *Adjustment with a Human Face,* Oxford: Clarence Press.

Government of India (2001). *National Human Development Report (India),* Planning Commission.

Government of India (2007). *Select Health Parameters: A Comparative Analysis across the National Sample Survey Organisation 42nd, 52nd and 60th Rounds,* March, 10, Retrieved from: http://www.whoindia.org/LinkFiles/Health_Finance_NSSO_Report.pdf.

Government of India (various issues). *Indian Public Finance Statistics,* Ministry of Finance, Department of Economic Affairs, Economic Division, New Delhi.

Government of India (various issues). *RBI State Finance: A Study of State Budget,* Ministry of Finance. Government of India, New Delhi. Retrieved from: https://www.rbi.org.in/scripts/AnnualPublications.aspx

Government of India (2011, December). *Annual Report to the People on Health, Ministry of Health and Family Welfare,* Department of Health and Family Welfare, New Delhi. February, 12. Retrieved from http: // www.earth.columbia.edu

Joshi, Seema (2006, January 28). Impact of Economic Reforms on Social Sector Expenditure in India, *Economic and Political Weekly*, XLI (04): 123-134.

Lalitha, N. and Samira Guennif (2007). A Status Paper on the Pharmaceutical Industry in France, Gujarat Institute of Development Research, Working Paper No. 1980.

Narayana, D. (2008). Adjustment and health sector reforms: the solution to low public spending on health care in India? In: Haddad S., Baris E., Narayana D., editors. *Safeguarding the Health Sector in Times of Macroeconomic Instability*. New Jersey and Ottawa: Africa World Press and International Development Research Centre.

Nirupam, B. and Sangeeta, G. (2005, April 25). *Financing Health for All in India*, CGSD Working Paper No. 25, Working Papers Series Centre on Globalization and Sustainable Development, February, 12. Retrieved from http: // www.earth.columbia.edu.

Panchamukhi, P.R. (1965, January-March). Educational Capital in India, *Indian Economic Journal*, 13(3): 26-41.

Panchamukhi, P.R. (2000, March 4). Social Impact of Economic Reforms in India: A Critical Appraisal, *Economic and Political Weekly*, XXXV (10), Special Issue, 23-42.

Panchamukhi, P.R. (1965, January-March). Educational Capital in India, *Indian Economic Journal*, 13(3): 26-41.

Prabhu, K. Seeta. (1994, April 16). The Budget and Structural Adjustment with Human Face, *Economic and Political Weekly*, XXIX (16-17): 342-35.

Qadeer, I. (2000). Health Care Systems in Transition III. India, Part I. The Indian Experience, *Journal of Public Health Medicine*, 22(1): 25-32.

Sarkar, A.K., and Gupta, S.P. (1994, March 26). Fiscal Correction and Human Resource Development: Expenditure at Central and State Levels. *Economic and Political Weekly*, XXIX (13): 256-269.

Uko Tsujita. (2005, June). *Economic Reform and Social Sector Expenditure: A Study of Fifteen Indian States 1980/81-1999/2000*, Institute of Developing Economies, Japan External Trade Organisation (JETRO), Discussion Paper, 31, Retrieved from: http://ir.ide.go.jp/dspace/handle/2344/175.

World Bank (1993). Investing in Health, *World Bank Report*, Oxford University Press.

# 3
# High Risk and Testing Behaviours of HIV/AIDS among Female Sex Workers
## Survey in Rajshahi City, Bangladesh

*Sheikh Moin Uddin, Ismail Hossain* and
*Md. Golam Hossain*

## Introduction

Female sex workers (FSWs) and their clients are the risk group for spreading HIV/AIDS infection. Female sex workers (FSWs) are considered to be an important at risk group for HIV infection in Bangladesh (Uddin *et al.*, 2014). HIV/AIDS is one of the major concerns for health authorities in worldwide because it generally affects the young and reproductive sectors of a population. Bangladesh is a densely populated nation with a fast growing urban population with a growth rate of about 6 per cent every year. Most of the FSWs are trading sex in urban areas.

Rajshahi is one of the divisions and big city in Bangladesh, which is situated at the western border of Bangladesh, separated from India by a big river Padma (*Encyclopaedia Britannica*, 2009). Many young people travel regularly across the border for various purposes such as education, business, and wok. India has the greatest number of HIV/AIDS cases in Asia (AIDS Epidemic Update, WHO, 2007). The behavioural patterns of at-risk populations in the border city would be of interest to authorities involved in HIV/AIDS prevention.

Information on the rate of HIV testing in high risk groups like injecting drug users (IDUs) and female sex workers (FSWs) will assist with prevention measures of this epidemic. Disease transmission can be potentially reduced by early treatment of those already infected, and providing support for vulnerable groups (Leta *et al.*, 2012).

Some studies have been carried out in regard to HIV testing behaviour among FSWs. Hong *et al.* (2012) investigated the factors related to HIV testing behaviour among FSWs in Southwest China, and they reported that FSWs who never had HIV testing were more likely to engage in high risk behaviours. They also identified a number of psychological and structural barriers to HIV testing. Tsereteli *et al.* (2013) studied HIV testing behaviour among FSWs in Georgia and they established the relationship between epidemiological factors and HIV testing behaviours.

Due to the extensive range of the spread of HIV/AIDS through FSWs and their clients, it is, therefore, essential to be able to investigate HIV testing behaviours and observe the epidemiological factors such as age, residence, education level, marital status, economic condition, sex trading place, use condoms while having sex, asking HIV testing for new client, in order to ensure that corrective measures can be undertaken.

We designed this study to assess the awareness of FSWs and to investigate epidemiological factors associated with HIV testing behaviours among FSWs in Rajshahi city, Bangladesh.

## Materials and Methods

There is no legal brothel in Rajshahi city, and most of the female sex workers (FSW) are trading sex based on hotels or residence or side of street. The number of hotel, residence and street based FSW had been estimated to be 1135 and 450 respectively (BBS, 2011), but getting the contacts of these sex workers would not be easy. Due to frequent checking by law and enforcement agency and harassments of landlords, neighbours and clients, these sex workers change their address and contact frequently. For those who came from other parts of the country, many of them would be transferred to other cities after duration of 7 to 10 days.

We designed the study based on principles of Good Clinical Practice. With the co-operation of a few organizations that worked for the welfare FSW in Rajshahi city, we managed to obtain hand-phone contacts of 500 sex workers among them 250 contacts were randomly selected and eventually 200 of them agreed for an interview. From February to September 2012, we conducted the interviews based on standard questionnaires designed in local language (Bengali). Most of the interviews were conducted at a venue suggested by the respondents, and written consents were obtained from all them before we started the interview. Information collected included socio-demographic data, general and specific knowledge about HIV/AIDS and related issues.

**Statistical Analysis:** Pearson chi-square test was utilized to establish the association between testing behaviour of HIV and socio-economic variables among FSWs. Multiple logistic regression was used to find the effect of socio-economic factors on HIV testing behaviours. Statistical analyses were carried out using the Statistical Package for the Social Sciences software (SPSS version 15).

## Results and Discussions

In this study, 200 female sex workers (FSWs) were considered, and they were selected by randomly from Rajshahi city, Bangladesh. The mean age of FSW was 24.52 ± 6.27 years (range 16 to 41 years), while age of client was 29.43 ± 5.87 years (range 16 to 42 years). The mean age of FSWs at the time of first sexual contact was 15.01 ± 1.14 years with range 12 to 18 years (Table 3.1).

**Table 3.1:** Descriptive Statistics for some Characteristics of Sex Workers with their Clients

| *Descriptive* | *N* | *Minimum* | *Maximum* | *Mean* | *S.D.* |
|---|---|---|---|---|---|
| Female sex workers age | 200 | 16 | 41 | 24.52 | 6.27 |
| Clients age | 200 | 16 | 42 | 29.43 | 5.87 |
| Age of female sex workers at the time of first sexual contact | 200 | 12 | 18 | 15.01 | 1.14 |

*Source:* Field Survey.

Among the 200 FSWs interviewed, 68 per cent had already been tested for HIV, while 32 per cent had not (Table 3.2).

There were several socio demographic studies on FSWs and their commercial sex activities in Bangladesh (Uddin *et al.*, 2014). However, study on rate of HIV testing behaviour and factors related to willingness to undergo the test have not been reported. It was noted that only 68 per cent of FSWs in Rajshahi city have been tested HIV. Although, that rate is relatively high when

**Table 3.2:** Frequency Distribution of HIV testing Behaviour (Yes or No)

| | | *Frequency* | *Percentage* |
|---|---|---|---|
| Did you test HIV? | Yes | 136 | 68.00 |
| | No | 64 | 32.00 |
| | **Total** | **200** | **100.0** |

*Source:* Field Survey.

compared to the 48 per cent reported in a study based on the cities of Guilin and Beihai in China (Hong *et al.*, 2012). It is still an alarmingly high figure considering that Bangladesh is very densely populated country with very limited resources to counter the negative outcome of HIV/AIDs on the population. Moreover, Bangladesh is also a major source of labour for many other developing countries including India and other South-East Asian nations; thus, problems with HIV/AIDS would also adversely affect the productivity of those younger populations.

Slightly less than half (45%) of the FSWs interviewed were between 21-30 years old, and about the same percentage (45%) were from a slum environment. Only 42.5 per cent of the FSWs had secondary and higher education, while 12 per cent were uneducated (Table 3.3). Most of them (84.5%) were married and were living with their husband. Most (67.5%) of the FSWs were considered to be rich, and about 77 per cent FSWs had been tested for STI testing before. Many FSWs (40.5%) had traded sex at hotels, followed by private residence (39%) and the streets (20.5%). Among the 200 FSWs, 80.5 per cent were interested in using condoms while having sex with their clients, but only 10.5 per cent of them routinely asked their new clients about their HIV status. The $\chi^2$-test was used to detect the presence of an association between HIV testing behaviour and the selected factors. $\chi^2$-test demonstrated that the association between HIV testing behaviour and sex trading place with client ($p<0.05$), age group ($p<0.01$), sexually transmitted infections (STIs) testing behaviour ($p<0.01$), informed about HIV test to client ($p<0.01$), education level ($p<0.010$), social Status ($p<0.05$), interest to condom use having sex ($p<0.01$), and ask new client about his HIV testing behaviour ($p<0.01$) (Table 3.3) were statistically significant, while the other selected variables were not significantly associated with HIV testing behaviour of FSWs.

**Table 3.3:** Association between HIV Testing Behaviour and Selected Socio-Economic Factors

| Variable | Group | HIV testing behaviour | | | |
|---|---|---|---|---|---|
| | | Yes | No | $\chi^2$-value | p-value |
| Sex trading place with client | Street (20.5) | 21 (51.2) | 20 (48.8) | 10.281 | p<0.05 |
| | Hotel (40.5) | 53 (65.4) | 28 (34.6) | | |
| | Residence (39) | 62 (79.5) | 16 (20.5) | | |
| Age | Age?20 (36.5) | 45 (61.6) | 28 (38.4) | 14.933 | p<0.01 |
| | 21 ?Age?30 (45) | 73 (81.1) | 17 (18.9) | | |
| | 31 ?Age?41 (18.5) | 18 (48.6) | 19 (51.4) | | |
| Sexually transmitted infections (STIs) test? | Yes (77) | 120 (77.9) | 34 (22.1) | 30.293 | p<0.01 |
| | No (23) | 16 (34.8) | 30 (65.2) | | |
| Have you informed about HIV test? | Yes (83.5) | 132 (79.0) | 35 (21.0) | 56.710 | p<0.01 |
| | No (16.5) | 4 (12.1) | 29 (87.9) | | |
| Education Level of Female sex workers | No education (12) | 7 (29.2) | 17 (70.8) | 28.737 | p<0.01 |
| | Primary education (45.5) | 57 (62.6) | 34 (37.4) | | |
| | Secondary and higher education (42.5) | 72 (84.7) | 13 (15.3) | | |
| Marital Status | Married (84.5) | 118 (69.8) | 51 (30.2) | 1.664 | 0.197 |
| | Single (15.5) | 18 (58.1) | 13 (41.9) | | |
| Social Status | Poor (32.5) | 38 (58.5) | 27 (41.5) | 4.026 | p<0.05 |
| | Rich (67.5) | 98 (72.6) | 37 (27.4) | | |
| Are you are interested to use condom for safe sex? | Yes (80.5) | 120 (74.5) | 41 (25.5) | 16.200 | p<0.01 |
| | No (19.5) | 16 (41.0) | 23 (59.0) | | |
| Do you ask new client about his HIV testing? | Yes (10.5) | 19 (90.5) | 2 (9.5) | 5.447 | p<0.05 |
| | No (89.5) | 117 (65.4) | 62 (34.6) | | |

*Note:* Figures in the parentheses represent percentage.
*Source:* Field Survey.

Only the significantly associated variables were considered as independent variables for multiple logistic regression analysis. Multiple logistic regression model demonstrated that FSWs who were 21-30 years old were more likely to undergo HIV testing than those who were less than 20 years ($p<0.01$, OR = 0.374; CI: 0.184-0.760) and those who were between 31-41 years old ($p<0.01$, OR = 0.221; CI: 0.096-0.508). FSWs with secondary or higher education were more likely to undergo HIV testing, 0.074 ($p<0.01$) and 0.303 ($p<0.01$) times higher than uneducated and primary educated counterparts respectively (Table 3.4). FSWs who came from rich family background were 0.531 ($p<0.05$) times more likely to have HIV testing done compared to those from poor family background. FSWs who had previously been tested for STI were also more likely to have HIV testing compared those who had no history of STI testing ($p<0.01$, OR=0.151; CI: 0.074-0.309). Sex trade on residence based FSWs were more likely to have HIV testing than street based ($p<0.01$, OR =0.217; CI: 0.119-0.617) and hotel based ($p<0.01$, OR=0.488; CI: 0.239-0.999) FSWs. Those who practiced use of condom during sex with their clients were more likely to have HIV testing than their counterparts ($p<0.01$, OR= 0.238; CI: 0.115-0.493) (Table 3.4), and a similar tendency was also noted for those who routinely asked their new clients about their HIV testing status ($p<0.05$, OR = 0.199; CI: 0.045-0.881) (Table 3.4).

This study has demonstrated that sex traded at residence and hotel-based FSWs were more likely to have HIV testing than street-based FSWs. Higher percentage of street-based FSWs were from slum or rural areas, and many received little or only a primary level of education. Lack of knowledge and time were considered as the main reasons for low rate of HIV testing among street-based FSWs (Mondal *et al.*, 2008). In Rajshahi city, this group of FSWs is more likely to spread HIV/AIDS infection because their potential clients are mainly rickshaw pullers, day labourers, and transport workers who may also be unaware about HIV/AIDS. FSWs aged 21-30 years old were generally more aware and willing to undergo HIV testing, while those above 30 years of age may have a false sense of security because they have survived over the years as reported in another study (Uddin *et al.*, 2014).

Awareness programmes on availability and importance of HIV testing, and behaviour change communication (BCC) programmes should be organized for all FSWs in all major cities of Bangladesh including Rajshahi. Risk of HIV/AIDS among FSWs in low and middle income countries like Bangladesh, China, India and Nepal is about 14 times higher than the global population in general (Baral

**Table 3.4:** Effect of Socio-economic Factors on HIV Testing Behaviour among Female Sex Workers

| *Variable* | *Group* | *Coefficient* | *S.E.* | *Wald* | *df* | *p-value* | *Odds ratio (OR)* | *95% CI for OR* | |
|---|---|---|---|---|---|---|---|---|---|
| | | | | | | | | Lower | Upper |
| Sex trading place | | | | 9.857 | 2 | p<0.01 | | | |
| | Street *Vs* Residence | –1.306 | 0.420 | 9.674 | 1 | p<0.01 | 0.271 | 0.119 | 0.617 |
| | Hotel *Vs* Residence | –0.716 | 0.365 | 3.853 | 1 | p<0.05 | 0.488 | 0.239 | 0.999 |
| Age | | | | 14.036 | 2 | p<0.01 | | | |
| | Age ? 20 *Vs* 21?Age?30 | –0.983 | 0.361 | 7.404 | 1 | p<0.01 | 0.374 | 0.184 | 0.760 |
| | 31?Age?41 *Vs* 21?Age?30 | –1.511 | 0.425 | 12.639 | 1 | p<0.01 | 0.221 | 0.096 | 0.508 |
| STI test | No *Vs* Yes | –1.890 | 0.365 | 26.734 | 1 | p<0.01 | 0.151 | 0.074 | 0.309 |
| Informed HIV | No *Vs* Yes | –3.308 | 0.566 | 34.139 | 1 | p<0.01 | 0.037 | 0.012 | 0.111 |
| Education of Female sex workers | | | | 24.469 | 2 | p<0.01 | | | |
| | No *Vs* Secondary and higher | –2.599 | 0.541 | 23.094 | 1 | p<0.01 | 0.074 | 0.026 | 0.215 |
| | Primary *Vs* Secondary and higher | –1.195 | 0.371 | 10.366 | 1 | p<0.01 | 0.303 | 0.146 | 0.627 |
| Social Status | Poor *Vs* Rich | –0.632 | 0.317 | 3.975 | 1 | p<0.05 | 0.531 | 0.285 | 0.989 |
| Use condom having sex | No *Vs* Yes | –1.437 | 0.372 | 14.884 | 1 | p<0.01 | 0.238 | 0.115 | 0.493 |
| Asking HIV testing of new client | No *Vs* Yes | –1.616 | 0.760 | 4.525 | 1 | p<0.05 | 0.199 | 0.045 | 0.881 |
| | Constant | 3.55 | 1.04 | 11.495 | 1 | p<0.01 | 34.827 | | |

*Source:* Field Survey.

*et al.*, 2012). Frequent change in place of stay and migration between cities were some of the barriers for FSWs to gain proper information about HIV/AIDs and HIV testing (Uddin *et al.*, 2014). Eighty-three per cent of all FSWs in the current study were aware about HIV testing. Females were noted to be four times more vulnerable than men to be infected with HIV/AIDS, and this should serve as a strong reason for them to protect themselves (UNICEF, 2009).

One of the major factors that influence the effort towards prevention of HIV/AIDS is education. In Rajshahi, rate of HIV testing among FSWs with secondary level or higher education was higher than FSWs who were uneducated and those with primary education. Educated FSWs were closer to mainstream of the society, and they have more exposed to information related to health in the form of electronic and print media.

The study showed that most of the FSWs were married and were living with their spouses. Most (61.7%) married women in Bangladesh preferred to use oral contraceptive pills, and the use of condoms (21.4%) was less popular (Ferdousi *et al.*, 2010). In Bangladesh, oral contraceptive pills were being distributed through health clinics by Governmental and Non-governmental Organizations (NGOs). This is provides a good opportunity where awareness on HIV/AIDS and availability of HIV testing can be disseminated. However, unmarried FSWs were generally more hesitant to attend these clinics due to social barriers and, so, they may not have access to this information. Clients of FSWs are the most important source and mode of spread for HIV/AIDS. This study showed that most of the FSWs did not ask new clients about their HIV testing status. FSWs that had already undergone HIV testing were more interested to know about the HIV testing status of their new clients. In Rajshahi city the sex trade is based on the sexual act and not on the time spent. Young FSWs are keen to look for new customers and may not have time to discuss matters like HIV/AIDS testing. Use of condoms is an effective method to reduce or control the HIV/AIDS epidemic (Hong *et al.*, 2012). This study showed that FSWs who had HIV testing done generally prefer the use of condoms during the sex trade, while those who had not been tested were less likely to do so. Increasing awareness on the infection prevention and promoting the use condoms should contribute towards reduction and control of HIV/AIDS.

In the present study only the HIV testing behaviours and factors associated with HIV testing among FSWs were investigated. Thus, it is essential to estimate the prevalence and investigate the epidemiological factors associated with HIV/AIDS patients among FSWs in Rajshahi and other big cities in Bangladesh. Clearly, more research will be required with FSWs in Bangladesh.

## Conclusion

The study showed that 68 per cent of FSWs in Rajshahi city had been tested for HIV. Factors associated with higher rate of HIV testing included age between 21-30, higher level of education, richer family background and history of STI testing. FSWs that had been tested for HIV were more likely to use condoms and asked their new clients on their HIV testing status. This information will help the health authorities to target groups of FSWs who have not undergone HIV testing. This should contribute towards better control of HIV/AIDS, which is at epidemic levels in this country.

**Acknowledgments:** We would like to thank Rajshahi City Corporation, Population Services and Training Centre (PSTC), Urban Primary Health Care Project (UPHCP), Khulna Mukti Seba Sanstha (KMSS), Urban Primary Health Care Project (UPHCP), Tilottoma-Smiling Sun Franchising Project (SSFP), and other Non-Government Organizations (NGOs) who are implementing programmes to fight against HIV/AIDS at Rajshahi City in Bangladesh.

**Ethical Approach:** Female sex workers were not listed/ registered in Rajshahi city and they were not interested to expose themselves socially as a sex worker for a lot of social factors. Due to this, ethical approach should be questionable. To overcome this problem we approached to get interview with our questionnaire and it maintained strictly confidential to only use data for research purpose. After their consent, those female sex workers were asked as a respondent with name, address and signature.

**Limitation of Research:** Female sex workers were always moving from one place to another. Most of them were guided by broker, client and Mokkhirani (team leader). Most of female sex workers had multiple identifications such as; name, address, contact number. To overcome this problem, firstly, the current hand phone number of female sex workers was collected from difference Governmental and Non-Governmental Organizations (NGOs) which were working with sex workers at Rajshahi city, then corresponded with them and identified their address and finally we contacted them.

## References

Bangladesh Bureau of Statistics (BBS). Population Census-2011. Retrieved from < http://www.bbs.gov.bd/userfiles/Image/RptPop Cen.pdf >. (Accessed on 3-5-2015)

Baral, S., Beyrer, C., Muessig, K., Poteat, T., Wirtz, A.L., Decker, M.R., Sherman, S.G., and Kerrigan, D. (2012). Burden of HIV among female sex workers in low-income and middle-income countries: a systematic review and meta-analysis. *Lancet Infectious Diseases, 12*(7): 538-549.

*Encyclopedia Britannica* (2009). Rajshahi. Encyclopedia Britannica Online. Available at <http: //global.britannica.com/EBchecked/topic/490171/ Rajshahi> accepted 18, 2009.

Ferdousi, S.K., Jabbar, M.A., Hoque, S.R., Karim, S.R., Mahmood, A.R., Ara, R., and Khan, N.R. (2010). Unmet need of family planning among rural women in Bangladesh. *Journal* of the *Dhaka Medical College, 19*: 11-15.

Hong, Y., Zhang, C., Li, X., Fang, X., Lin, X., Zhou, Y, Liu W. (2012). HIV Testing Behaviours among Female Sex Workers in Southwest China. *AIDS* and *Behaviour, 16*(1): 44-52.

Leta, T·H., Sandøy, I.F., and Fylkesnes, K. (2012). Factors affecting voluntary HIV counselling and testing among men in Ethiopia: a cross-sectional survey. BMC Public Health, 15 June, 12438. doi: 10.1186/ 1471-2458-12-438. Available at http://www.ncbi.nlm.nih.gov/pubmed/ 22703550 (Accessed on 15 June, 2015).

Tsereteli, N., Chikovani, I., Chkhaidze, N., Goguadze, K., Shengelia, N., and Rukhadze, N. (2013). HIV testing uptake among female sex workers and men who have sex with men in Tbilisi, Georgia. HIV Medicine, 14 Suppl. 3, 29-32. doi: 10.1111/hiv.12065.

Mondal, N.I., Hossain, K., Islam, R., and Mian, A.B. (2008). Sexual behaviour and sexually transmitted diseases in street-based female sex workers in Rajshahi City, Bangladesh. *Brazilian Journal of Infectious Diseases*, 12(4), 287-92.

Uddin, S.M., Hossain, M.G., Islam, M.A., Islam, M.N., Aik, S., and Kamarul, T. (2014). High Risk Behaviour of HIV/AIDS among Females Sex Workers in Bangladesh: Survey in Rajshahi City. *Japanese Journal of Infectious Diseases, 67*(3), 191-196.

UNICEF (2009). *HIV and AIDS in Bangladesh*, Page-1, March, 2009.

United Nations.Asia (2007), AIDS Epidemic Update. Regional Summary. Geneva: Joint United Nations Programme on HIV/AIDS/World Health Organization.

# 4
# Demographic and Socio-Economic Factors Affecting Variation at Levels of Fertility in Odisha
## A District Level Analysis

*Bisworanjan Behuria*

### Introduction

Higher rate of fertility has been considered as the main reason for the rapid population growth in Developing countries including India. The population of India in the last seven decade is increasing at a great pace because of the decreasing death rate, which is the cause of more availability of healthcare facilities. Among the demographic variables affecting the growth of population in India, the birth rate is of obvious importance owing to the potential possibility, it holds for lowering the rate of population growth. India's one-third of the districts has Crude Birth Rate of 25 and more and 174 out of 621 have today fertility levels below 2.1 and the regional patterns of fertility at district level vary from the low fertility in the South to high fertility in the North (Gulmoto and Rajan, 2013).

It is widely acknowledged all across the world that age at marriage has a significant influence on fertility, particularly in countries where childbearing occurs within marriage. The importance of marriage age on fertility variation is evident from its inclusion as one of the four proximate determinants of fertility as proposed by Bongaarts (Bongaarts, 1982). In many societies, as Coale (1992) observed, the relationship between late marriage and low fertility is the result of higher control levels of marital fertility among the populations that marry late. Marriage rates in India have been remarkably stable for more than a century, with universal marriage being the norm. However, the marriage age has undergone a gradual, but steady increase: singulate mean age at marriage increased from 16.8 to 21.2 years for women between 1961 and 2011 (Registrar General, India, 2011). Over the last few decades, fertility rates have been falling. The 2001 and 2011 census, gives a clear indication that India is passing through the last phase of fertility transition, moving towards moderate to low fertility. Fertility decline have not been uniform across the country and the differential rates are mainly responsible for the differentials in population growth rates across the states and UTs. One of the important changes taking place in relatively less developed regions is the rapid decline in fertility defying conventional theories and beliefs. One such example is Odisha, socio-economically backward states of India. The trends in fertility in Odisha as indicated by Crude Birth Rate (CBR) and Total Fertility Rate (TFR) based on Sample Registration System (SRS), National Family Health Survey and Census show a declining trend, which is a positive sign for the coming generations. Based on the SRS estimates of 2001 the Crude Birth Rate and Total Fertility Rate of Odisha were 23.5 and 2.6 which is declined to 19.6 and 2.1 for the same in SRS 2014. The NFHS data also shows a declining trend in CBR and TFR for Odisha in NFHS I (1992-93) the CBR and TFR was 26.5 and 2.9 and it decline to 24.3 and 2.4 in NFHS II (1998-99), it further declined to 22.1 and 2.3 in NFHS III (2005-06).

## Statement of the Problem

Though, the fertility of Odisha is not among the highest, still, the decline is not significant as the western and southern states. The fertility decline in Odisha—a socio-economically lagging state of India contradicts itself and many researchers failed to understand the puzzle of low social development, large proportion of population living Below Poverty Line (47.15%), low level of urbanization (17%) and moderately high rate of infant mortality (61 per 1000 live births in 2010) with the much lower Total Fertility Rate than what is predicted for the socio-economic situations. A number of problems also associated with this study like the availability and reliability of data, because the SRS, NFHS and Census data, which is used in this study, is conducted by taking some of the samples so these data may not have reliability. The broad aim of the study is to examine the temporal and spatial variations in fertility level and find out the demographic and socio-economic factors affecting the variations.

## A Brief Review of Literature

### *Levels and Trends of Fertility*

Fertility decline is the most important social change that has occurred in India in recent years. After a slow decline in 1970s, the pace of decline began to accelerate since 1980s. There has been a clear decline in fertility since then (Visaria and Visaria, 1994). The most important features of this accelerated decline is that in many parts of India it has embraced all sections of society—rich and poor, educated and illiterate, upper caste and lower caste and so on and is well documented particularly in the south Indian states (Dev *et al.*, 2002; James, 1999; James and Subramanian, 2005; Kishore, 1994; Sekher *et al.*, 2005 and Srinivasan *et al.*, 1991). While (Skirbark, 2008) discussed the fertility and social statuses were inversely related with each other and particularly education depresses fertility from early in the twentieth century as long as this relation is observed. Whereas (Bacci, 1977) studied three Italian cities from the fifteenth to eighteenth centuries and found a positive relation between status and child bearing outcomes for all of them (Bardet, 1983) studied two lower classes and three higher classes from 1670 to 1789 in Rouen, France and found these classes substantially decreased their fertility. (Kondel, 1988) noted that wives of village leaders got married when they were 2.1 years younger than wives of non-village leaders in a study of German villages from 1700-1899.

### *Regional Variation of Fertility*

There are regional variation of fertility rate persist in India with higher fertility in the north to the lower fertility in the Western and the Southern parts and when we say fertility Transition in religious level Hindus are quite ahead of Muslims (Rajan, 2005; Guilmoto and Rajan, 2002). While (James and Nair, 2005) find that Muslim Fertility in India follows nearly the same pace transition as that of Hindus, particularly in the period of accelerated fertility decline. (Kumar and Satyanarayana, 2012) pointed out that fertility is not affected by migration and fertility of migrants and non-migrants do not differ and found that India is undergoing a fertility transition, yet around one-third of districts have a birth rate of 25 or more. The districts which were counted as a high fertility district now days show a pace of faster decline. In Indian context fertility at district level is very low in Kerala as followed by Tamil Nadu and Andhra Pradesh (Bhat, 1996). (Ramesh, 2003) stated that the caste differentials are notable in rural areas and at the lower levels of socio-economic status, but in urban areas and higher levels of socio-economic status, the differentials are narrow. Fertility has been much higher and contraceptive use much lower among Scheduled Castes and Scheduled Tribes compared to other castes.

### *Factors Affecting Fertility*

Many studies have done in India and it was found that in Kerala the print media and socio-economic variables played a crucial role, in Tamil Nadu, and to some extent in Andhra Pradesh, the access to electronic media and motivational programmes was crucial in explaining fertility decline (Bhat, 1996 and Manna, 1998). (Saha and Verma, 2000) noted that early marriage, low birth interval, strong preference for male child, lack of knowledge about family planning methods were the cause of high TFR among ST population of undivided MP which was higher than the average TFR of the country. Similar studies conducted in TN and found that the availability or road facilities and infant mortality are the most important factors influencing fertility (Savitri, 1994) whereas fertility declined has been faster in southern and coastal region of Karnataka with a high literacy, high female age at marriage, better health infrastructure and high status of women as comparable to the backward northern districts (Sekhar *et al.*, 2001). Educational levels of women, sex preference, delay in marriage, household income of women infant death and exposure to mass media have significant effects on the use of contraception, which is the cause of decline in fertility in many parts of India and particularly the southern states (Sahoo, 2007; Premchand and Agadjanian, 2009; Visaria, 2003; Chauhan and Singh, 2012; Dreez and Murthi, 2001; Unisa, 2000, Jain, 1985 and Paul, 2000).

## Objectives

The broad objective of the study is to examine the temporal and spatial variations in fertility level and factors affecting the variations. The specific objectives are as follows:

1. To analyse the trends of fertility in Odisha over last few decades.
2. To examine the inter-district variation in fertility in Odisha and its changing patterns.
3. To find out the demographic, economic and social factors affecting variation at district level in fertility in Odisha.

## Data Source and Methodology

The data is obtained mainly from three sources, i.e. from the census 2001 and 2011; NFHS 1 (1992-93), NFHS-2 (1998-99), and NFHS-3 (2005-06); SRS 1971-2011. Besides, data from DLHS-2 (2002-03) and DLHS-3 (2007-08), Annual Health Survey (2010-11) and Economic Survey-Odisha, 2009-10 and 2012-13. To map district level patterns of Fertility in Odisha, districts have been categorized into three groups. Range method is used to group the districts into three categorized; low, medium and high. Class interval is carried out by a formula; Class interval equals to (Highest value-lowest value)/ Number of required groups. Decadal rate of change is calculated by the formula, Current year- base year/base year x 100. Coefficient of Variation is calculated by Standard Deviation/ Mean x 100. Correlation and Regression techniques are employed to observe the relative effects of socio-economic indicators such as female literacy rate, female work participation rate, and workers in non-agricultural sector, Sex Ratio, level of urbanization, SC population and ST population in Odisha, Per Capita NDDP, Contraceptive Prevalence Rate and Infant Mortality Rate on Crude Birth Rate and Total Fertility Rate in Odisha.

## Levels and Trends of Fertility in Odisha

Fertility as measured by Crude Birth Rate (CBR) and Total Fertility Rate (TFR) has been declining in Odisha since the 1970s and it is on a level lower than the national average Till the mid of 1980s the fertility decline was not so rapid, but the CBR and TFR was started falling consistently after that point. Table 4.1 shows state-wise comparable figures of CBR and TFR for 2001 and 2011.

**Table 4.1:** State-wise Crude Birth Rate and Total Fertility Rate in India from 2001 and 2011 Census

| | *2001* | | *2011* | |
|---|---|---|---|---|
| **States and UTs** | **CBR** | **TFR** | **CBR** | **TFR** |
| **India** | **25.9** | **3.1** | **21.2** | **2.7** |
| Andaman & Nicobar | 20 | 2.3 | 15.7 | 1.7 |
| Andhra Pradesh | 20.4 | 2.3 | 16.2 | 1.8 |
| Arunachal Pradesh | 29.9 | 3.9 | 23.7 | 3.3 |
| Assam | 27 | 3.1 | 23.7 | 2.9 |
| Bihar | 33.4 | 4.5 | 29.7 | 4.2 |
| Chandigarh | 20 | 2.2 | 17.4 | 2 |
| Chhattisgarh | 28.6 | 3.6 | 23.2 | 3 |
| Dadra Nagar & Haveli | 31.8 | 3.6 | 25.1 | 3.1 |
| Daman & Diu | 21.7 | 2.4 | 28.3 | 2.1 |
| Delhi | 23.4 | 2.6 | 18.7 | 2.2 |
| Goa | 15.9 | 1.7 | 14.3 | 1.5 |
| Gujarat | 22.6 | 2.5 | 20.1 | 2.4 |
| Haryana | 25.9 | 3.2 | 21.2 | 2.7 |
| Himachal Pradesh | 20.5 | 2.3 | 17.6 | 2 |
| Jammu & Kashmir | 24.5 | 2.9 | – | – |
| Jharkhand | 29.9 | 4 | 25.8 | 3.5 |
| Karnataka | 20.9 | 2.4 | 17.8 | 2 |
| Kerala | 17.1 | 1.7 | 14.7 | 1.6 |
| Lakshadweep | 22.6 | 2.6 | 16.6 | 2.1 |
| Madhya Pradesh | 30.7 | 3.8 | 24.3 | 3.2 |
| Maharashtra | 21.7 | 2.5 | 17.9 | 2.2 |
| Manipur | 21 | 2.5 | 20 | 2.5 |
| Meghalaya | 33.6 | 4.4 | 31.3 | 4.3 |
| Mizoram | 27.3 | 3.3 | 24.1 | 2.9 |
| Nagaland | 24.1 | 3.1 | 21.1 | 2.8 |
| **Odisha** | **23.6** | **2.8** | **19.7** | **2.4** |
| Pondicherry | 18.1 | 1.8 | 16.4 | 1.7 |
| Punjab | 20.1 | 2.4 | 16.6 | 2.1 |
| Rajasthan | 32.1 | 4.2 | 25.5 | 3.4 |
| Sikkim | 23.7 | 3 | 15.5 | 1.9 |
| Tamil Nadu | 17.2 | 1.8 | 14.9 | 1.6 |
| Tripura | 21.2 | 2.4 | 18.9 | 2.2 |
| Uttar Pradesh | 31.4 | 4.3 | 24.8 | 3.6 |
| Uttarakhand | 26.1 | 3.6 | 21 | 2.6 |
| West Bengal | 22.6 | 2.0 | 17.3 | 2 |

*Sources:* 1. Christophe Z. Guilmoto, S. Irudaya Rajan, 2002, District level Estimates of Fertility from India's 2001 Census, *Economic and Political Weekly*, pp. 668-670.

2. Christophe Z. Guilmoto, S. Irudaya Rajan, 2013, Fertility at District level in India: Lessons from the 2011 census, Working Papers DU CEPED, June 30, pp. 1-32.

As per the 2001 estimates based on census information, the Crude Birth Rate and the Total Fertility Rate were extremely high in states such as, Bihar, Uttar Pradesh, Rajasthan, Madhya Pradesh, Jharkhand and Meghalaya. It means that fertility rates were substantially high in the BIMARU states. Among the UTs, Dadra & Nagar Haveli were recorded to have the highest Crude Birth Rate and Total Fertility Rate (31.8 and 3.6% respectively). TFR in the southern and coastal states, along with Punjab, Himachal Pradesh, Tripura and Manipur was lower than 3 children per woman. Below replacement level TFR was observed in states such as Tamil Nadu, Kerala, Karnataka, Andhra Pradesh and Goa. Among the UTs, Pondicherry and Chandigarh had low levels of TFR.

Regional picture of fertility has changed between the year 2001 and 2011. In 2011, fertility data reveal that Total Fertility Rate has gone below the replacement level of 2.1 children per woman in no less than 12 states and UTs in the country. State level figures indicate that few states such as Kerala, Tamil Nadu and Goa have recorded fertility levels close to 1.5 children per woman. On the other hand, Bihar and Meghalaya are the only states where average fertility still stands at above four children per woman. Apart from these two states several other states which have high fertility are Rajasthan, Madhya Pradesh, Uttar Pradesh and Jharkhand. Again, 2011 data also brings out the picture of BIMARU states as the high fertility zone of India. These are also the areas where fertility decline has proceeded at a faster pace during the inter-censal period (a decline by around 0.6 children in ten years). Unlike Bihar, several "Empowered Action Group" states such as Rajasthan, Uttar Pradesh and Madhya Pradesh emerge as states with the fastest speed of fertility decline during previous decade. The largest number of states lies between these two extremes, with fertility ranging from replacement level to four children per woman. However, TFR in Odisha is relatively low; lower than BIMARU states. And TFR figure is lower than Haryana, a developed state of India.

Fertility Rate has declined significantly in Odisha from 34.6 (CBR) in 1971 to 19.6 (CBR) in 2013 and 4.7 (TFR) in 1971 to 2.1 (TFR) in 2013. Compared to this state's average, India's Crude Birth Rate declined from 36.9 in 1971 to 21.4 in 2013, and Total Fertility Rate declined from 5.2 in 1971 to 2.3 in 2013. If we compare the trend line of India (both CBR and TFR), it can observed that the pace of decline in fertility rate in Odisha has been slightly slower than the average decline in the country (Figs. 4.1 and 4.2).

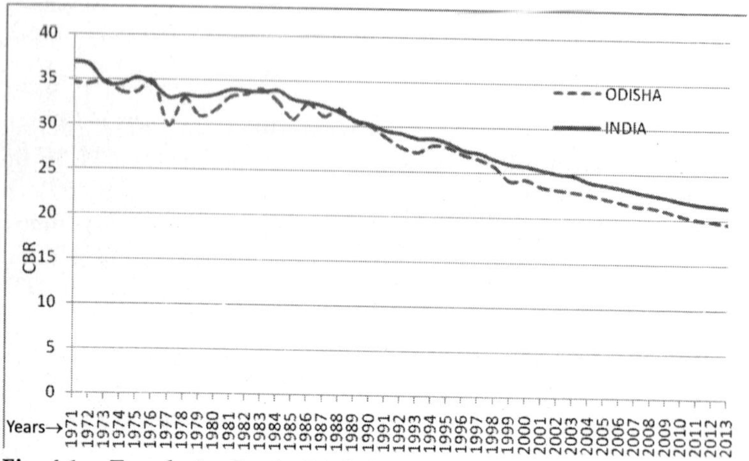


**Fig. 4.1:** Trends in Crude Birth Rate in Odisha Based on Annual Estimates, 1971-2013

*Source:* Based on SRS data given in the Appendix 1.

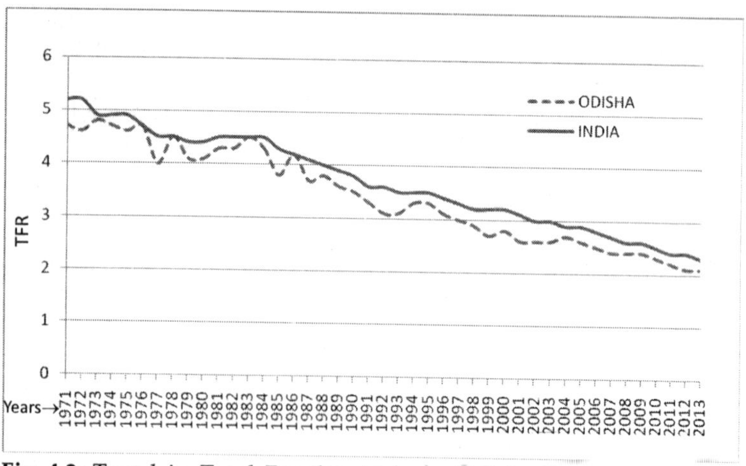


**Fig 4.2:** Trend in Total Fertility Rate in Odisha Based on Annual Estimates 1971-2013

*Source:* Based on SRS data given in the Appendix 1.

If one looks at the data on the CBR and TFR in Odisha over the last four decades, one can find some significant up and down movements particularly in the 1970s, 1980s and 1990s. Even when one takes three-year moving averages to smooth annual fluctuations, one finds similar fluctuations in the 1970s and 1980s (Figs. 4.3 and

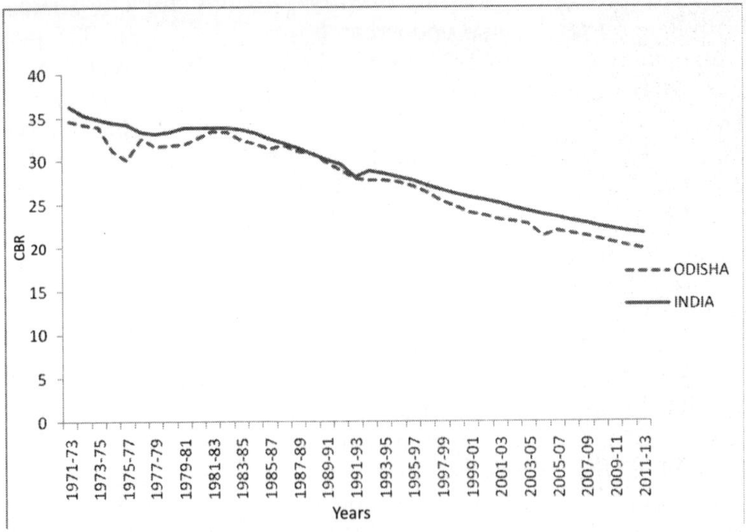


**Fig. 4.3:** Trends in Crude Birth Rate in Odisha Based on Three Years Moving Average, 1971-2013.

*Source:* Based on SRS data given in the Appendix 2.

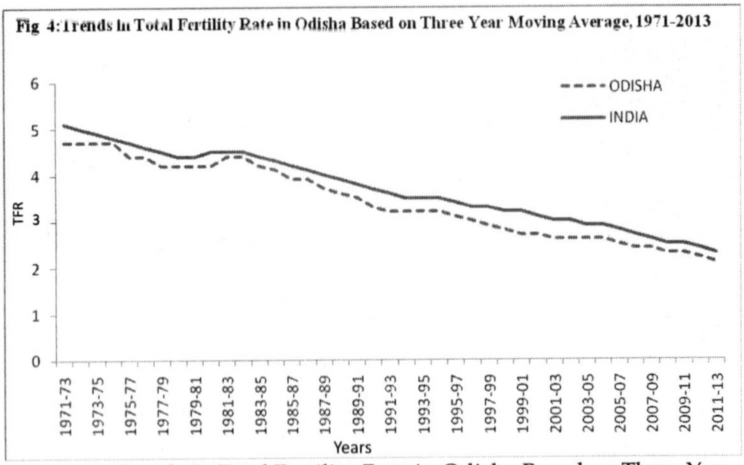


**Fig. 4.4:** Trends in Total Fertility Rate in Odisha Based on Three Years Moving Average, 1971-2013.

*Source:* Based on SRS data given in the Appendix 2.

4.4). From the three years moving average of CBR and TFR for the state, Odisha and the country India, it was observed that India's CBR and TFR in case of total or rural or urban is higher than Odisha's three year average. So, starting from 1971-73 for Odisha the Crude Birth Rate for total, Rural and urban it was 34.7, 34.8 and 32.5 per cent, in this period the CBR for total, rural and urban was 36.3, 37.7 and 30.0 per cent. The TFR in this same period for Odisha was 4.7, 4.8 and 4.2 per cent for total, rural and urban while the TFR of India was 5.1, 5.3 and 4.0 per cent for the same respectively. Though the state have achieved the replacement level of 2.1 per cent, the country have not achieved yet, in 2011-13 Odisha's TFR for total is 2.1 per cent and India's TFR for total is 2.3 per cent. Though many countries have now achieved the replacement level of fertility (*see* appendix for both annual and three year moving average data).

Two rounds of National Family Health Surveys were conducted in 1990's, first in 1992-93 and the second in 1998-99. The Third round of NFHS III was conducted in 2005-06. Data from this source can be utilized to look into the change in Fertility Rate in the recent past. Throughout the NFHS-I, NFHS-II and NFH-III the crude Birth rate and the Total fertility rate is declining in Odisha. During the period between first and second survey (1992-93 and 1998-99), CBR declined by 22 points and TFR declined by 5 points. CBR and TFR reduced by 22 points and 1 point in Odisha during the second inter-survey period (1998-99) and third survey (2005-06). It is evident from these figures that the decline for CBR during (NFHS-I and NFHS-II) and (NFHS-II and NFHS-III) was same but for TFR the decline was much faster during the first inter-survey period (NFHS-I and NFHS-II) than later (NFHS-II and NFHS-III) one in Odisha. From the NFHS data it is clear that Odisha will achieve soon the replacement level of fertility of 2.1 (*see* Table. 4.2).

**Table 4.2:** Trend in Fertility Rate in Odisha for the Five-year Period Preceding the Survey: Evidences from NFHS Surveys

| | *Odisha* | |
|---|---|---|
| | *CBR* | *TFR* |
| NFHS-1 (1992-93) | 26.5 | 2.9 |
| NFHS-2 (1998-99) | 24.3 | 2.4 |
| NFHS-3 (2005-06) | 22.1 | 2.3 |

*Source:* IIPS and ORC Macro, "National Family Health Surveys Odisha". 2005-06.

## District Level Patterns of Fertility in Odisha

The district level variations in fertility persist across districts of Odisha. The Crude Birth Rate declined from 23.4 in 2001 to 19.6 in

2011. Similarly, the Total Fertility Rate reduced from of 2.8 in 2001 to 2.4 in 2011. The decadal rates of decline in CBR and TFR were 16.9 per cent and 14.2 per cent respectively (*see* Table 4.3).

**Table 4.3:** District level Estimates of Fertility from India's 2001 and 2011 Census

| *State and Districts* | *CBR* | | *Difference* | *Decadal change in percentage in CBR* | *TFR* | | *Difference* | *Decadal change in percentage in TFR* |
|---|---|---|---|---|---|---|---|---|
| | *2001* | *2011* | | | *2001* | *2011* | | |
| Odisha | 23.6 | 19.6 | 4.0 | –16.9 | 2.8 | 2.4 | 0.4 | –14.2 |
| Bargarh | 20.6 | 16.8 | 3.8 | –18.4 | 2.5 | 2.1 | 0.4 | –16 |
| Jharsuguda | 21.1 | 16.9 | 4.2 | –19.9 | 2.6 | 2.1 | 0.5 | –19.2 |
| Sambalpur | 21.2 | 17.7 | 3.5 | –16.5 | 2.6 | 2.1 | 0.5 | –19.2 |
| Debagarh | 25.5 | 20.5 | 5 | –19.6 | 3.1 | 2.5 | 0.6 | –19.3 |
| Sundergarh | 22.8 | 19.3 | 3.5 | –15.3 | 2.7 | 2.3 | 0.4 | –14.8 |
| Kendujhar | 25.3 | 23.1 | 2.2 | –8.6 | 3.0 | 2.8 | 0.2 | –6.6 |
| Mayurbhanj | 26.0 | 21.4 | 4.6 | –17.6 | 3.0 | 2.7 | 0.3 | –10 |
| Baleshwar | 25.2 | 19.1 | 6.1 | –24.2 | 2.9 | 2.3 | 0.6 | –20.6 |
| Bhadrak | 24.8 | 18.9 | 5.9 | –23.7 | 2.9 | 2.3 | 0.6 | –20.6 |
| Kendrapara | 21.8 | 17.0 | 4.8 | –22.0 | 2.6 | 2.0 | 0.6 | –23.0 |
| Jagatsingpur | 18.8 | 14.3 | 4.5 | –23.9 | 2.3 | 1.7 | 0.6 | –26.0 |
| Cuttack | 19.6 | 15.4 | 4.2 | –21.4 | 2.4 | 1.8 | 0.6 | –25 |
| Jajpur | 21.8 | 18.1 | 3.7 | –16.9 | 2.6 | 2.2 | 0.4 | –15.3 |
| Dhenkanal | 21.8 | 18.1 | 3.7 | –16.9 | 2.7 | 2.1 | 0.6 | –22.2 |
| Anugul | 23.4 | 10.5 | 4.9 | –20.9 | 2.9 | 2.2 | 0.7 | –24.1 |
| Nayagarh | 20.9 | 17.2 | 3.7 | –17.7 | 2.5 | 2.1 | 0.4 | –16 |
| Khurdha | 20.3 | 16.2 | 4.1 | –20.1 | 2.4 | 1.9 | 0.5 | –20.8 |
| Puri | 20.2 | 15.8 | 4.4 | –21.7 | 2.4 | 1.8 | 0.6 | –25 |
| Ganjam | 24.0 | 18.4 | 5.6 | –23.3 | 2.9 | 2.2 | 0.7 | –24.1 |
| Gajapati | 27.6 | 24.1 | 3.5 | –12.6 | 3.3 | 2.9 | 0.4 | –12.1 |
| Kandhamal | 30.8 | 24.7 | 6.1 | –19.8 | 3.6 | 3.0 | 0.6 | –16.6 |
| Boudh | 27.4 | 22.6 | 4.8 | –17.5 | 3.2 | 2.8 | 0.4 | –12.5 |
| Subarnapur | 22.7 | 19.2 | 3.5 | –15.4 | 2.8 | 2.5 | 0.3 | –10.7 |
| Balangir | 22.9 | 21.2 | 1.7 | –7.4 | 2.8 | 2.7 | 0.1 | –3.5 |
| Nuapada | 25.9 | 23.1 | 2.8 | –10.8 | 3.0 | 2.9 | 0.1 | –3.3 |
| Kalahandi | 26.8 | 23.0 | 3.8 | –14.1 | 3.2 | 2.8 | 0.4 | –12.5 |
| Rayagada | 28.5 | 25.1 | 3.4 | –11.9 | 3.3 | 2.9 | 0.4 | –12.1 |
| Nabarangpur | 30.0 | 28.6 | 1.4 | –4.6 | 3.4 | 3.5 | –0.1 | 2.9 |
| Koraput | 27.3 | 26.2 | 1.1 | –4.0 | 3.1 | 3.0 | 0.1 | –3.2 |
| Malkangiri | 28.8 | 30.0 | –1.2 | 4.1 | 3.3 | 3.5 | –0.2 | 6.0 |

*Sources:* 1. CBR and TFR values are from; Christophe Z. Guilmoto, S. Irudaya Rajan. 2002, District level Estimates of Fertility from India's 2001 Census, *Economic and Political Weekly*, pp. 668-670; Christophe Z. Guilmoto, S. Irudaya Rajan, 2013, Fertility at District level in India: Lessons from the 2011 census, Working Papers DU CEPED, June 30 pp. 1-32.

2. Values of differences and decadal rate of change in percentage are author's calculation.

### Crude Birth Rate (CBR)

This analysis in Table 4.3 reveals that the CBR is very high in Rayagada, Koraput, Nabarangpur and Malkangiri and lowest in Jagatsingpur, Puri, Cuttack, Khorda, Kendrapara etc. The data reveals that high rate of CBR particularly seen in the southern parts of Odisha and low in coastal parts of Odisha (*see* Table 4.4, Fig. 4.5 and Maps 4.1 and 4.2).

**Table 4.4:** Difference in Crude Birth Rate and change in percentage across districts of Odisha

| | |
|---|---|
| Low (14.3-19.5) | Jagatsingpur (14.3), Cuttack (15.4), Puri (15.8), Khurda (16.2), Bargarh (16.8), Jharsuguda (16.9), Kendrapara (17.0), Nayagarh (17.2), Sambalpur (17.7), Jajpur (18.1), Dhenkanal (18.1), Ganjam (18.4), Anugul (18.5), Bhadrak (18.9), Baleswar (19.1), Subarnapur (19.2), Sundergarh (19.3) |
| Medium (19.6-24.8) | Debagarh (20.5), Balangir (21.2), Mayurbhanj (21.4), Boudh (22.6), Kalahandi (23.0), Keonjhar (23.1), Nuapada (23.1) Gajapati (24.1), Kandhamal (24.7) |
| High (24 9-30.0) | Rayagada (25.1), Koraput (26.2), Nabarangpur (28.6), Malkangiri (30.0) |

*Source:* Based on Table 4.3.

**Table 4.5:** Differences in Decadal Change in Percentage in CBR Across Districts in Odisha

| | |
|---|---|
| High rate of decline | Balasore (–24.2), Jagatsingpur (–23.9), Bhadrak (–23.7), Ganjam (–23.3), Kendrapara (–22), Puri (–21.7), Cuttack (–21.4), Angul (–20.9), Khordha (–20.1), Jharsuguda (–19.9) |
| Moderate rate of decline | Kandhamal (–19.8), Deogarh (–19.6), Bargarh (–18.4), Nayagarh (–17.7), Mayurbhanj (–17.6), Boudh (–17.5), Jajpur (–16.9), Dhenkanal (–16.9), Sambalpur (–16.5), Subarnapur (–15.4) |
| Low rate of decline | Sundergarh (–15.3), Kalahandi (–14,1), Gajapati ( 12.0), Rayagada (–11.9), Nuapada (–10.8), Kendujhar (–8.6), Balangir (–7.4), Nabarangpur (–4.6), Koraput (–4) |
| Increase | Malkangiri (4.1) |

*Source:* Based on Table 4.3.

It has been found from Table 4.5 that the high rate of decline in CBR across the districts of Odisha is in Balasore, Jagatsingpur.

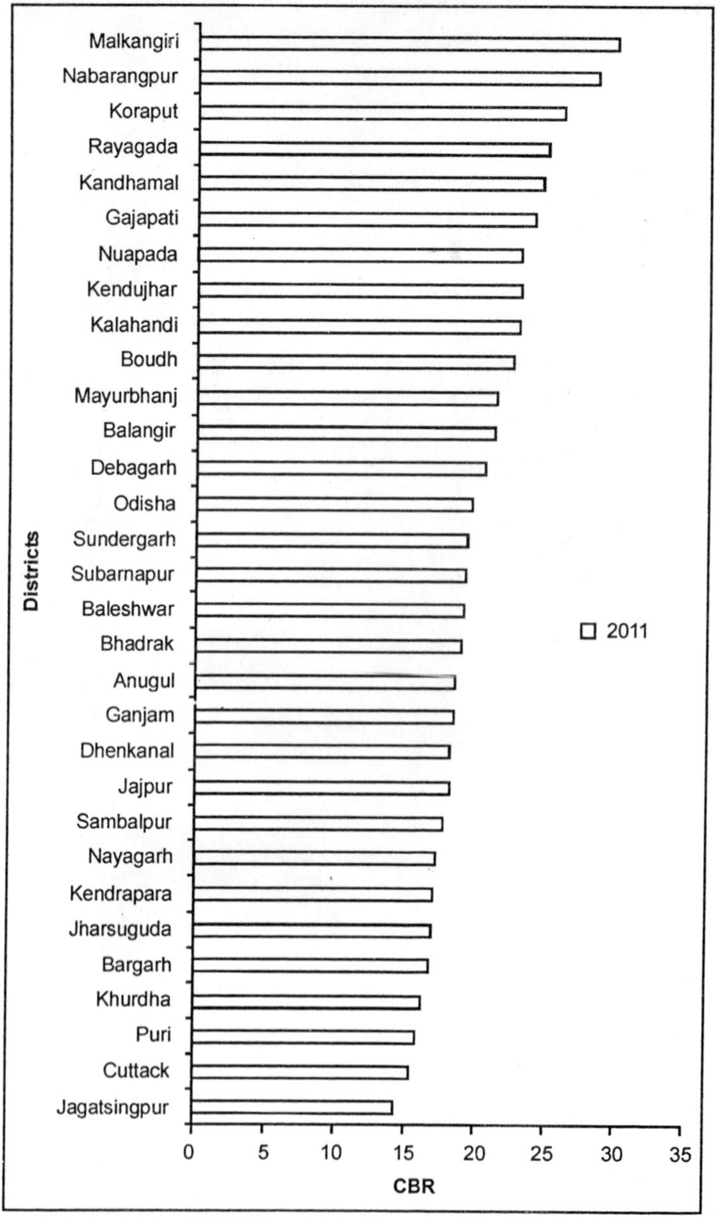


**Fig. 4.5:** District level Variations in Crude Birth Rate in Odisha, 2011 Census

*Source:* Based on Table 4.3.

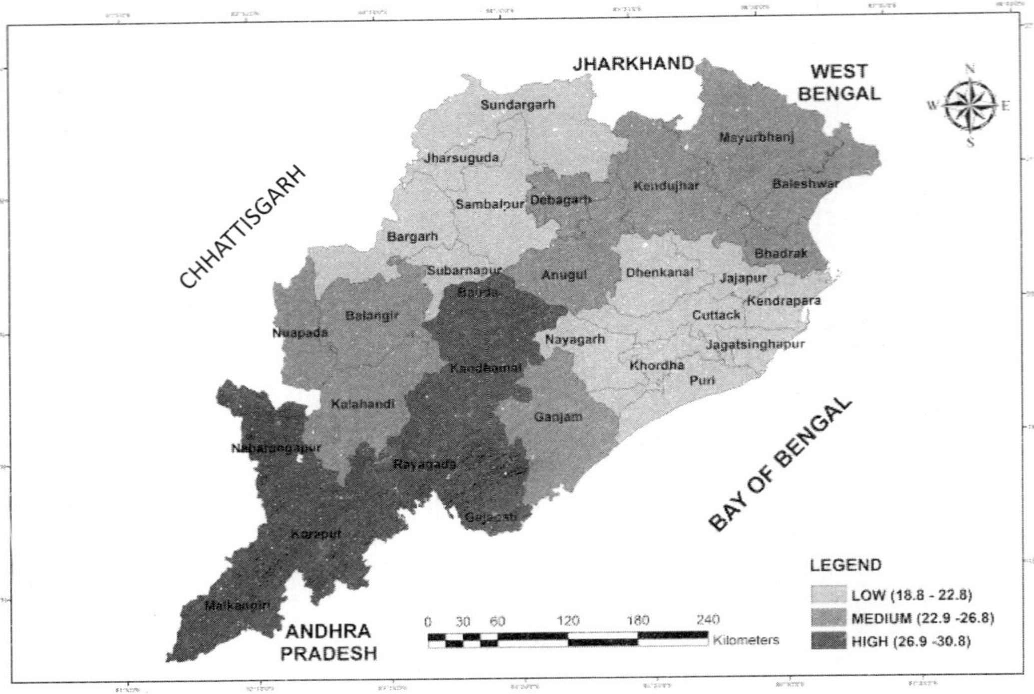


**Map 4.1:** Distributions of Districts by Crude Birth Rate, 2001.

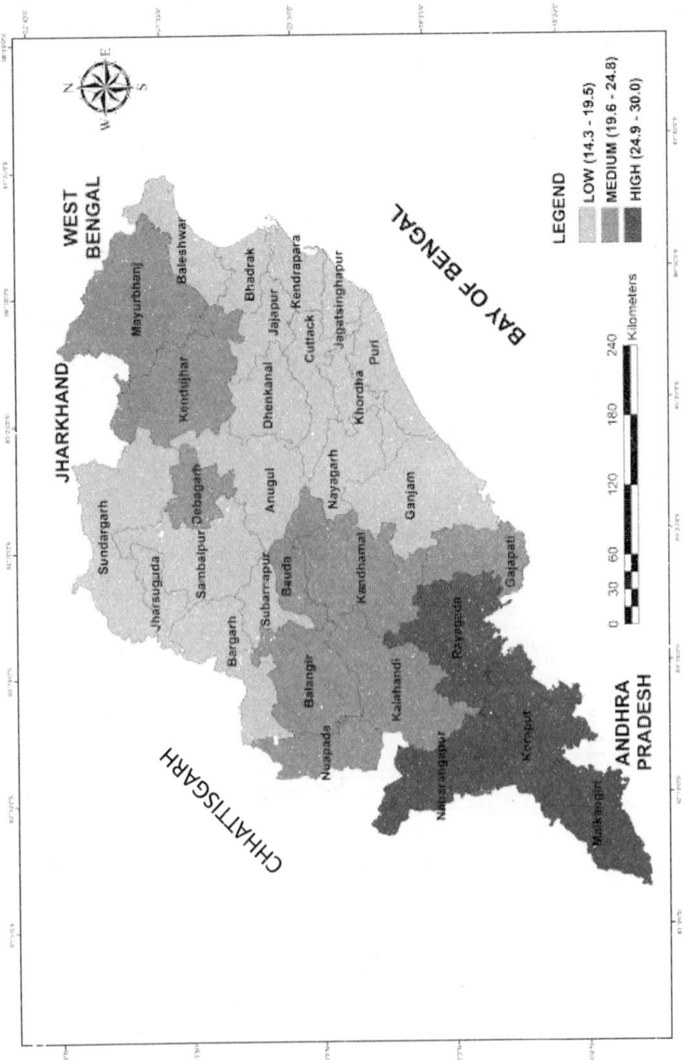


**Map 4.2:** Distributions of Districts by Crude Birth Rate, 2011.

*Source:* Based on Table 4.3.

The districts where the rate of decline in CBR (2001-11) is moderate are Kandhamal, Deogarh, Bargarh, Nayagarh. Low rate of decline in CBR districts are Sundergarh, Kalahandi, Gajapati, Rayagada, Nuapada, Nabarangpur, Koraput etc. And finally the exceptional case i.e. the district which shows the rate of change in increasing is Malkangiri.

### *Rate of Change in CBR (2001-11)*

The rate of change (decline) is highest in the coastal districts of Odisha such as Balasore, Jagatsingpur, Bhadrak, Ganjam, Kendrapara, Puri, Cuttack, Angul and Khordha and lowest in southern and south-western Koraput, Nabarangpur, Balngir, Kendujhar, Nuapada, Rayagada, Gajapati, Kalahandi, sudergarh etc with Malkangir showing increase in percentage in CBR.

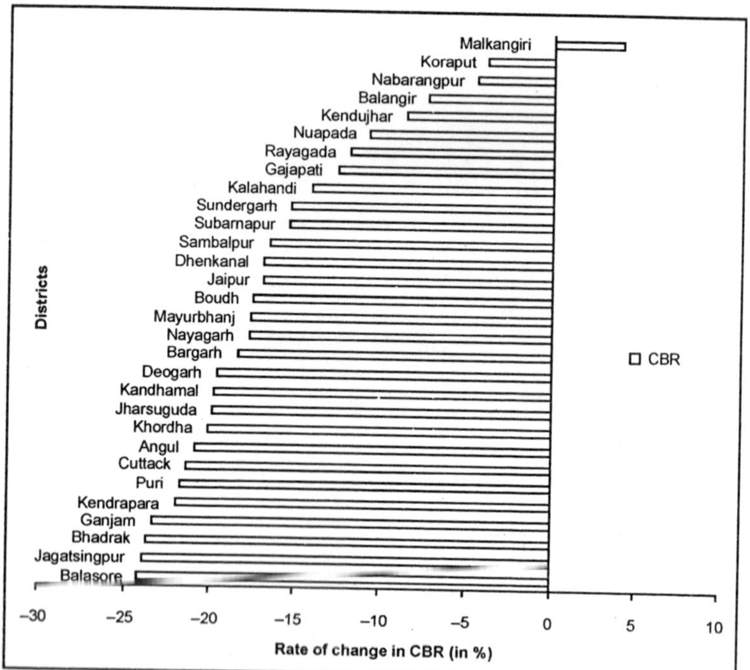


**Fig. 4.6:** Rate of Change in Crude Birth Rate (CBR) in Odisha, 2001-11.
*Source:* Based on Table 4.3.

### *Total Fertility Rate (TFR)*

The analysis in Table 4.6 reveals that the districts with highest TFR rate are Kandhamal, Koraput, Nabarangpur and Malkangiri and lowest in Jagatsingpur, Cuttack, Puri, Khorda, Kendrapara etc. It also states that the low rate of TFR is seen in Coastal parts of Odisha where as high rate is seen mainly in the southern districts.

**Table 4.6:** Difference in Total Fertility Rate and Change in Percentage Across Districts of Odisha

| *TFR* | |
|---|---|
| | **2011** |
| Low (1.7-2.3) | Jagatsingpur (1.7), Cuttack (1.8), Puri (1.8), Khurda (1.9), Kendrapara (2.0), Bargarh (2.1), Jharsuguda (2.1), Dhenkanal (2.1), Nayagarh (2.1), Sambalpur (2.1), Angul (2.2), Ganjam (2.2), Jajpur (2.2), Baleswar (2.3), Bhadrak (2.3), Sundergarh (2.3) |
| Medium (2.4-2.9) | Debagarh (2.5), Subarnapur (2.5), Balangir (2.7), Mayurbhanj (2.7), Boudh (2.8), Kalahandi (2.8), Keonjhar (2.8), Gajapati (2.9), Nuapada (2.9), Rayagada (2.9) |
| High (3.0-3.5) | Kandhamal (3.0), Koraput (3.0), Nabarngpur (3.5) Malkangiri (3.5) |

*Source:* Based on Table 4.3.

There are large scale variations of fertility of population from one district to another in Odisha. In 2011 census when Malkangiri have 30 Birth Rate, Jagatsingpur have only 14.3. In case of Number of children per woman in 2011 Malkangiri tops the rank by 3.5 children per woman, Jagatsingpur have only 1.7 children per woman. The variation of fertility is classified into following categories.

**Areas of low Fertility:** Districts having Crude Birth Rate of 14.3 to 19.5 and Total Fertility Rate having 1.7 to 2.3 are included in this category for 2011 population census. These districts are Jagatsingpur, Cuttack, Puri, Khurda, Kendrapara etc. in case of CBR and Jagatsingpur, Cuttack, Puri, Khurda and Kendrapara, Bargarh, Jharsuguda, Sundergarh in case of TFR.

**Areas of medium Fertility:** This class includes those districts which are having CBR 19.6 to 24.8 and TFR having 2.4 to 2.9. The average for whole of Odisha also falls in this class. In case of CBR

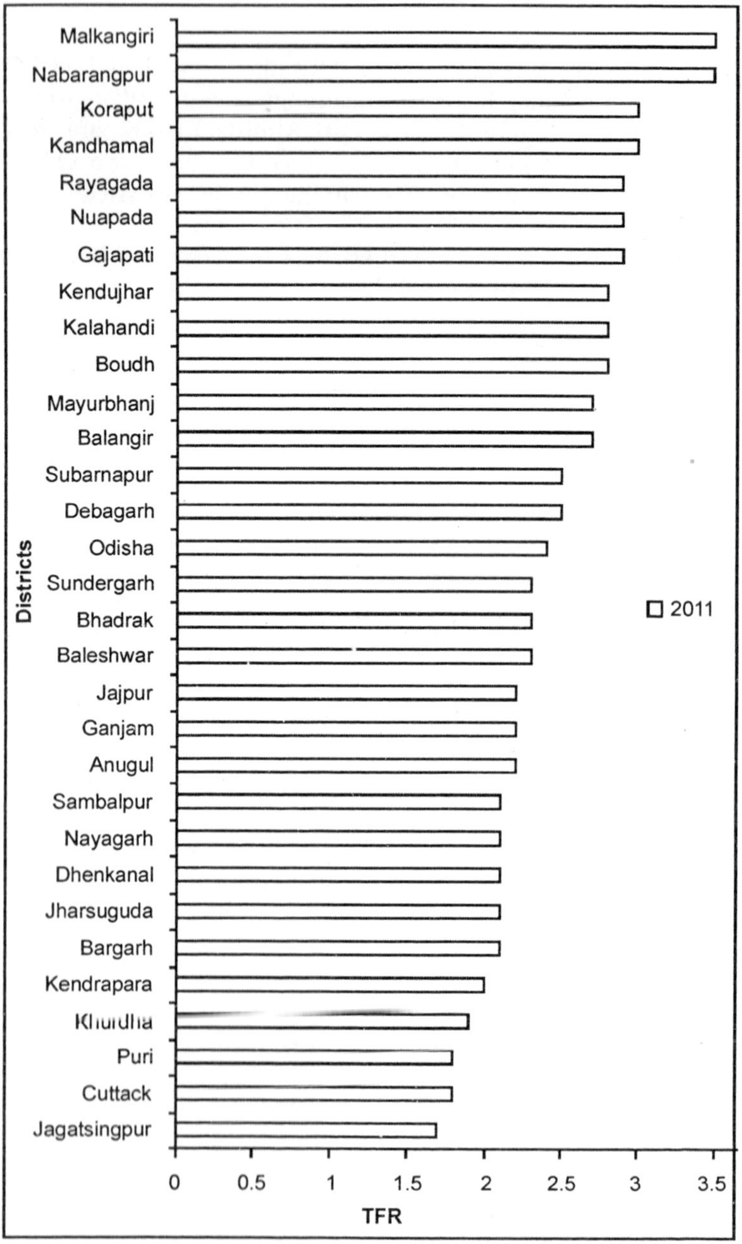


**Fig. 4.7:** District Level Variations in Total Fertility Rate in Odisha, 2011 Census

*Source:* Based on Table 4.3.

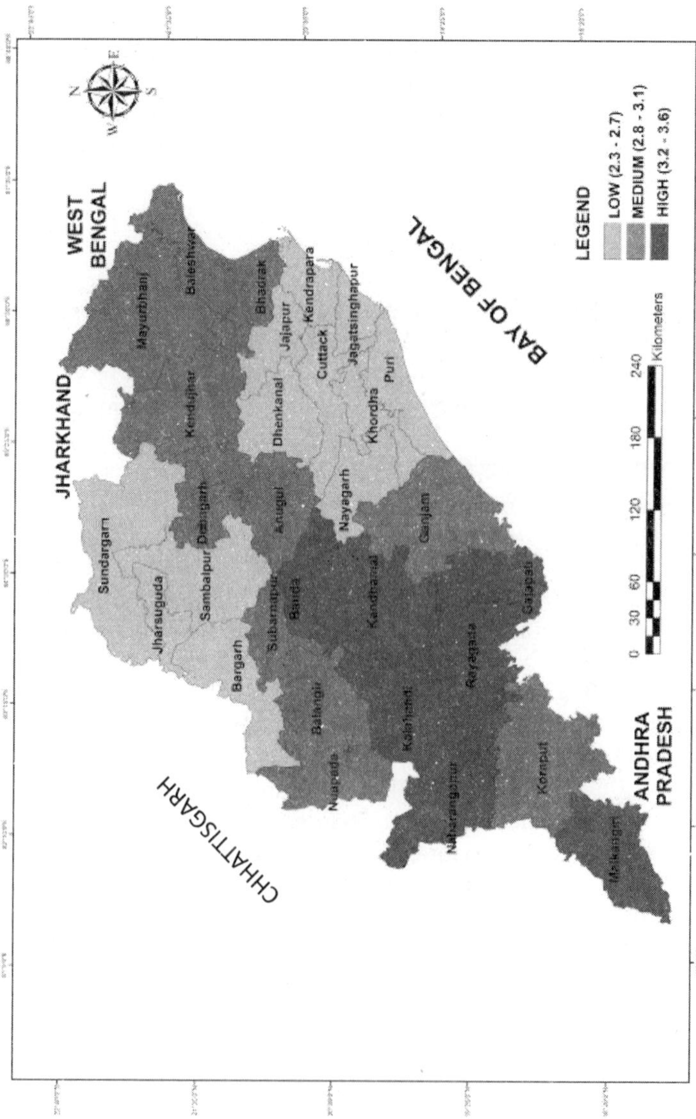


**Map 4.3:** Distributions of Districts by Total Fertility Rate, 2001

*Source:* Based on Table 4.3.

the districts are Debagarh, Balangir, Mayurbhanj, Boudh, Kalahandi, Keonjhar, Nuapada etc. and in case of TFR the districts are Debagarh, Subarnapur, Balangir, Kalahandi, Gajapati, Nuapada, Rayagada etc.

**Areas of High Fertility:** These are districts having fertility CBR 24.9-30.0 and TFR 3.0-3.5 children per woman. In case of CBR the districts are Rayagada, Koraput, Nabarangpur, Malkangiri and in case of TFR the districts are Kandhamal, Koraput, Nabarngpur and Malkangiri.

### *Rate of Change in TFR (2001-11)*

The rate of decline in TFR is highest in the coastal districts such as Jagatsingpur, Puri, Cuttack, Ganjam, Kedrapara, Khordha, Balasore, Bhadrak etc. and lowest rate of decline is seen in southern,western and also some districts of northern areas such as Koraput, Nuapada, Balangir, Kendujhar, Mayurbhanj, Subarnapur, Rayagada, Gajapati, Kalahandi etc. with two districts Nabarangpur and Malkangiri shows increase in rate of change from 2001-11.

As per census data 2001 and 2011, for CBR the Coefficient of variation is 13.59 in 2001 which is increased to 19.45, the change in percentage is 69.8. Similarly for TFR the Coefficient of Variation is 12.67 in 2001 which is increased to 19.10, the change in percentage is 66.3. The regional pattern of CBR and TFR as Correlation coefficient value shows both are strongly correlated (*See* Map 4.4 and Table 4.7).

From Table 4.7 it is clear that the high rate of decline in TFR across districts are Jagatsingpur, 56 Puri, Cuttack, Angul, Ganjam (–24.1), Kendrapara, Balasore, Bhadrak etc.The districts where TFR moderately decline are Deogarh, Jharsuguda, Sambalpur, Kandhamal etc. The districts with low rate of decline in TFR are Gajapati, Rayagada, Subarnapur, Mayurbhanj, Balangir (–3.5), Nuapada, Koraput etc. Two districts Nabarangpur, Malkangiri shows increase in rate of change in percentage (*see* Fig. 4.8).

From this analysis it is concluded that though the fertility rate is declined in Odisha it is the district level variation still persist. The Crude Birth Rate is high in southern districts such as Malkangiri, Nabarangpur, Koraput, Rayagada etc. and low in the coastal districts such as Jagatsingpur, Cuttack, Puri, and Khorda

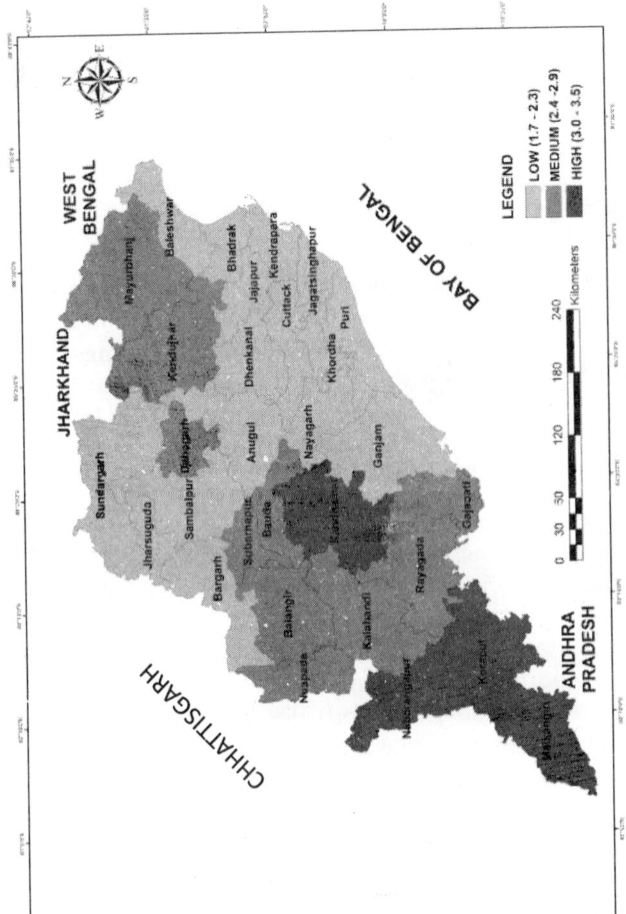


**Map 4.4:** Distributions of Districts by Total Fertility Rate, 2011

*Source:* Based on Table 4.3.

**Table 4.7:** Differences in Decadal Change in Percentage in Total Fertility Rate Across Districts in Odisha

| | |
|---|---|
| **High rate of decline** | Jagatsingpur (–26), Puri (–25), Cuttack (–25), Angul (–24.2), Ganjam (–24.1), Angul (–24.2), Kendrapara (–23), Dhenkanal (–22.2), Khordha (–20.8), Balasore (–20.6), Bhadrak (–20.6) |
| **Moderate rate of decline** | Deogarh (–19.3), Jharsuguda (–19.2), Sambalpur (–19.2), Kandhamal (–16.6), Bargarh (–16), Nayagarh (–16), Jajpur (–15.3), Sundergarh (–14.8), Boudh (–12.5), Kalahandi (–12.5) |
| **Low rate of decline** | Gajapati (–12.1), Rayagada (–12.1), Subarnapur (–10.7), Mayurbhanj (–10), Kendujhar (–6.6), Balangir (–3.5), Nuapada (–3.3), Koraput (–3.2) |
| **Increase** | Nabarangpur (2.9), Malkangiri (6) |

*Source:* Based on Table 4.3.

etc. Total Fertility Rate also have the same with the Southern and some south-western districts have high rate of fertility and Coastal distiсts with low rate of fertility. The rate of decadal change (2001-11) in percentage shows coastal districts has the highest decline than the southern and some south-western districts of Odisha.

## Correlates of Fertility Rate in Odisha

In this section, an attempt is made to look at the correlates of variations in fertility across districts. Different socio-economic indicators like Crude Birth Rate, Total Fertility Rate, Female literacy rate, Female work Participation Rate, Workers in Non-agricultural sectors, Percentage of Urban Population, Proportion of SC population, Proportion of ST population, Sex-Ratio, Contraceptive Prevalence Rate (any modern method), per capita NDDP at current prices and Infant mortality rate are taken into account to assess the significant correlates of Total Fertility Rate and Crude Birth Rate. Female Literacy Rate and Female work Participation Rate can be treated as a proxy for women's autonomy. Population engaged in Non-agricultural activity and per capita NDDP at current prices show the average economic condition. Sex-Ratio (number of females per 1000 males), proportion of urban population, SC population and ST population, and IMR reflects the demographic condition. Contraceptive Prevalence Rate (any modern method) can be treated as a programme indicator. Mean, Standard Deviation and Coefficient of Variation of different variables used in the analysis are given in Table 4.12.

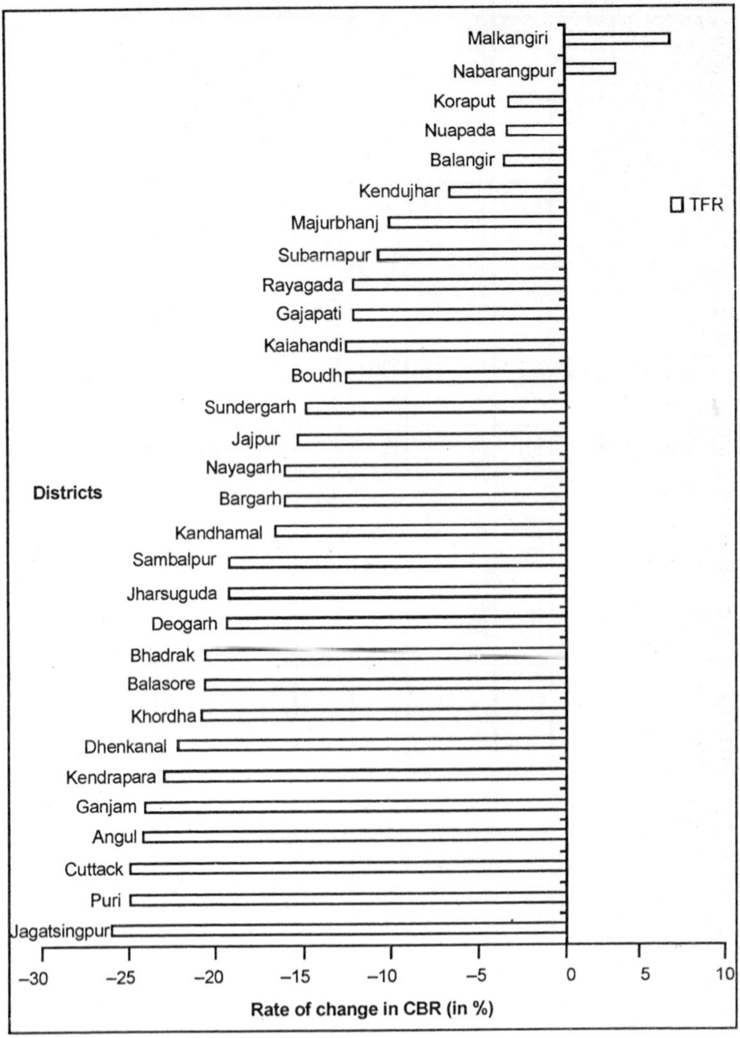


**Fig. 4.8:** Rate of Change in Total Fertility Rate (TFR) in Odisha, 2001-11

*Source:* Based on Table 4.3.

The Correlation coefficients values for the year 2001 are shown in Table 4.8. It has been found that variables Female Literacy Rate, Workers in Non-agricultural sectors, percentage of urban population and contraceptive prevalence rate have negative statistically significant correlation with TFR. Statistically significant

**Table 4.8:** Inter-correlations among Fertility Rate and Socio-economic Conditions of 2001

| *Socio-economic Indicators* | | *X1* | *X2* | *X3* | *X4* | *X5* | *X6* | *X7* | *X8* | *X9* | *X10* | *X11* | *X12* | *X13* |
|---|---|---|---|---|---|---|---|---|---|---|---|---|---|---|
| Total Fertility Rate | X1 | 1 | .931** | –.794** | .716** | –.695** | .591** | –.410* | –0.265 | .735** | 0.312 | –.548** | –0.045 | .667** |
| Crude Birth rate | X2 | | 1 | –.853** | .743** | –.714** | .671** | –.399* | –0.272 | .720** | .395* | –.584** | –0.15 | .696** |
| Female literacy rate | X3 | | | 1 | –.885** | .775** | –.706** | .369* | 0.341 | –.781** | –0.064 | .540** | 0.127 | –.557** |
| Female work participation rate | X4 | | | | 1 | –.650** | .630** | –0.188 | –.421* | .816** | 0.031 | –.505** | 0.113 | .441* |
| Workers in non agricultural sectors | X5 | | | | | 1 | –.758** | .744* | 0.023 | –.460* | 0.112 | .548** | .423* | –.519** |
| Sex-Ratio | X6 | | | | | | 1 | –.541** | –0.123 | .500** | –0.141 | –.510** | –.387* | .636* |
| Percentage Urban Population | X7 | | | | | | | 1 | –0.26 | –0.022 | 0.174 | 0.344 | .596** | –.387* |
| Percentage Scheduled Caste | X8 | | | | | | | | 1 | –.631** | 0.006 | 0.084 | –0.178 | –0.085 |
| Percentage Scheduled Tribe | X9 | | | | | | | | | 1 | 0.129 | –.418* | 0.133 | .368* |
| Decadal Growth Rate | X10 | | | | | | | | | | 1 | –0.182 | 0.133 | 0.16 |
| Contraceptive Prevalence Rate | X11 | | | | | | | | | | | 1 | 0.031 | –0.336 |
| Net District Domestic Product | X12 | | | | | | | | | | | | 1 | –0.25 |
| Infant Mortality Rate | X13 | | | | | | | | | | | | | 1 |

*Note:* ** Correlation is significant at the 0.01 level (2-tailed), * Correlation is significant at the 0.05 level (2-tailed)
*Source:* Based on Table 4.3.

Positive relations are found in case of four variables such as Female Work Participation Rate, Sex-Ratio, Percentage of ST population and IMR. The correlations coefficients are not statistically significant for percentage of SC and Net District Domestic Product (both are negatively correlated with TFR) .

Similarly for the year 2011, same set of indicators were used to see the degree and extent association of TFR and CBR with socio-economic development and population composition. Correlation coefficient values are shown in Table 5.2. It is observed Female Literacy Rate, Workers in Non-agricultural sectors, percentage of urban population and contraceptive prevalence rate have negative statistically significant correlation with TFR. Positive relations are found in case of three variables such as Female Work Participation Rate, Sex Ratio and ST population. All these three indicators have statistically significant association with TFR. However, the correlation coefficients are not statistically significant for percentage of SC, Net District Domestic Product and IMR (all are negatively related with TFR). The above discussion shows that the correlates of TFR in 2001 and 2011 are almost same with the exception of IMR. It is to be noted that IMR was found to have positive statistically significant correlation with TFR in 2001 (Tables 4.9 to 4.12).

Multiple regressions model has been employed to ascertain the relative contribution of each of the independent variables. The partial regression Coefficient (standardized or unstandardized) for the variables in an analysis of areal units such as states and districts measures the effect of differences between districts. As per the findings based on 2001 TFR data, IMR, Sex-Ratio and ST Population are significant factors affecting TFR. Female literacy, Female Work Participation Rate, Non-agricultural workers and Contraceptive Prevalence Rate are not found to have statistically significant effect on TFR.

Analysis of 2011 data reveals that female literacy rate, female work participation rate, and proportion of workers in Non-agricultural sector have strong statistically significant effect on TFR. It is also observed that Contraceptive prevalence (modern method) has also negative effect on TFR. Concentration of ST population has positive effect on TFR.

The Correlation Coefficient and Multiple regression models using CBR as dependent variable yielded similar results as

**Table 4.9:** Inter-correlations among Fertility Rate and Socio-economic Conditions of 2011

| *Socio-economic Indicators* | | *X1* | *X2* | *X3* | *X4* | *X5* | *X6* | *X7* | *X8* | *X9* | *X10* | *X11* | *X12* | *X13* |
|---|---|---|---|---|---|---|---|---|---|---|---|---|---|---|
| Total Fertility Rate | X1 | 1 | .985** | –.927** | .742** | –.722** | .768** | –.368* | –0.283 | .795** | .558** | –.627** | –0.135 | –0.055 |
| Crude Birth rate | X2 | | 1 | –.932** | .772** | –.761** | .751** | –.408* | –0.272 | .776** | .583** | –.672** | –0.152 | –0.055 |
| Female literacy rate | X3 | | | 1 | –.839** | .722** | –.796** | 0.335 | .390* | –.817** | –.471** | .653** | 0.152 | 0.029 |
| Female work participation rate | X4 | | | | 1 | –.665** | .667** | –0.242 | –0.341 | .776** | 0.35 | –.667** | –0.004 | –0.074 |
| Workers in Non-Agricultural sectors | X5 | | | | | 1 | –.672** | .804** | –0.031 | –.444* | –0.316 | –566** | .531** | 0.098 |
| Sex-Ratio | X6 | | | | | | 1 | –.393* | –0.29 | .693** | 0.169 | –.535** | –0.174 | 0.02 |
| Percentage Urban Population | X7 | | | | | | | 1 | –0.244 | –0.054 | –0.012 | .409* | .604** | 0.014 |
| Percentage Scheduled Caste | X8 | | | | | | | | 1 | –.634** | 0.054 | 0.163 | –0.214 | –0.061 |
| Percentage Scheduled Tribe | X9 | | | | | | | | | 1 | 0.27 | –.471** | 0.166 | –0.117 |
| Decadal Growth Rate | X10 | | | | | | | | | | 1 | –0.318 | –0.144 | 0.213 |
| Contraceptive Prevalence Rate | X11 | | | | | | | | | | | 1 | 0.007 | –0.073 |
| Net District Domestic Product | X12 | | | | | | | | | | | | 1 | 0.004 |
| Infant Mortality Rate | X13 | | | | | | | | | | | | | 1 |

*Note:* ** Correlation is significant at the 0.01 level (2-tailed), * Correlation is significant at the 0.05 level (2-tailed).

*Source:* Based on Table 4.3.

**Table 4.10:** Determinants of District level Variations in Crude Birth Rate: Findings from Multiple Regression Analysis

| *Socio-economic Variables* | *CBR (2001)* | *CBR (2011)* |
|---|---|---|
| | *Standardized Coefficients* | *Standardized Coefficients* |
| Female literacy | –.425 | –.645* |
| Female work participation rates | –.105 | –.391** |
| Non-agricultural workers | –.096 | –.454*** |
| Sex-Ratio | –.110 | –.016 |
| Level of Urbanization | –.059 | .187 |
| Scheduled Tribe population | .292*** | .324** |
| Infant Mortality Rate | .343* | .004 |
| Contraceptive Prevalence Rate | –.153 | –.142 |
| $R^2$ | .842 | .900 |
| F | 13.949 | 23.695 |
| N | 3 | 30 |

*Notes:* *** Significant at 10 per cent level of significance, ** Significant at 5 per cent level of significance.
* Significant at 1 per cent level of significance.

*Source:* Based on Appendix 3 and 4.

**Table 4.11:** Determinants of District level Variations in Total Fertility Rate: Findings from Multiple Regression Analysis

| *Socio-economic Variables* | *TFR (2001)* | *TFR (2011)* |
|---|---|---|
| | *Standardized Coefficients* | *Standardized Coefficients* |
| Female literacy | –.071 | –.615* |
| Female work participation rates | –.012 | –.319** |
| Non-agricultural workers | –.229 | –.511* |
| Sex-Ratio | –.305*** | –.088 |
| Level of Urbanization | –.169 | .188 |
| Scheduled Tribe population | .530* | .279*** |
| Infant Mortality Rate | .404* | .007 |
| Contraceptive Prevalence Rate | –.131 | –.185*** |
| $R^2$ | .827 | .913 |
| F | 12.513 | 27.658 |
| N | 30 | 30 |

*Notes:* *** Significant at 10 per cent level of significance.
** Significant at 5 per cent level of significance.
* Significant at 1 per cent level of significance.

*Source:* Based on Appendix 3 and 4.

**Table 4.12:** Mean, Standard Deviation and Coefficient of Variation of Different Variables based on 2001 and 2011 Census data

| | 2001 | | | 2011 | | | |
|---|---|---|---|---|---|---|---|
| *Characteristics (N=30)* | *Mean* | *Std. Deviation* | *Coefficient of Variations (CV)* | *Mean* | *Std. Deviation* | *Coefficient of Variations (CV)* | *Change in Percentage in CV* |
| Crude Birth Rate | 24.12 | 3.28 | 13.59 | 20.35 | 3.96 | 19.45 | 69.8 |
| Total Fertility Rate | 2.84 | 0.36 | 12.67 | 2.46 | 0.47 | 19.10 | 66.3 |
| Female Literacy Rate | 47.50 | 15.79 | 33.24 | 62.11 | 14.00 | 22.54 | 147.4 |
| Female Work Participation Rate | 27.16 | 13.29 | 48.93 | 29.89 | 13.43 | 44.93 | 108.9 |
| Proportion of Non-agricultural workers | 33.73 | 12.57 | 37.26 | 36.46 | 13.78 | 37.79 | 101.4 |
| Sex-Ratio | 976.76 | 28.53 | 2.92 | 983.3 | 33.79 | 3.43 | 85.1 |
| Proportion of Urban Population | 13.35 | 10.14 | 75.95 | 14.84 | 10.87 | 73.24 | 103.7 |
| Proportion of Scheduled Caste Population | 16.71 | 4.29 | 25.67 | 17.4 | 4.77 | 27.41 | 93.6 |
| Proportion of Scheduled Tribe Population | 25.39 | 20.76 | 81.76 | 25.89 | 21.12 | 81.57 | 100.2 |
| Decadal Growth Rate | 15.95 | 3.44 | 21.56 | 14.30 | 3.71 | 25.94 | 83.1 |
| Contraceptive Prevalence Rate | 41.57 | 4.61 | 11.09 | 38.92 | 7.20 | 18.49 | 59.9 |
| Net District Domestic Product | 10807.07 | 3595.07 | 33.26 | 33218.97 | 11772.12 | 35.43 | 93.8 |
| Infant Mortality Rate | 83.36 | 11.92 | 14.29 | 62.10 | 11.68 | 18.80 | 76.0 |

*Source:* Calculated Based on data provided in Appendix 3 and 4.

observed in the case of TFR. This is true for both the time points; 2001 and 2011. This is because of the fact that TFR and CBR are highly correlated.

From the multiple regression analysis, it can stated that the district level variation or regional variation in fertility in Odisha is primarily because of the role Women's Agency (female education and female work participation), Economic Prosperity and concentration of Scheduled Tribes population.

## Conclusion

An attempt has been made in this work to look at trends and regional patterns of fertility rate in Odisha. Data from the SRS, the NFHS and the census have been used in this work. Findings show a declining trend of Crude Birth Rate and Total Fertility Rate in Odisha. The rate of decline was more consistent in 1990s and in the first decade of twenty first century as contrast to 1970s and 1980s. Regional divide in fertility rate is also persistent in Odisha. In fact, it is revealed that the degree regional differences in CBR and TFR have increase over time. The Crude Birth Rate is particularly high in the southern districts like Rayagada, Koraput, Nabarangpur and Malkangiri. Total Fertility Rate is also high in the southern districts such as Kandhamal, Koraput, Nabarangpur and Malkangiri.

Almost all districts have recorded decline in fertility between 2001 and 2011 in Odisha with one or two exceptions. For example, in Malkangiri CBR increased during 2001 and 2011. During the same time period Malkangiri and Nabarangpur recorded increase in TFR. The highest Decadal rate of change (decline) is seen in the costal districts of Odisha in case of both CBR and TFR. The lowest rate of decline is seen in southern and south-western districts in case of both CBR and TFR. Bivariate analysis results indicate that Female Literacy Rate, Female Work Participation Rate, Workers in Non-Agricultural sectors, and Contraceptive Prevalence Rate are negatively correlated with fertility while concentration of ST population and higher proportion of females are associated with high fertility rate.

Multiple Regression analysis indicate an increasing role of Female Literacy Rate, Female work Participation Rate (Women's Agency), Non-Agricultural Workers (Economic Prosperity) and use of modern contraceptives in influencing fertility in the state. These variables have fertility reducing effects. On the other hand, concentration of ST population leads to higher fertility rate.

Women's education is most important because educated mother likely to be more aware of information about family planning programmes and can use contraceptives more effectively. On the other hand, educated mothers may also take better care of the children increasing the chances of child survival leading to low birth rate (Manna, 1998). The effect of female work participation Rate, especially in the developing countries is not well supported by empirical evidences. Still it has major importance in Odisha's context; it is observed that controlling other factors female work participation has fertility reducing effects. The regional variation of fertility rate is also due to the concentration of ST population because of mainly biological factors and some cultural practices in Odisha (Roth *et al.*, 1983). Hence, effort should be made to identify the factors affecting fertility among tribes and to design policies accordingly to reduce fertility rate among tribes. The Bi-variate as well as multivariate analysis reveal that programme indicator, i.e. Contraceptive Prevalence Rate (CPR) has strongly associated with variations in fertility indicators. However, multiple regression analysis reveals no such strong significant effect of CPR (only modern method) on fertility (only 2011 census data shows some effect of CPR on fertility which is significant at 10% level of significance). This is probably due to the fact that literacy and CPR are strongly related. As per National Family Health Survey-3 (2005-06), the Contraceptive Prevalence Rate (modern) among illiterate women (39.1%) was substantially lower than among females with primary education (51.4%). Economic prosperity is also found to have net effect on fertility in Odisha. In Odisha, as per recent round of NSS (2009-10) around 37 per cent of populations are below poverty line (Government of India, 2012). It is also observed that poverty rate is substantially high in southern region as compared to other parts of the state. The ongoing effort to reduce poverty and to accelerate the process of industrialization in the state would lead to further decline in fertility.

There is a need to bring down the fertility rate in high fertility districts of the state in order to reduce overall fertility rate of the state to replacement level. Therefore, there is a need to bring socio-economic transformations in those regions by accelerating the implementation of various government-sponsored programmes such as poverty reduction, employment guarantee and universalisation of education. Socio-economic upliftment of the women is very important to reduce fertility as this study observes the significant effect of womens' agency on fertility. To Conclude, it can be said that well articulated and well planned programmes are needed for the speedy decline in fertility rate in Odisha.

## References

Bhat, P. N. M. (1994). Levels and trends in Indian fertility, *Economic and Political Weekly, 17* (24): 3273-3280.

Dev, M. S, K. S. James and B. Sen. (2002). Causes of fertility decline in India and Bangladesh: role of community, *Economic and Political Weekly, 37* (43): 4447-54.

Dreze, J. and M. Murthi. (2001). Fertility education and development: evidence from India, *Population and Development Review, 27* (1): 33-63.

Economic Survey. (2009-10). Odisha, Planning and Coordination Department, Directorate of Economics and Statistics, Government of Odisha, http://www.odisha.gov.in

Economic Survey. (2012-13). Odisha, Planning and Coordination Department, Directorate of Economics and Statistics, Government of Odisha, http://www.odisha.gov.in

Guilmoto, C.Z., and S. Irudaya Rajan. (2013). Fertility at district level in India: lessons from the 2011 census, Working Papers DU CEPED, 1-32, http://www.ceped.org/wp

Guilmoto, C.Z., and S.I. Rajan. (2002). District level estimates of fertility from India's 2001 census, *Economic and Political Weekly, 37* (7): 665-672.

India, Registrar General. (2009). General Population Tables, Odisha, Census of India 2001, New Delhi: Office of the Registrar General and Census Commissioners.

India, Registrar General. (2011). Provisional population totals, Odisha, Census of India, 2011, Series 22, New Delhi: Office of the Registrar General and Census Commissioners.

India, Registrar General. (2010). Compendium of Fertility and Mortality Report, 1971-2007, Delhi.

International Institute of Population Sciences and ORC Macro. (1994). *National Family Health Survey (NFHS-1)*, 1992-93.

International Institute of Population Sciences and ORC Macro. (2000). *National Family Health Survey (NFHS-2)*, 1998-99.

Jain, A.K. (1985). The impact of development and population policies on fertility in India, *Studies in Family Planning, 16* (4): 181-198.

James, K.S. and S.V. Subramaniam. (2005). Decline in fertility in Andhra Pradesh: a re-examination of conflicting arguments in C.Z. Guilmoto and S. I. Rajan (eds.), *Fertility Transition in South India*, New Delhi: Sage Publications.

James, K. S. (1999). Fertility decline in Andhra Pradesh: a search for alternative hypothesis, *Economic and Political Weekly, 34* (8): 491-99.

James, K. S. and S. B. Nair. (2005). Accelerated decline in fertility in India since the 1980s: trends among Hindus and Muslims, *Economic and Political Weekly, 40* (5): 375-383.

Kishore, S. (1994). Fertility decline in Tamil Nadu, India, in Bernel Ergo (ed.), *Undertanding Reproductive Change: Kenya, Tamil Nadu, Punjab and Costa Rica*, Lund: Lund University Press.

Knodel, J. (1988), Demographic behaviour in the past: a study of fourteen German village populations in the eighteenth and nineteenth centuries, Cambridge: Cambridge University Press.

Kumar, S. and K. M. Sathyanarayana. (2012). District-level estimates of fertility and implied sex-ratio at birth in India, *Economic and Political Weekly, 47* (33): 66-72.

Manna, M. (1998). Factors affecting fertility decline and fertility variation in 1990s: an interstate analysis, *Economic and Political Weekly, 33* (52): 3280-3284.

Premchand, D. and V. Agadjanian. (2009). India's north-south divide ad theories of fertility change, *Journal of Population Research, 26*: 249-272.

Rajan, S.I. (2005). District level fertility estimates for Hindus and Muslims, *Economic and Political Weekly, 40* (5): 437-446.

Saha, K.B. and A. Verma. (2006). High fertility among scheduled tribes of Madhya Pradesh, *Indian J. Med. Res.*, 89-90.

Sahoo, H. (2007). Determinants of contraceptive use in Odisha: an analysis from national family health survey III, *Health and Population Perspective and Issues, 30* (3): 208-221.

Sekhar, T.V., K.N.M. Raju and M. N. Sivakumar. (2001). Fertility transition in Karnataka: Levels, trends and implications, *Economic and Political Weekly*, 22: 4742-4752.

Skirbekk, V. (2008). Fertility trends by social status, *Demographic Research, 18* (5): 145-180.

Srinivasan, K., *et al.* (1991). The effects of family planning components on contraceptive acceptance in four Indian states, *International Family Planning Perspectives, 1*: 14-24.

Unisa, S. (2000). Education and son preference in India: a study based on NFHS data, *South Asian Anthropologists, 21* (1): 23-35.

Visaria, P. and Visaria, L. (1994). Demographic transition: accelerating fertility decline during the 1980s, *Economic and Political Weekly, 29* (51 and 52): 3281-3292.

## Appendix 1

*Annual Estimates of Crude Birth Rate and Total Fertility Rate by Residence, 1971-2013*

| Years | ODISHA | | | | | | INDIA | | | | | |
|---|---|---|---|---|---|---|---|---|---|---|---|---|
| | Crude Birth Rate | | | Total Fertility Rate | | | Crude Birth Rate | | | Total Fertility Rate | | |
| | Total | Rural | Urban | Total | Rural | Urban | Total | Rural | Urban | Total | Rural | Urban |
| 1971 | 34.6 | 34.7 | 33 | 4.7 | 4.8 | 4.3 | 36.9 | 38.9 | 30.1 | 5.2 | 5.4 | 4.1 |
| 1972 | 34.5 | 34.7 | 31.7 | 4.6 | 4.7 | 4 | 36.6 | 38.4 | 30.5 | 5.2 | 5.4 | 4.3 |
| 1973 | 34.8 | 35 | 32.7 | 4.8 | 4.9 | 4.2 | 34.6 | 35.9 | 28.9 | 4.9 | 5.2 | 3.7 |
| 1974 | 33.6 | 33.9 | 30.5 | 4.7 | 4.7 | 4.1 | 34.5 | 35.9 | 28.4 | 4.9 | 5.2 | 3.7 |
| 1975 | 33.6 | 33.8 | 30.7 | 4.6 | 4.7 | 4.1 | 35.2 | 36.7 | 28.5 | 4.9 | 5.2 | 3.7 |
| 1976 | 34.8 | 35.3 | 29.1 | 4.7 | 4.8 | 3.8 | 34.4 | 35.8 | 28.4 | 4.7 | 5 | 3.6 |
| 1977 | 29.9 | 30.2 | 26 | 4 | 4.1 | 3.4 | 33 | 34.3 | 27.8 | 4.5 | 4.8 | 3.4 |
| 1978 | 32.9 | 33.3 | 28.9 | 4.5 | 4.5 | 3.7 | 33.3 | 34.7 | 27.8 | 4.5 | 4.8 | 3.4 |
| 1979 | 31 | 31 | 30.5 | 4.1 | 4.1 | 3.9 | 33.1 | 34.3 | 28.3 | 4.4 | 4.7 | 3.4 |
| 1980 | 31.6 | 31.9 | 29 | 4.1 | 4.2 | 3.7 | 33.3 | 34.6 | 28.1 | 4.4 | 4.7 | 3.4 |
| 1981 | 33.1 | 33.4 | 29.3 | 4.3 | 4.3 | 3.7 | 33.9 | 35.6 | 27 | 4.5 | 4.8 | 3.3 |
| 1982 | 33.4 | 33.7 | 30.9 | 4.3 | 4.4 | 3.8 | 33.8 | 35.5 | 27.6 | 4.5 | 4.9 | 3.4 |
| 1983 | 34 | 34.4 | 30.5 | 4.5 | 4.6 | 3.7 | 33.7 | 35.3 | 28.3 | 4.5 | 4.9 | 3.4 |
| 1984 | 32.7 | 33 | 29.8 | 4.3 | 4.4 | 3.6 | 33.9 | 35.3 | 29.4 | 4.5 | 4.8 | 3.5 |
| 1985 | 30.7 | 30.9 | 28.3 | 3.8 | 3.9 | 3.3 | 32.9 | 34.3 | 28.1 | 4.3 | 4.6 | 3.3 |
| 1986 | 32.5 | 33.2 | 26.8 | 4.2 | 4.3 | 3.1 | 32.6 | 34.2 | 27.1 | 4.2 | 4.5 | 3.1 |

(Contd.)

| Years | ODISHA | | | | | | INDIA | | | | | |
|---|---|---|---|---|---|---|---|---|---|---|---|---|
| | Crude Birth Rate | | | Total Fertility Rate | | | Crude Birth Rate | | | Total Fertility Rate | | |
| | Total | Rural | Urban | Total | Rural | Urban | Total | Rural | Urban | Total | Rural | Urban |
| 1987 | 31 | 31.6 | 25.7 | 3.7 | 3.8 | 3 | 32.2 | 33.7 | 27.4 | 4.1 | 4.4 | 3.2 |
| 1988 | 31.9 | 32.5 | 26.5 | 3.8 | 3.9 | 3 | 31.5 | 33.1 | 26.3 | 4 | 4.3 | 3.1 |
| 1989 | 30.5 | 31.1 | 25 | 3.6 | 3.7 | 2.7 | 30.6 | 32.2 | 25.2 | 3.9 | 4.2 | 2.8 |
| 1990 | 30 | 30.7 | 23.7 | 3.5 | 3.6 | 2.6 | 30.2 | 31.7 | 24.7 | 3.8 | 4.1 | 2.8 |
| 1991 | 28.8 | 29.6 | 21.6 | 3.3 | 3.4 | 2.3 | 29.5 | 30.9 | 24.3 | 3.6 | 3.9 | 2.7 |
| 1992 | 27.8 | 28.5 | 21.4 | 3.1 | 3.2 | 2.3 | 29.2 | 30.9 | 23.1 | 3.6 | 3.9 | 2.6 |
| 1993 | 27.2 | 27.8 | 23.2 | 3.1 | 3.2 | 2.7 | 28.7 | 30.4 | 23.7 | 3.5 | 3.8 | 2.8 |
| 1994 | 28 | 28.8 | 22.7 | 3.3 | 3.4 | 2.5 | 28.7 | 30.5 | 23.1 | 3.5 | 3.8 | 2.7 |
| 1995 | 27.8 | 28.5 | 22 | 3.3 | 3.4 | 2.4 | 28.3 | 30 | 22.7 | 3.5 | 3.9 | 2.6 |
| 1996 | 27 | 27.7 | 21.3 | 3.1 | 3.3 | 2.3 | 27.5 | 29.3 | 21.6 | 3.4 | 3.7 | 2.4 |
| 1997 | 26.5 | 27.2 | 21.3 | 3 | 3.1 | 2.2 | 27.2 | 28.9 | 21.5 | 3.3 | 3.6 | 2.4 |
| 1998 | 25.7 | 26.4 | 20.9 | 2.9 | 3 | 2.3 | 26.5 | 28 | 21.1 | 3.2 | 3.5 | 2.4 |
| 1999 | 24.1 | 24.6 | 20.3 | 2.7 | 2.8 | 2.2 | 26 | 27.5 | 20.8 | 3.2 | 3.5 | 2.3 |
| 2000 | 24.3 | 24.9 | 20.1 | 2.8 | 2.9 | 2.1 | 25.8 | 27.6 | 20.7 | 3.2 | 3.5 | 2.3 |
| 2001 | 23.5 | 24 | 19.7 | 2.6 | 2.7 | 2.1 | 25.4 | 27.1 | 20.3 | 3.1 | 3.4 | 2.3 |
| 2002 | 23.2 | 23.7 | 19.6 | 2.6 | 2.7 | 2 | 25 | 26.6 | 20 | 3 | 3.3 | 2.2 |
| 2003 | 23 | 23.5 | 19.4 | 2.6 | 2.6 | 2 | 24.8 | 26.4 | 19.8 | 3 | 3.2 | 2.2 |
| 2004 | 22.7 | 23.6 | 17.3 | 2.7 | 2.8 | 1.9 | 24.1 | 25.9 | 19 | 2.9 | 3.3 | 2.1 |
| 2005 | 22.3 | 23.2 | 16.3 | 2.6 | 2.7 | 1.7 | 23.8 | 25.6 | 19.1 | 2.9 | 3.2 | 2.1 |
| 2006 | 21.9 | 22.8 | 16.2 | 2.5 | 2.6 | 1.7 | 23.5 | 25.2 | 18.8 | 2.8 | 3.1 | 2 |

(Contd.)

| Years | ODISHA | | | | | | INDIA | | | | | |
|---|---|---|---|---|---|---|---|---|---|---|---|---|
| | Crude Birth Rate | | | Total Fertility Rate | | | Crude Birth Rate | | | Total Fertility Rate | | |
| | Total | Rural | Urban | Total | Rural | Urban | Total | Rural | Urban | Total | Rural | Urban |
| 2007 | 21.5 | 22.4 | 16.1 | 2.4 | 2.5 | 1.7 | 23.1 | 24.7 | 18.6 | 2.7 | 3 | 2 |
| 2008 | 21.4 | 22.2 | 16 | 2.4 | 2.5 | 1.6 | 22.8 | 24.4 | 18.5 | 2.6 | 2.9 | 2 |
| 2009 | 21 | 21.9 | 15.7 | 2.4 | 2.5 | 1.6 | 22.5 | 24.1 | 18.3 | 2.6 | 2.9 | 2 |
| 2010 | 20.5 | 21.4 | 15.2 | 2.3 | 2.4 | 1.6 | 22.1 | 23.7 | 18 | 2.5 | 2.8 | 1.9 |
| 2011 | 20.1 | 21 | 14.7 | 2.2 | 2.3 | 1.5 | 21.8 | 23.3 | 17.6 | 2.4 | 2.7 | 1.9 |
| 2012 | 19.9 | 20.8 | 14.6 | 2.1 | 2.3 | 1.4 | 21.6 | 23.1 | 17.4 | 2.4 | 2.6 | 1.8 |
| 2013 | 19.6 | 20.5 | 14.4 | 2.1 | 2.2 | 1.4 | 21.4 | 22.9 | 17.3 | 2.3 | 2.5 | 1.7 |

*Sources:* 1. Compendium of Fertility and Mortality Report, 1971-2007.

2. Sample Registration System Statistical Report 2011, Office of the Registrar General India, Ministry of Home Affairs, Government of India, New Delhi.
3. Sample Registration System Statistical Report 2012, Office of the Registrar General India, Ministry of Home Affairs, Government of India, New Delhi.
4. Sample Registration System Statistical Report 2013, Office of the Registrar General India, Ministry of Home Affairs, Government of India, New Delhi.

## Appendix 2

*Three Year Moving average of Crude Birth Rate and Total Fertility Rate by residence, 1971-2013*

| Periods | ODISHA | | | | | | INDIA | | | | | |
|---|---|---|---|---|---|---|---|---|---|---|---|---|
| | Crude Birth Rate | | | Total Fertility Rate | | | Crude Birth Rate | | | Total Fertility Rate | | |
| | Total | Rural | Urban | Total | Rural | Urban | Total | Rural | Urban | Total | Rural | Urban |
| 1971-73 | 34.7 | 34.8 | 32.5 | 4.7 | 4.8 | 4.2 | 36.3 | 37.7 | 30 | 5.1 | 5.3 | 4 |
| 1972-74 | 34.3 | 34.5 | 31.7 | 4.7 | 4.8 | 4.1 | 35.3 | 36.7 | 29.4 | 5 | 5.3 | 3.9 |
| 1973-75 | 34 | 34.3 | 31.3 | 4.7 | 4.8 | 4.1 | 34.8 | 36.2 | 28.6 | 4.9 | 5.2 | 3.7 |
| 1974-76 | 31.2 | 31.3 | 30.1 | 4.7 | 4.7 | 4 | 34.4 | 36.1 | 28.4 | 4.8 | 5.1 | 3.7 |
| 1975-77 | 30.1 | 30.2 | 28.5 | 4.4 | 4.5 | 3.8 | 34.2 | 35.6 | 28.5 | 4.7 | 5 | 3.6 |
| 1976-78 | 32.6 | 33 | 28 | 4.4 | 4.5 | 3.6 | 33.3 | 34.9 | 27.6 | 4.6 | 4.9 | 3.5 |
| 1977-79 | 31.7 | 32 | 28.5 | 4.2 | 4.2 | 3.7 | 33.1 | 34.5 | 27.9 | 4.5 | 4.8 | 3.4 |
| 1978-80 | 31.8 | 32.1 | 29.5 | 4.2 | 4.3 | 3.8 | 33.3 | 34.5 | 28.1 | 4.4 | 4.7 | 3.4 |
| 1979-81 | 31.9 | 32.1 | 29.6 | 4.2 | 4.2 | 3.8 | 33.8 | 35.3 | 27.5 | 4.4 | 4.7 | 3.4 |
| 1980-82 | 32.7 | 33 | 29.7 | 4.2 | 4.3 | 3.7 | 33.8 | 35.4 | 27.6 | 4.5 | 4.8 | 3.4 |
| 1981-83 | 33.5 | 33.8 | 30.3 | 4.4 | 4.4 | 3.7 | 33.8 | 35.4 | 27.8 | 4.5 | 4.9 | 3.4 |
| 1982-84 | 33.4 | 33.7 | 30.4 | 4.4 | 4.5 | 3.7 | 33.8 | 35.3 | 28.6 | 4.5 | 4.9 | 3.4 |
| 1983-85 | 32.5 | 32.8 | 29.6 | 4.2 | 4.3 | 3.5 | 33.6 | 35 | 28.6 | 4.4 | 4.8 | 3.4 |
| 1984-86 | 32 | 32.4 | 28.3 | 4.1 | 4.2 | 3.3 | 33.2 | 34.6 | 28.2 | 4.3 | 4.6 | 3.3 |

(Contd.)

| Periods | ODISHA | | | | | | INDIA | | | | | |
|---|---|---|---|---|---|---|---|---|---|---|---|---|
| | Crude Birth Rate | | | Total Fertility Rate | | | Crude Birth Rate | | | Total Fertility Rate | | |
| | Total | Rural | Urban | Total | Rural | Urban | Total | Rural | Urban | Total | Rural | Urban |
| 1985-87 | 31.4 | 31.9 | 26.9 | 3.9 | 4 | 3.1 | 32.6 | 34.1 | 27.5 | 4.2 | 4.5 | 3.2 |
| 1986-88 | 31.8 | 32.4 | 26.3 | 3.9 | 4 | 3 | 32.1 | 33.6 | 26.9 | 4.1 | 4.4 | 3.1 |
| 1987-89 | 31.1 | 31.7 | 25.7 | 3.7 | 3.8 | 2.9 | 31.5 | 33 | 26.3 | 4 | 4.3 | 3 |
| 1988-90 | 30.8 | 31.4 | 25.1 | 3.6 | 3.7 | 2.8 | 30.8 | 32.3 | 25.4 | 3.9 | 4.2 | 2.9 |
| 1989-91 | 29.8 | 30.5 | 23.4 | 3.5 | 3.6 | 2.5 | 30.1 | 31.6 | 24.7 | 3.8 | 4.1 | 2.8 |
| 1990-92 | 28.9 | 29.6 | 22.3 | 3.3 | 3.4 | 2.4 | 29.6 | 31.2 | 24 | 3.7 | 4 | 2.7 |
| 1991-93 | 27.9 | 28.6 | 22.2 | 3.2 | 3.3 | 2.4 | 28.1 | 30.7 | 23.7 | 3.6 | 3.9 | 2.7 |
| 1992-94 | 27.7 | 28.4 | 22.5 | 3.2 | 3.3 | 2.5 | 28.8 | 30.6 | 23.3 | 3.5 | 3.8 | 2.7 |
| 1993-95 | 27.7 | 28.4 | 22.6 | 3.2 | 3.3 | 2.5 | 28.5 | 30.3 | 23.1 | 3.5 | 3.8 | 2.7 |
| 1994-96 | 27.5 | 28.3 | 21.9 | 3.2 | 3.4 | 2.4 | 28.1 | 29.9 | 22.4 | 3.5 | 3.8 | 2.6 |
| 1995-97 | 27.1 | 27.8 | 21.5 | 3.1 | 3.3 | 2.3 | 27.7 | 29.4 | 21.9 | 3.4 | 3.7 | 2.5 |
| 1996-98 | 26.4 | 27.1 | 21.2 | 3 | 3.2 | 2.3 | 27.1 | 28.7 | 21.4 | 3.3 | 3.6 | 2.4 |
| 1997-99 | 25.4 | 26.1 | 20.8 | 2.9 | 3 | 2.2 | 26.6 | 28.1 | 21.1 | 3.3 | 3.6 | 2.4 |
| 1998-00 | 24.7 | 25.3 | 20.5 | 2.8 | 2.9 | 2.2 | 26.1 | 27.7 | 20.9 | 3.2 | 3.5 | 2.4 |
| 1999-01 | 24 | 24.5 | 20.1 | 2.7 | 2.8 | 2.1 | 25.7 | 27.4 | 20.6 | 3.2 | 3.5 | 2.3 |
| 2000-02 | 23.7 | 24.2 | 19.8 | 2.7 | 2.8 | 2.1 | 25.4 | 27.1 | 20.3 | 3.1 | 3.4 | 2.3 |
| 2001-03 | 23.2 | 23.7 | 19.6 | 2.6 | 2.7 | 2.1 | 25.1 | 26.7 | 20 | 3 | 3.3 | 2.2 |
| 2002-04 | 23 | 23.6 | 18.8 | 2.6 | 2.7 | 2 | 24.6 | 26.3 | 19.6 | 3 | 3.3 | 2.2 |

| Periods | ODISHA | | | | | | INDIA | | | | | |
|---|---|---|---|---|---|---|---|---|---|---|---|---|
| | Crude Birth Rate | | | Total Fertility Rate | | | Crude Birth Rate | | | Total Fertility Rate | | |
| | Total | Rural | Urban | Total | Rural | Urban | Total | Rural | Urban | Total | Rural | Urban |
| 2003-05 | 22.7 | 23.4 | 17.7 | 2.6 | 2.7 | 1.9 | 24.2 | 26 | 19.3 | 2.9 | 3.2 | 2.1 |
| 2004-06 | 21.3 | 23.2 | 16.6 | 2.6 | 2.7 | 1.8 | 23.8 | 25.6 | 19 | 2.9 | 3.2 | 2.1 |
| 2005-07 | 21.9 | 22.8 | 16.2 | 2.5 | 2.6 | 1.7 | 23.5 | 25.2 | 18.8 | 2.8 | 3.1 | 2 |
| 2006-08 | 21.9 | 22.4 | 16.1 | 2.4 | 2.5 | 1.6 | 23.1 | 24.7 | 18.6 | 2.7 | 3 | 2 |
| 2007-09 | 21.5 | 22.1 | 15.9 | 2.4 | 2.5 | 1.6 | 22.8 | 24.4 | 18.4 | 2.6 | 2.9 | 2 |
| 2008-10 | 21.4 | 21.8 | 15.6 | 2.3 | 2.4 | 1.6 | 22.4 | 24 | 18.2 | 2.5 | 2.8 | 1.9 |
| 2009-11 | 21 | 21.4 | 15.2 | 2.3 | 2.4 | 1.5 | 22.1 | 23.7 | 17.9 | 2.5 | 2.8 | 1.9 |
| 2010-12 | 20.1 | 21 | 14.8 | 2.2 | 2.3 | 1.5 | 21.8 | 23.3 | 17.6 | 2.4 | 2.7 | 1.8 |
| 2011-13 | 19.8 | 20.7 | 14.5 | 2.1 | 2.2 | 1.4 | 21.6 | 23.1 | 17.4 | 2.3 | 2.6 | 1.8 |

*Sources:* 1. Compendium of Fertility and Mortality Report 1971-2007.

2. Sample Registration System Statistical Report 2011, Office of the Registrar General India, Ministry of Home Affairs, Government of India, New Delhi.
3. Sample Registration System Statistical Report 2012, Office of the Registrar General India, Ministry of Home Affairs, Government of India, New Delhi.
4. Sample Registration System Statistical Report 2013, Office of the Registrar General India, Ministry of Home Affairs, Government of India, New Delhi.

## Appendix 3

### *Demographic and Socio-economic indicators based on 2001 census data*

| State and Districts | FL | FWPR | NAW | SR | UP | SC | ST | CBR | TFR | CPR | NDDP | IMR |
|---|---|---|---|---|---|---|---|---|---|---|---|---|
| Odisha | 55.4 | 26.7 | 41.7 | 941 | 13.9 | 17.2 | 11.7 | 23.4 | 2.9 | 40.3 | 23471 | 76 |
| Anugul | 39.5 | 28.4 | 28.9 | 984 | 11.54 | 16.9 | 20.6 | 22.9 | 2.8 | 38.9 | 9745 | 76 |
| Balangir | 58.9 | 11.4 | 32.9 | 953 | 10.89 | 18.8 | 11.3 | 25.2 | 2.9 | 44.8 | 8212 | 77 |
| Baleshwar | 50.3 | 31.3 | 24.6 | 976 | 7.69 | 19.4 | 19.4 | 20.6 | 2.5 | 41.9 | 10259 | 69 |
| Bargarh | 62.8 | 8.1 | 32.4 | 974 | 10.58 | 21.5 | 1.9 | 24.8 | 2.9 | 44.2 | 6848 | 83 |
| Bhadrak | 39 | 35.5 | 22 | 984 | 4.83 | 21.9 | 12.5 | 27.4 | 3.2 | 41.6 | 9250 | 90 |
| Boudh | 66.9 | 13.8 | 56.8 | 938 | 27.39 | 19.1 | 3.6 | 19.6 | 2.4 | 50 | 11723 | 82 |
| Cuttack | 47.2 | 38.6 | 21.5 | 980 | 7.33 | 15.4 | 33.6 | 25.5 | 3.1 | 34 | 12120 | 93 |
| Debagarh | 57.9 | 15.1 | 39.9 | 961 | 8.71 | 18.5 | 12.8 | 21.8 | 2.7 | 51.2 | 9705 | 83 |
| Dhenkanal | 28.4 | 49.7 | 22.1 | 1031 | 10.19 | 7.5 | 50.8 | 27.6 | 3.3 | 42.8 | 10011 | 104 |
| Gajapati | 46.4 | 30.9 | 36.7 | 998 | 17.6 | 18.6 | 2.9 | 24 | 2.2 | 40 | 8957 | 82 |
| Ganjam | 69.3 | 11.5 | 45.4 | 963 | 9.87 | 21.1 | 0.8 | 18.8 | 2.3 | 45.6 | 9336 | 76 |
| Jagatsingpur | 61.8 | 6.8 | 43.9 | 972 | 4.49 | 23 | 7.8 | 21.8 | 2.6 | 38.2 | 8440 | 77 |
| Jajpur | 58.3 | 22.9 | 53.3 | 946 | 36.1 | 17.1 | 31.5 | 21.1 | 2.6 | 43.5 | 19933 | 61 |
| Jharsuguda | 29.3 | 35.9 | 20.1 | 1001 | 7.5 | 17.7 | 28.6 | 26.8 | 3.2 | 33.9 | 9569 | 97 |
| Kalahandi | 35.9 | 42.2 | 30.6 | 1008 | 6.8 | 16.9 | 52 | 30.8 | 3.6 | 34.9 | 11869 | 112 |
| Kandhamal | 66.8 | 10 | 32.5 | 1014 | 5.69 | 20.5 | 0.5 | 21.8 | 2.6 | 35.9 | 7266 | 85 |

(Contd.)

| State and Districts | FL | FWPR | NAW | SR | UP | SC | ST | CBR | TFR | CPR | NDDP | IMR |
|---|---|---|---|---|---|---|---|---|---|---|---|---|
| Kendrapara | 46.2 | 28.1 | 30.7 | 977 | 13.64 | 11.6 | 44.5 | 25.3 | 3 | 42 | 10876 | 82 |
| Kendujhar | 70.4 | 8.8 | 69.8 | 902 | 42.92 | 13.5 | 5.2 | 20.3 | 2.4 | 44.1 | 14230 | 73 |
| Khurdha | 24.3 | 40.4 | 27.3 | 999 | 16.81 | 13 | 49.6 | 27.3 | 3.1 | 42 | 11503 | 95 |
| Koraput | 20.9 | 42.3 | 16.7 | 997 | 6.87 | 21.4 | 57.4 | 28.8 | 3.3 | 38.1 | 10037 | 95 |
| Malkangiri | 37.8 | 39.9 | 33.7 | 980 | 7 | 7.7 | 56.6 | 26 | 3 | 40.4 | 8385 | 61 |
| Mayurbhanj | 20.7 | 42.4 | 16.9 | 991 | 5.78 | 14.1 | 55 | 30 | 3.4 | 37.7 | 8511 | 96 |
| Nabarangpur | 57.6 | 11 | 37.5 | 938 | 4.29 | 14 | 5.9 | 20.9 | 2.5 | 44 | 7218 | 85 |
| Nayagarh | 25.8 | 36.8 | 19.6 | 1007 | 5.66 | 13.6 | 34.7 | 25.9 | 3 | 38.9 | 9963 | 86 |
| Nuapada | 50.5 | 24.7 | 35.2 | 972 | 14.99 | 16.5 | 22.1 | 23.6 | 2.8 | 41.9 | 10567 | 82 |
| Puri | 67.5 | 7.7 | 39.9 | 968 | 13.58 | 18.2 | 0.3 | 20.2 | 2.4 | 51.8 | 8896 | 85 |
| Rayagada | 24.6 | 41.3 | 24.8 | 1028 | 13.89 | 13.9 | 55.8 | 28.5 | 3.3 | 38.7 | 10175 | 99 |
| Sambalpur | 55.2 | 35.6 | 46.5 | 969 | 27.27 | 17 | 34.4 | 21.2 | 2.6 | 47.4 | 14584 | 77 |
| Subarnapur | 46.2 | 32.8 | 22.7 | 966 | 7.39 | 23.6 | 9.8 | 22.7 | 2.8 | 40.7 | 8635 | 71 |
| Sundergarh | 53.9 | 28.9 | 40.6 | 957 | 34.37 | 8.6 | 50.2 | 22.8 | 2.7 | 39.6 | 14485 | 73 |

*Note:* FL–Female Literacy, FWPR–Female Work Participation Rate, NAW–Non-Agricultural Workers, SR–Sex-Ratio, UP–Urban Population, SC–Scheduled Caste, ST-Scheduled Tribe, CBR–Crude Birth Rate, TFR–Total Fertility Rate, CPR–Contraceptive Prevalence Rate.

*Source:* Registrar General of India, 2001.

## Appendix 4

***Demographic and Socio-economic indicators based on 2011 census data***

| *State and Districts* | *FL* | *FWPR* | *NAW* | *SR* | *UP* | *SC* | *ST* | *CBR* | *TFR* | *CPR* | *NDDP* | *IMR* |
|---|---|---|---|---|---|---|---|---|---|---|---|---|
| Odisha | 64.36 | 27.2 | 38.2 | 978 | 16.68 | 17.1 | 22.8 | 19.6 | 2.4 | 39.6 | 33029 | 62 |
| Anugul | 70.44 | 26.8 | 46.9 | 942 | 16.23 | 18.8 | 14.1 | 18.5 | 2.2 | 37.5 | 57824 | 50 |
| Balangir | 53.77 | 30.6 | 31.6 | 983 | 11.96 | 17.9 | 21.1 | 21.2 | 2.7 | 37.2 | 29894 | 100 |
| Baleshwar | 72.95 | 21.9 | 30.6 | 957 | 10.92 | 20.6 | 11.9 | 19.1 | 2.3 | 53.5 | 24928 | 49 |
| Bargarh | 65.84 | 39.4 | 24 | 976 | 10.12 | 20.2 | 19 | 16.8 | 2.1 | 44.4 | 24734 | 66 |
| Bhadrak | 76.49 | 7.9 | 34.4 | 981 | 12.33 | 22.2 | 2 | 18.9 | 2.3 | 50.4 | 23665 | 55 |
| Boudh | 60.44 | 42.7 | 23.3 | 991 | 4.65 | 23.8 | 12.5 | 22.6 | 2.8 | 27.1 | 29671 | 64 |
| Cuttack | 77.64 | 13.7 | 58.6 | 955 | 27.94 | 19 | 3.6 | 15.4 | 1.8 | 48.7 | 38043 | 63 |
| Debagarh | 63.66 | 47.3 | 24.4 | 976 | 7.16 | 16.7 | 35.3 | 20.5 | 2.5 | 33.5 | 29621 | 58 |
| Dhenkanal | 71.4 | 16.4 | 46.1 | 947 | 9.83 | 19.6 | 13.6 | 18.1 | 2.1 | 46.4 | 31307 | 76 |
| Gajapati | 43.59 | 46.8 | 25.7 | 1042 | 12.25 | 6.8 | 54.3 | 24.1 | 2.9 | 32.7 | 30812 | 65 |
| Ganjam | 61.84 | 29.2 | 43.3 | 981 | 21.78 | 19.5 | 3.4 | 18.4 | 2.3 | 38.9 | 30714 | 61 |
| Jagatsingpur | 80.88 | 14 | 45.1 | 967 | 10.2 | 21.8 | 0.7 | 14.3 | 1.7 | 42 | 33123 | 56 |
| Jajpur | 73.37 | 7.3 | 44.4 | 972 | 7.39 | 23.7 | 8.3 | 18.1 | 2.2 | 42.2 | 29517 | 53 |
| Jharsuguda | 70.05 | 26.8 | 60.6 | 951 | 39.89 | 18.1 | 30.5 | 16.9 | 2.1 | 44.9 | 64191 | 51 |
| Kalahandi | 47.27 | 38.6 | 22.7 | 1003 | 7.75 | 18.2 | 28.5 | 23 | 2.8 | 29 | 26309 | 59 |

(*Contd.*)

| State and Districts | FL | FWPR | NAW | SR | UP | SC | ST | CBR | TFR | CPR | NDDP | IMR |
|---|---|---|---|---|---|---|---|---|---|---|---|---|
| Kandhamal | 52.46 | 43.4 | 31.9 | 1037 | 9.86 | 15.8 | 53.3 | 24.7 | 3 | 25.6 | 55599 | 88 |
| Kendrapara | 79.51 | 11.1 | 37.2 | 1006 | 5.8 | 21.5 | 0.7 | 17 | 2 | 36.8 | 21933 | 64 |
| Kendujhar | 58.7 | 30 | 33.7 | 987 | 14.04 | 11.6 | 45.4 | 23.1 | 2.8 | 38.3 | 54044 | 58 |
| Khurdha | 82.06 | 13.5 | 73.6 | 925 | 48.11 | 13.2 | 5.1 | 16.2 | 1.9 | 44.9 | 43561 | 76 |
| Koraput | 38.92 | 44.1 | 28.2 | 1031 | 16.37 | 14.2 | 50.6 | 26.2 | 3 | 36.6 | 34003 | 56 |
| Malkangiri | 38.95 | 45.3 | 17.1 | 1016 | 7.97 | 22.6 | 57.8 | 30 | 3.5 | 33.2 | 22998 | 55 |
| Mayurbhanj | 53.18 | 41.6 | 34 | 1005 | 7.67 | 7.3 | 58.7 | 21.4 | 2.7 | 39.7 | 24868 | 53 |
| Nabarangpur | 37.22 | 43.5 | 17.9 | 1018 | 7.2 | 14.5 | 55.8 | 28.6 | 3.5 | 33.4 | 20004 | 54 |
| Nayagarh | 71.08 | 12.8 | 40.9 | 916 | 8.29 | 14.2 | 6.1 | 17.2 | 2.1 | 34.4 | 21399 | 67 |
| Nuapada | 45.21 | 44.5 | 19.9 | 1020 | 5.61 | 13.5 | 33.8 | 23.1 | 2.9 | 31.6 | 26352 | 56 |
| Puri | 78.67 | 14.8 | 45.8 | 963 | 15.63 | 19.1 | 0.4 | 15.8 | 1.8 | 53 | 24047 | 80 |
| Rayagada | 39.87 | 42.2 | 25.6 | 1048 | 15.36 | 14.4 | 56 | 25.1 | 2.9 | 36 | 30771 | 65 |
| Sambalpur | 68.47 | 37.5 | 51 | 973 | 29.81 | 18.4 | 34.1 | 17.7 | 2.1 | 41.4 | 41749 | 56 |
| Subarnapur | 63.63 | 35.2 | 25.5 | 959 | 7.66 | 25.6 | 9.4 | 19.2 | 2.5 | 33.3 | 25266 | 54 |
| Sundergarh | 65.93 | 28 | 49.9 | 971 | 35.5 | 9.2 | 50.7 | 19.3 | 2.3 | 41.1 | 45622 | 55 |

*Note:* FL–Female Literacy, FWPR–Female Work Participation Rate, NAW–Non-Agricultural Workers, SR–Sex-Ratio, UP–Urban Population, SC–Scheduled Caste, ST–Scheduled Tribe, CBR–Crude Birth Rate, TFR–Total Fertility Rate, CPR–Contraceptive Prevalence Rate.

*Source:* Registrar General of India, 2011.

# PART 2
# Socio-Economic Factors and Health Issues

# 5

# Influencing Socio-Demographic and Anthropometric Factors on Caesarean Deliveries among Bangladeshi Women

## Survey in Rajshahi City

*Farhana Hasan, Md. Sabiruzzaman* and *Md. Golam Hossain*

## Introduction

The delivery system of child birth is a spontaneous process, which works in two ways such as natural or vaginal and caesarean. Vaginal delivery is known as the best, but unfortunately because of development of caesarean section (C-section), the prevalence of vaginal delivery is declined in recent years (Clark & Taffeles, 1997). World Health Organization suggested that C-section rates should not exceed 15 per cent (Bailey *et al.*, 2009), but it has increased worldwide in the last three decades. Based on recent studies, this rate is about 22 per cent in USA, 25 per cent in Brazil, 27 per cent in Chili and also is about 17-40 per cent in 19 countries in Latin America (Hopkins, 2000). A recent analysis of Demographic and Health Survey (DHS) data in 26 South Asian and sub-Saharan African countries found that rates were highest among the 'urban rich' in all countries, and lowest among the 'rural poor' in 18 (Betrán *et al.*, 2007). In all countries, fewer than 5 per cent of mothers in the poorest wealth quintile delivered by caesarean (Cavallaro *et al.*, 2013). In Bangladesh prior to 1970, C-section was an uncommon procedure. Based on Bangladesh Demographic Health Survey (BDHS), during the period 2003-2004, mean C-section rate was only 2.5 per cent. Currently 12.2 per cent of births were delivered by C-section (BMMS, 2010) and now a days C-section has become more common in Bangladesh like in most other comparable countries (Ravindran, 2008).

C-section delivery reduced the risk of foetal death in breech presentations and the risk of intrapartum foetal death in cephalic presentations. On the other hand, C-sections increased the risk of severe maternal and neonatal morbidity and mortality in cephalic presentations (Villar *et al.*, 2007). A multi-country study based on the World Health Organization (WHO), Global Survey on Maternal and Perinatal Health found that risks for adverse short-term maternal outcomes (death, intensive care unit admission, blood transfusion and hysterectomy) increased among women undergoing C-sections without medical indication in all three continents where the survey was conducted – the Americas, Africa and Asia (Souza *et al.*, 2010). Increasing C-section rates have been reported in several South Asian countries over the past decade. In Bangladesh, rates rose from 2 per cent (2000) to 17 per cent (2011); in India, from 3 per cent (1992) to 11 per cent (2006); and in Nepal, from 1 per cent (2000) to 5 per cent (2011) (Corsi *et al.*, 2012).

Lack of knowledge of caesarean delivery and misinformation about natural childbirth is important factors for caesarean section (Arjmandi & Farzin, 2007). On the other hand, maternal satisfaction from the previous childbirth experience has tremendous impact on the type of delivery which is based on maternal deciding. Also, the results of the studies showed that fear, anxiety and pain have important role in the choice of delivery type. The increase in caesarean deliveries has been attributed to multiple factors ranging from maternal, socio-demographic and institutional factors. Caesarean delivery rates are known to vary widely among different population groups, with known risk factors including maternal age, baby weight, place of residence, socio-economic status, high levels of maternal education, previous C-section, obstetric complications, maternal request (refers to a primary caesarean delivery per-formed because the mother requests this method of delivery in the absence of conventional medical or obstetrical indications), high income level and physicians' choices especially within private hospitals. A large number of studies have stressed that as the age of a mother increases, so does the likelihood of caesarean birth (Khawaja *et al.*, 2004). Age at marriage is also a significant cause of caesarean birth rates in the developing countries.

In view of increasing C-section rates in Bangladesh, there are growing concerns about its indiscriminate use. The aim of this study is to explore the prevalence and risk factors in the tendency of women to caesarean section delivery.

## Material and Methods

### *Study Area*

The trials were conducted with 194 women who had either caesarean or non-caesarean delivery at three private and one public hospital maternity wards in the northern region of Bangladesh. Among the 194 delivery cases, 150 were caesarean and the remaining 44 were non-caesarean.

### Study Design

A cross sectional study was conducted where the data were collected by direct interviews. For calculating the sample size we follow the published papers of Rahman *et al.*, 2014. We have to get the prevalence in our study which was 75 per cent. We consider 80 per cent power of study and 5 per cent level of significance. The formula provided that 192 was the significant sample size in our present study. The participants were selected by consecutive sampling technique. Most of the questions were close-ended and the answers chosen by the respondents were indicated by tick mark. All interviews were conducted within 24 to 48 hours of post-delivery.

### Measures Used

Webster *et al.*, 1992 suggested that women with medical complications near delivery are more likely to undergo C-section in order to improve their survival prospects as well as their newborns. Therefore, maternal factors (clinical) were considered as risk factors in the present study which includes previous C-section, swollen leg, breathing difficulty, child aborted around delivery time, birth control process, mother's height, weight and food habit. Previous works also suggested that a thorough understanding of decisions to perform C-section should recognize many non-medical factors as playing important part in such decisions. In order to investigate the non-medical determinants of C-section, a set of socio-demographic factors such as maternal age at birth, age at marriage, birth order, mother's educational level, mother's occupation, family income was identified. Padmadas *et al.* (2000) and Misra *et al.* (2002) have also found that there is a strong association between C-section and place of residence.

### Statistical Analyses

Initially, a bivariate logistic regression analysis was used to identify the significant association between the process of child birth (caesarean *vs* non-caesarean) and a series of independent variables. Dichotomous variables were analysed by the $\chi^2$-test or Fisher's exact test, where appropriate. Some risk factors which were associated with the C-section was isolated by performing multiple logistic regression analysis. The birth process was the dependent variable and it was taken to be dichotomous in nature (coded by the value 1 if the respondents undergo caesarean deliveries and 0 otherwise). In brief to determine risk factors, let $Y_i$ denote a binary variable that equals 1 with probability P and 0 with probability 1-P. For a logistic regression

$$\begin{aligned}\text{Log}\,[p/(1-p)] &= \beta_0 + \beta_1 X_1 + \beta_2 X_2 + \beta_3 X_3 + \beta_4 X_4 + \beta_5 X_5 + \beta_6 X_6 + \beta_7 X_7 + \beta_8 X_8 + \beta_9 X_9 \\ &= \beta_0 + \Sigma \beta_i X_i\end{aligned}$$

where, p = the probability of caesarean delivery (coded 1)

1-p = the probability of non-caesarean delivery (coded 0)

$X_1$ = Residence

$X_2$ = Mother's education

$X_3$ = Age group

$X_4$ = Age at first marriage

$X_5$ = Senseless in pregnancy

$X_6$ = Food habit

$X_7$ = Birth control

$X_8$ = Family income and

$X_9$ = BMI (kg/m$^2$)

$\beta_0$ = Intercept term

$\beta_i$ = the coefficient of independent variables (i=

1,2,3,.......,9).

The parameter $\beta_i$ refers to the effect of $X_i$ on the log odds such that Y=1, controlling the other $X_i$. Finally, results of the regression analyses have been presented by odds ratios (OR) with 95 per cent confidence interval (C.I.) with significance level $p < 0.05$. All statistical analyses in this study were performed by Statistical Package for Social Sciences (SPSS) version IBM 20.

## Results

A total of 194 mothers with the aggregate caesarean and non-caesarean rates among the participants were 77.3 per cent (150) and 22.7 per cent (44) respectively. Table 5.1 presents the prevalence and association of women reporting caesarean and non-caesarean delivery by patient characteristics and their significance level. Table 5.1 also shows that out of 19 variables examined, 12 were statistically significant while the remaining eight were statistically not associated with the birth process. The significant proportion rate were highest among women having previous C-section (p<0.001), BMI (p<0.001), height (p<0.001), senselessness in pregnancy (p<0.01), weight (p<0.01), age group (p<0.01), and food habit (p<0.01). Maternal age and their educations showed a positive association with birth process. The same pattern was also observed in age at marriage and family income. Urban women compared to their rural counterparts, were more likely to choose C-section for childbirth. Birth control also found to be statistically significant (p<0.05). Table 5.2 shows the prevalence of caesarean section, with the results multivariate logistic regression analysis. For multiple logistic regressions, we only use the significant variables. The results revealed that, when other socioeconomic factors were held constant, maternal age, senseless in pregnancy, birth control and BMI were found to have significant effect on caesarean delivery.

As shown in Table 5.2, the adjusted OR (with 95% confidence intervals) for a C-section in overall delivery cases increases significantly with maternal age, senseless in pregnancy, birth control and BMI. The highest odds ratios for caesarean delivery were seen in women aged 20-25 years (OR=0.198, 95% CI, 0.066-0.600) as compared to those aged 20 years and below. Over weighted women were more likely to get caesarean delivery than

**Table 5.1:** Association between Maternal, Socio-Economic and Demographic Behaviour Factor by Type of Delivery and their Significance level N= 194

| *Selected variables* | *Total n (%) n = 194* | *Birth Process* | | $\chi^2$ | *p-value* |
|---|---|---|---|---|---|
| | | *Non-Caesarean number (%) = 44 (22.7)* | *Caesarean number (%) = 150 (77.3)* | | |
| (1) | (2) | (3) | (4) | (5) | (6) |
| **Age group** | | | | | |
| 15–20 | 31 (16.0) | 12 (38.7) | 19 (61.3) | 12.057 | 0.002 |
| 20–25 | 77 (39.7) | 22 (28.6) | 55 (71.4) | | |
| 25+ | 86 (44.3) | 10 (11.6) | 76 (88.4) | | |
| **Residence** | | | | | |
| Urban | 107 (55.2) | 30 (28.0) | 77 (72.0) | 3.904 | 0.035 |
| Rural | 87 (44.8) | 14 (16.1) | 73 (83.9) | | |
| **Height (cm)** | | | | | |
| <150 | 57 (29.4) | 2 (4.5) | 55 (36.7) | 16.917 | 0.0001 |
| 150+ | 137 (70.6) | 42 (95.5) | 95 (63.3) | | |
| **Weight (kg)** | | | | | |
| <51 | 78 (40.2) | 9 (11.5) | 79 (88.5) | 9.235 | 0.002 |
| 51+ | 116 (59.8) | 35 (30.2) | 81 (69.8) | | |
| **Educational qualification** | | | | | |
| Primary | 51 (26.3) | 19 (37.3) | 32 (62.7) | 8.381 | 0.015 |
| Secondary | 69 (35.6) | 12 (17.4) | 57 (82.6) | | |
| Higher Secondary | 74 (38.1) | 13 (17.6) | 61 (82.4) | | |
| **Occupation** | | | | | |
| Housewife | 129 (66.5) | 30 (23.3) | 99 (76.7) | 1.301 | 0.729 |
| Service | 26 (13.4) | 4 (15.4) | 22 (84.6) | | |
| Students | 26 (13.4) | 6 (23.1) | 20 (76.9) | | |
| others | 13 (6.7) | 4 (30.8) | 9 (69.2) | | |
| **Husband's occupation** | | | | | |
| Service | 67 (34.5) | 11 (16.4) | 66 (83.0) | 2.826 | 0.419 |
| Agriculture | 51 (26.3) | 13 (25.5) | 38 (74.5) | | |
| Business | 61 (31.4) | 15 (74.6) | 46 (75.4) | | |
| Others | 15 (7.7) | 5 (33.3) | 10 (66.7) | | |
| **Age at marriage** | | | | | |
| 10–15 | 15 (7.7) | 8 (53.3) | 7 (46.7) | 9.030 | 0.011 |
| 15–20 | 150 (77.3) | 29 (19.3) | 121 (80.7) | | |
| 20+ | 29 (14.9) | 7 (24.1) | 22 (75.9) | | |

*(Contd. ...)*

| (1) | (2) | (3) | (4) | (5) | (6) |
|---|---|---|---|---|---|
| **Family Income** | | | | | |
| <12000 | 127 (65.5) | 34 (26.8) | 93 (73.2) | 3.510 | 0.043 |
| 12000+ | 67 (34.5) | 10 (14.9) | 57 (85.1) | | |
| **Malnutrition** | | | | | |
| Yes | 52 (26.8) | 8 (15.4) | 44 (84.6) | 2.156 | 0.099 |
| No | 142 (73.2) | 36 (25.4) | 106 (74.6) | | |
| **Food habit** | | | | | |
| As usual | 82 (42.3) | 11 (13.4) | 71 (86.6) | 6.594 | 0.006 |
| Nutritious | 112 (57.7) | 33 (29.5) | 79 (70.5) | | |
| **Senseless in pregnancy** | | | | | |
| Yes | 98 (50.5) | 31 (31.6) | 67 (68.4) | 9.051 | 0.002 |
| No | 96 (49.5) | 13 (13.5) | 83 (86.5) | | |
| **Birth control** | | | | | |
| Yes | 131 (67.5) | 36 (27.5) | 95 (72.5) | 5.301 | 0.015 |
| No | 63 (32.5) | 8 (12.7) | 55 (87.3) | | |
| **Previous C-section** | | | | | |
| Yes | 54 (27.8) | 2 (3.7) | 52 (96.3) | 15.366 | 0.0001 |
| No | 140 (72.2) | 42 (30.0) | 98 (70) | | |
| **Pregnancy induced swollen leg** | | | | | |
| Yes | 117 (60.3) | 25 (21.4) | 92 (78.6) | 0.290 | 0.356 |
| No | 77 (39.7) | 19 (24.7) | 58 (75.3) | | |
| **Child abortion** | | | | | |
| Yes | 55 (28.4) | 10 (18.2) | 45 (81.8) | 0.886 | 0.229 |
| No | 139 (71.6) | 34 (24.5) | 105 (75.5) | | |
| **Child death in pregnancy** | | | | | |
| Yes | 60 (30.9) | 11 (18.3) | 49 (81.7) | 0.936 | 0.219 |
| No | 134 (69.1) | 33 (24.6) | 101 (75.4) | | |
| **Multiple birth** | | | | | |
| Yes | 21 (10.8) | 7 (33.3) | 14 (66.7) | 1.524 | 0.168 |
| No | 173 (89.2) | 37 (21.4) | 136 (78.6) | | |
| **Birth order** | | | | | |
| 0–2 | 146 (75.3) | 32 (21.9) | 114 (78.1) | 0.197 | 0.396 |
| 2+ | 48 (24.7) | 12 (25) | 36 (75) | | |
| **BMI** | | | | | |
| Under weight | 12 (6.2) | 4 (33.3) | 8 (66.7) | 18.004 | 0.0001 |
| Normal | 97 (50.0) | 33 (34.0) | 64 (66.0) | | |
| Over weight | 85 (43.8) | 7 (8.2) | 78 (91.8) | | |

*Note:* Figures in the parentheses represent percentage of the corresponding group.

*Source:* Data collected from Rajshahi City Corporation, Bangladesh.

normal weighted women (OR=0.073, $p<0.01$). It was found that women who have related complications around delivery (maternal age, senseless in pregnancy, birth control, BMI) have higher risk of C-section.

## Discussions

This study aimed to explore the socio-demographic factors affecting the prevalence and risk factors of caesarean delivery in Bangladesh. The C-section rates in the different health facilities had been of great concern. Past studies in different countries found that the rate of caesarean delivery in private hospitals is higher than public hospitals (Sufang *et al.*, 2007). It seems that the private practice of the doctors and the financial motive of the private hospitals may be playing some important role in determining the caesarean rates. There is also an ongoing debate on the causes for increasing C-section rates. Much has been written about why and how much mothers-to-be request their doctors for C-section. The reasons include fear of childbirth pain, along with the perception that C-sections are safe (Fenwick *et al.*, 2010) the view that they are a superior form of medical care since they are so common among the better-off women. Added to the fact that the caesarean delivery can be carried out in an hour or less, whereas a vaginal delivery requires several hours, there was a sharp increase in C-sections that was concentrated among middle class families that were social security users. Private Doctors providing care to better-off families charged more for C-sections than for vaginal deliveries. Consequently, C-sections also represented increased income, resulting in higher C-section rates for this group as well.

The result from the logistic regression analysis showed that maternal age, senselessness in pregnancy, birth control and BMI were important determinants of C-section. Furthermore, the association of these determinants with C-section varied by the different health facilities. Our results also confirmed by other studies (Kassak *et al.*, 2009). This study shows that mother's educational level has a strong association in choosing caesarean delivery. In the previous study, it was found that mother's education is a proxy of socio-economic variable and it is associated with C-section (Padmadas *et al.*, 2000).

**Table 5.2:** The Effects of Selected Factors on C-section

| *Variable* | *Coefficients* | *S.E.* | *p-value* | *OR* | *95% CI for Odds Ratio* | |
|---|---|---|---|---|---|---|
| | | | | | **Lower** | **Upper** |
| **Age Group** | | | | | | |
| 15–20 | –2.713 | 0.782 | 0.001 | 0.065 | 0.014 | 0.307 |
| 20–25 | –1.664 | 0.565 | 0.003 | 0.198 | 0.066 | 0.600 |
| 25+(Ref) | 0 | | | | | |
| **Residence** | | | | | | |
| Urban | 0.812 | 0.479 | 0.090 | 2.252 | 0.880 | 5.760 |
| Rural (Ref) | 0 | | | | | |
| **Mother's Education** | | | | | | |
| Primary | –1.485 | 0.734 | 0.043 | 0.227 | 0.054 | 0.956 |
| Secondary | 0.235 | 0.676 | 0.121 | 1.265 | 0.336 | 4.757 |
| Higher (Ref) | 0 | | | | | |
| **Family Income** | | | | | | |
| <12000 | 0.497 | 0.691 | 0.472 | 1.644 | 0.424 | 6.366 |
| 12000+(Ref) | 0 | | | | | |
| **Age at marriage** | | | | | | |
| 10–15 | –0.169 | 1.059 | 0.873 | 0.845 | 0.106 | 6.726 |
| 15–20 | 0.603 | 0.731 | 0.410 | 1.827 | 0.436 | 7.655 |
| 20+(Ref) | 0 | | | | | |
| **Senseless in pregnancy** | | | | | | |
| Yes | –1.094 | 0.512 | 0.032 | 0.335 | 0.123 | 0.913 |
| No (Ref) | 0 | | | | | |
| **Birth control** | | | | | | |
| Yes | –1.282 | 0.580 | 0.027 | 0.277 | 0.089 | 0.865 |
| No (Ref) | 0 | | | | | |
| **Food habit** | | | | | | |
| As usual | 0.415 | 0.510 | 0.416 | 1.515 | 0.558 | 4.115 |
| Nutritious (Ref) | 0 | | | | | |
| **BMI** | | | | | | |
| Under weight | –1.433 | 0.857 | 0.049 | 0.235 | 0.144 | 0.985 |
| Normal | –2.587 | 0.606 | 0.001 | 0.073 | 0.022 | 0.242 |
| Over weight (Ref) | 0 | | | | | |

*Source:* Data collected from Rajshahi City Corporation, Bangladesh.

It is also established that age of mother is closely related to C-section. (Nassar & Sullivan, 2001) suggested that age and parity (order of birth) alone account for most demographic changes because there is a high primary caesarean rate for first birth to women 30 years age and older. In our study we found that maternal age of 20-25 are more likely to have C-section in urban area.

Mothers with senselessness problem in pregnancy and low birth order, who undergo C-section, explained that the choice was made mainly because of their greater risk of pregnancy and delivery-related complications. Therefore, it has been imply that delivery by caesarean birth is a complicated health issue in a country level and also a global perspective. Padmadas *et al.* (2000) and Misra & Ramanathan (2002) have also found that there is a strong association between C-section and place of residence. It seems that women residing in urban areas of the northern region were more likely to undergo C-section in private hospitals. This also indicates the importance of social status in determining the type of delivery. Furthermore, mother's height and weight is also affecting the delivery system. As a point of view, food habit and birth control considered as independent variables and the study found that irregular intake of nutritious food and regular controlling birth are significant determinant for caesarean delivery. Among the risk factors, maternal factors seem to be less important in determining which women would have C-section in private hospitals; however, socio-demographic factors were the most important factors that influenced the decision to perform a C-section.

## Limitation of the Study

First, the findings of this study are only applicable to the northern part of Bangladesh, but not the whole of the country. Second, several risk factors have been mentioned in the literature (Mossialos *et al.*, 2005) all of which were not considered in this study. Another limitation is that although all the women expressed their desire in oral interviews to be involved in decisions on delivery option, they however did not feel "medically capable" of making a decision on elective and non-elective C-section. As a result, we could not include maternal choice directly as a factor in this study. Finally, patient's medical records were not examined to determine on what grounds the doctors opted for caesarean delivery; therefore, we did not look at the physician factor in relation to caesarean birth rates, although other researchers have studied this factor. Besides the selected clinical and socio-demographic factors which have been included in this analysis, a host of other programmatic factors, e.g. accessibility, quality, and costs of delivery services, religiosity, prejudices, women's role in decision-making process, and subordinate status of women are also likely to influence the delivery process of women.

## Conclusion

Considering drastic prevalence of caesarean delivery in our country the present study provided strong evidence on a well-established culture of C-sections. Therefore, this study demonstrates that the roles of selected risk factors are not the main source of influence on the rate of caesarean delivery. Consequently, some other unrecorded factors influence strongly the decision on whether or not to perform a C-section. Since C-section deliveries cost more than vaginal deliveries, both in terms of the number of days of hospitalization required and the financial costs, it is possible that this very useful surgical procedure is being misused for profit purposes in the private hospitals in the northern region of Bangladesh. Efforts to reduce C-section birth in developing countries, like the northern region of Bangladesh, will require a comprehensive approach that would address patients' variables, care giver practices and hospital policies. Considering the key reasons for caesarean prevalence including: previous caesarean, food habit, fear of birth pain and doctors recommendation, providing psychological interventions and education, raising public awareness, reorganizing obstetric care increase the quality of vaginal delivery services, appropriate culture, providing solutions and legislation which are preventing doctors from personal opinions can be an effective strategy to reduce the caesarean delivery rate in Bangladesh.

## References

Arjmandi, B., and Farzin, M. (2007). Assessment of the level of the pregnant women's knowledge towards the advantages and disadvantages of normal vaginal delivery and cesarean section, Tehran (2005). *Iranian Journal of Basic Medical Sciences, 14*(55): 13-22.

Bailey, P., Lobis, S., Maine, D., and Fortney, J. (2009). Monitoring emergency obstetric care: a handbook. *World Health Organization*. 25-30. Retrieved from whqlibdoc.who.int/pubiications/2009/9789241547734_eng.pdf (Accessed on 12-06-2015).

Betrán, A.P., Merialdi, M., Lauer, J.A., Bing-Shun, W., Thomas, J., Van Look, P., and Wagner, M. (2007). Rates of caesarean section: analysis of global, regional and national estimates. *Paediatr Perina Epidemiol, 21*(2): 98–113.

BMMS (2010). Bangladesh maternal mortality and health care survey 2010: Summary of key findings and implications, Dhaka, Bangladesh, (1-12).

Clark, S. C., and Taffeles, S. (1997). Caesarean rate decreasing. *Obstetrics and Gynaecology, 31*:10.

Cavallaro, F.L., Cresswell, J.A., França, G.V., Victora, C.G., Barros, A.J., and Ronsmans, C. (2013). Trends in caesarean delivery by country and wealth quintile: cross-sectional surveys in southern Asia and sub-Saharan Africa. *Bull World Health Organ,* 91(12): 914, 6.22D, doi: 10.2471/BLT.13.117598.

Corsi, D. J., Neuman, M., Finlay, J. E., and Subramanian, S. V. (2012). Demographic and health surveys: a profile. *International Journal of Epidemiology, 41*(6), 1602-1613.

Hopkins, K. (2000). Are Brazilian women really choosing to deliver by Caesarean? *Social Science and Medicine, 51*(5): 725-740.

Khawaja, M., Kabakian-Khasholian, T. and Jurdi, R. (2004). Determinants of Caesarean section in Egypt: evidence from the demographic and health survey. *Health Policy, 69* (3): 273-281.

Kassak, K.M., Mohammad, A.A. and Abdullah, A.M. (2009). Opting for a caesarean: what deter-mines the decision? *Public Administration and Management, 13*(3): 100-122.

Mishra, U.S., and Ramanathan, M. (2002). Delivery related complications and determinants of caesarean section rates in India. *Health Policy Planning, 17* (1): 90–98.

Mossialos, E., Allin, S., Karras, K., and Davaki, K. (2005). An investigation of Caesarean section in three Greek hospitals: the impact of financial incentives and convenience. *European Journal of Public Health, 15*(3): 288-295.

Nassar, N. and Sullivan, E.A. (2001). Australia's mothers and babies 1999. Australian Institute of Health and Welfare. 4-34. Retrieved from https://npesu.unsw.edu.au/sites/default/files/npesu/data_collection/Australia's%20mothers%20and%20babies%201999.pdf (Accessed on 12-06-2015).

Padmadas, S., Kumar, S., Nair, S., and Kumari, A. (2000). Caesarean section delivery in Kerala, India: evidence from a national family health survey. *Social Science and Medicine, 51*(4): 511–521.

Ravindran, J. (2008). Rising Caesarean section rates in public hospitals in Malaysia 2006. *Medical Journal of Malaysia, 63*(5): 434-435.

Rahman, M., Shariff, A.A., Shafie, A., Saaid, R., and Tahir, R.M. (2014). Determinants of Caesarean Risk Factor in Northern Region of Bangladesh: A Multivariate Analysis. *Iranian Journal of Public Health,* 43(1): 16-27.

Souza, J.P., Gülmezoglu, A., Lumbiganon, P., Laopaiboon, M., Carroli, G., Fawole, B., Ruyan, P., WHO Global Survey on Maternal and Perinatal Health Research Group (2010). Caesarean section without medical indications is associated with an increased risk of adverse short-term maternal outcomes: the 2004-2008 WHO Global Survey on Maternal and Perinatal Health. *BMC Medicine,* 8, 71. DOI: 10.1186/1741-7015-8-71.

Sufang, G., Padmadas, S.S., Fengmin, Z., Brown, J.J., and Stones, R.W. (2007). Delivery settings and Caesarean section rates in China. *Bulletin of World Health Organization, Geneva, 85*(10): 755-762.

Villar, J., Carroli, G., Zavaleta, N., Donner, A., Wojdyla, D., Faundes, A., Velazco, A., Bataglia, V., Langer, A., Narváez, A., Valladares, E., Shah, A., Campodónico, L., Romero, M., Reynoso, S., de Pádua, K.S., Giordano, D., Kublickas, M., Acosta, A.; World Health Organization 2005 Global Survey on Maternal and Perinatal Health Research Group. (2007). Maternal and neonatal individual risks and benefits associated with caesarean delivery: multicentre prospective study. *BMJ*.2007; 335(7628):1025. DOI:10.1136/ bmj.39363.706956.55.

Webster, L., Daling, J., Mcfarlane, C., Ashley, D., and Warren, C. (1992). Prevalence and determinants of caesarean section in Jamaica. *Journal of Biosocial Science, 24*(4): 515-525.

# 6
# Utilisation of Maternal and Child Health Care Services among the Thadou-Kuki of Senapati District, Manipur

*Hoineilam Kipgen* and *B. T. Langstieh*

## Introduction

In our attempt to relate to the theme of this seminar on poverty, inequality and health in India with special reference to North East India, this chapter attempts to address the issue on maternal health, healthcare services and development among the Thadou-Kuki of Senapati District, Manipur. From an anthropological perspective a micro-level critical analysis on maternal health issues with reference to determinants of utilisation, healthcare services provided and health outcomes was examined on 560 ever married women aged between 15 – 49 years respectively.

Globally maternal health advancement and healthcare improvements have been key topical issues to address preventable maternal and child deaths overall staging for a conscious effort to address and adopt 'safe motherhood' programmes worldwide. The evidences of improvement have been supported by WHO (2012) reports that states that maternal mortality worldwide has dropped by 47 per cent since 1990. At the national scenario, preventing deaths to mothers associated with pregnancy and childbirth has been one of the greatest challenges before our nation in this twenty first century. Women are the prime caretakers of family and bearers of children and any repercussion on their health affects the family as a whole. Women in India face constraints not only in obtaining health services, but also in expressing health needs (Modi, Moitra, Patel, Kapadia, and Kantharia, 2013).

In North East India, except for the NFHS 1, 2 and 3 data, which provide a broad macro-level estimation on maternal and child health parameters regionally represented by politically demarcated eight states; very few but limited studies are available from the region relating to the population-specific and/or ethnic group related to micro-level understanding on culture, language and communication, behaviour, beliefs and local health practices, besides the role of other applied factors – education, socio-economic, political, chronic under development accompanied in times of social unrest and/or ethnic conflicts resulting in population displacement, affecting group social relations, perhaps contributing to the unequal distribution of development projects in the region.

Thus, as a population-specific micro-level case study on the utilisation of maternal and child health care services from the Thadou-Kuki representing the second largest tribe in Manipur preceded only by the Meitei or Manipuris, from Manipur (Census 2011), we examined our fieldwork empirical data under the following heads:

(i) Determinants of utilisation
(ii) Services provided
(iii) Health outcomes

**Land and People**

The study area, i.e. Tuilang-hom Block falls in the hilly region of Senapati district, Manipur. It is located in the northern most part of the state. The lush green district of Senapati covers an area of 3256.62 sq.km and is home to 3, 54, 972 persons recording a literacy rate of 75 per cent (Census of India, 2011).

Thadou-Kuki is one of the sub-tribes of Kuki who inhabit mainly in the hilly areas of the North Eastern states in India. They are one of the major tribes in Manipur (Haokip, 2012). It may be noted that various tribes of Kuki has in common, regarding their culture, tradition, language, food habits, beliefs etc. They belong to Mongoloid stock and linguistically, they belong to Tibeto-Burman language family (Goswami, 1985). It is Patrilineal-Patrilocal residence. They practice Christianity. The staple food of the Thadou-Kuki is rice.

## Material and Method

The present study was conducted among 551 households of the Thadou-Kuki of Tuilang-hom Block in Senapati district, Manipur. The anthropological fieldwork was conducted on nine (9) villages namely, Chalwa, Gelnel, Tujang Vaichong, Kotlen, Songjang, Songpijang, Selsi, Govajang and Phoikon during the period of January 2013-February 2014. With the help of a structured schedule, data was collected and recorded by interviewing the 560 ever-married women aged 15-49 years.

**Data on Maternal Care and Child Health:** Data on maternal care which includes pregnancy and birth histories, details of antenatal care and delivery care received during their past pregnancies from married women was collected with the help of an interview schedule. These include information on the number of antenatal visits, stage of pregnancy at first abdominal check-up (first trimester, second trimester and third trimester), place of delivery, persons conducting delivery and reasons for no antenatal check-up etc. In addition, the respondents were whether they received tetanus toxoid injection and iron/folic acid tablets or syrup during their pregnancies.

**Data on Family Planning:** Data on Family Planning was collected from married woman with the help of an interview schedule. Apart from our own re-constructed population specific schedule, reference was also made with the updated schedule of the National Family Health Survey-3 (International Institute of Population Sciences and Macro International, 2007). Information was collected on social network characteristics pertaining to parental aspirations for their children's future besides, the transmission of information on contraceptive knowledge, its acceptance, access and usage as well as decision-making matters and women's choice/preference on family planning. Both ever use and age at first use plus current contraceptive use will be the outcome variables.

## Statistical Analysis

Data entry and compilation of the demographic data was done on MS Excel data sheets and the collected data was analysed using SPSS.

## Results and Discussion

### *A. Determinants of Utilisation*

In the following tables the determinants of utilisation of the available maternal child health (MCH) services are being assessed in order to understand the following:

1. Socio-behavioural background of mothers with their notion and attitude towards conception and childbirth.
2. Awareness and priority towards safeguarding the maternal health.

Indirectly an assessment of MCH services and assistance provided that are available in the area will be known be it from government hospital (PHC, CHC and their subsidiary units) or Non-governmental aided agencies if any.

Table 6.1 show that the number of mothers who had reported undergoing the urine tests (as a confirmatory check-up for their pregnancy) was comparatively low at 38 per cent while the remaining 62 per cent of the mothers never took the test. However, the registration and ANC visits of the expectant mothers seems to be taken on a slightly serious note with a comparatively high number of 62 per cent overall cases of registration. These were done at the Government hospital (41%), Private Doctor's clinic (4%) and ASHA (17%). A sizeable number of mothers (38%) responded that they never got themselves registered at the time of pregnancy. One of the main reasons mentioned was basically due to ignorance and lack of knowledge from their part as reported in 30 per cent of the mothers while a sizeable 5 per cent do not feel the necessity of registration. From among those mothers who reside in remotely located villages lack of facility was the respond in 3 per cent cases.

Ante Natal Check-up (ANC) visits was reported by 55 per cent of the mothers which means that the remaining 45 per cent mothers never undertook this opportunity with reasons giventhat it was not necessary (26%), no time to go (9%), lack of knowledge (5%) and others (6%).

There is clear association between infant mortality rate and lack of poor quality antenatal care (Chandrasekhar, Rao, Nair, & Kutty, 1998). World Health Organisation has recommended a

**Table 6.1:** Pregnancy Test, Registration and ANC Visits of the Mothers

| | *No. of married women (n = 534)* | | | | | | |
|---|---|---|---|---|---|---|---|
| | *Pregnancy Test* | *Registration* | | | *ANC* | | |
| **Yes (%)** | 203 (38) | 331 (62) | Govt. Hospital | 217 (41) | 294 (55) | | |
| | | | Private | 21 (4) | | | |
| | | | ASHA | 93 (17) | | | |
| **No (%)** | 331 (62) | 203 (38) | Lack of knowledge | 159 (30) | 240 (45) | Not necessary | 139 (26) |
| | | | Do not feel necessary | 27 (5) | | No time to go | 47 (9) |
| | | | No facility | 17 (3) | | Lack of knowledge | 24 (5) |
| | | | | | | Others | 30 (6) |

*Source:* Field Survey.

minimum of 4 antenatal care visits for low risk pregnancy in women (Mathai, 2005). Most women who did not receive health care during pregnancy said this was because they thought it was unnecessary (International Institute of Population Sciences and Macro International, 2000). It is currently estimated that 16 per cent of the rural population lives more than 10 km from any medical facility (Bhalla, 1995).

Table 6.2 shows the characteristics of ANC visits by the 294 mothers who had availed the MCH services. It may be noted here that from the total number of 534 mothers taken for the present study, only 294 mothers (55%) have availed the ANC visits. The result depicted on Table 6.2 is inclusive of all mothers irrespective of the number of pregnancies per mother. Of mother's who attended ANC visits (51.7%) made their first ANC visits during the first trimester of pregnancy, 37.6 per cent in second trimester and 10.5 per cent in third trimester. The place where ANC visits was received were PHC (54.8%), CHC (29.6%) and private (15.6%). Table 6.2 further shows that majority of mothers (51.7%) had ANC visits for three times or more during their pregnancy.

Table 6.3 shows mother's awareness, source and adoption of family planning method. Out of the total number of 560 married women interviewed in the present study, the awareness on family planning measures was significantly high as 541 women (96.6%)

**Table 6.2:** ANC utilisation by 294 Mothers who had Availed the MCH services

| | *No. of mothers (n=294)* | *(%)* |
|---|---|---|
| **Period of ANC visits** | | |
| First trimester | 152 | 51.7 |
| Second trimester | 111 | 37.6 |
| Third trimester | 31 | 10.5 |
| **Frequency of antenatal check-up** | | |
| 1 time | 68 | 23.1 |
| 2 times | 77 | 26.2 |
| 3 times | 93 | 31.6 |
| 4 times | 37 | 12.6 |
| More than 5 times | 19 | 6.5 |
| **Place where antenatal care was received** | | |
| PHC | 161 | 54.8 |
| CHC | 87 | 29.6 |
| Private | 46 | 15.6 |

*Source:* Field survey.

responded to being aware of family planning methods. The main source of information regarding family planning is through 'friends' (57.5%) which seems to reflect that the close social networks among the women as an important factor in relating or sharing their knowledge in maternal well-being. However, a sizeable number of 17.9 per cent women reported that they had received awareness from the doctor(s), 15 per cent women from ASHA and 9.6 per cent from other sources.

It may be noted that though the percentage regarding awareness of family planning measures is as high as 96.6 per cent only 152 women (27.3%) reported to have had adopted family planning method. The reasons for non-adoption of family planning was due to want of more children (29.8%), husband/religious prohibition (18.2%), fear of side effects (8.8%) and other factors (16%). It was reported that the most commonly adopted method was intra-uterine device (14.8%), followed by pill (9.8%), injection (2%) and condom use (0.7%). The access and utilisation to family planning measures seems to be a self-motivated cause among 56.6 per cent women users though facilitating and providing access to the means was 11.2 per cent through doctors and medical practitioners, 21 per cent by the ASHA worker and procurement by other means from private sources in 11.2 per cent cases. It is interesting to note that the 'decision-making' and 'choice' to

Table 6.3: Awareness and Adoption of Family Planning

| Awareness | No. of mothers (n=560) | Per cent | Knowledge on FP | No. of mothers | Per cent |
|---|---|---|---|---|---|
| Yes | 541 | 96.6 | Doctor/ Nurse | 97 | 17.9 |
| | | | ASHA | 81 | 15.0 |
| | | | Friends | 311 | 57.5 |
| | | | Others | 52 | 9.6 |
| No | 19 | 3.4 | | | |
| **Ever use of FP** | | | **Method used** | | |
| Yes | 152 | 27.3 | Injection | 11 | 2.0 |
| | | | Pill | 55 | 9.8 |
| | | | Condom | 4 | 0.7 |
| | | | Intra-uterine device | 83 | 14.8 |
| No | 408 | 72.7 | **Reason for not adopting FP** | | |
| | | | Want more children | 167 | 29.8 |
| | | | Husband/Religious prohibition | 102 | 18.2 |
| | | | Fear of side effects | 49 | 8.8 |
| | | | Not necessary, costly, Lack of knowledge, etc. | 89 | 15.9 |
| **Source of FP among users** | | | | | |
| Doctor | 17 | 11.2 | | | |
| ASHA | 32 | 21.1 | | | |
| Self | 86 | 56.6 | | | |
| Others | 17 | 11.2 | | | |

*Source:* Field Survey.

adoption of family planning measures is mostly taken by the mothers in consultation with their spouses with an outcome that women have a big role to play on issues concerning the household in this patriarchal society.

### B. Services Provided

Access, Knowledge and Utilisation of any MCH services can also be gauge from the health parameter check-up that are made available and utilised during the ANC visits. Table 6.4 shows the battery of tests which were followed highlighting the sequence in order of importance examined among the 294 women who had availed the maternal health services provided. These include anthropometric measurements, physiological test functions and gynaecological and obstetric examination if any.

**Table 6.4:** Maternal Health Examination and Advice given to Mothers (N=294) during Antenatal Check-Up

| *Maternal health examination* | *No. of mothers* | *%* |
|---|---|---|
| (a) Abdomen examined | 289 | 98.3 |
| (b) Weight | 262 | 89.1 |
| (c) BP | 242 | 82.3 |
| (d) Delivery date told | 196 | 66.7 |
| (e) Nutrition advice given | 158 | 53.7 |
| (f) Blood test | 61 | 20.7 |
| (g) Ultrasound done | 58 | 19.7 |
| (h) Urine Test | 43 | 14.6 |
| (i) Breast examined | 14 | 4.8 |
| (j) Delivery advice given | 25 | 8.5 |
| **Advice given on:** | | |
| (a) Breastfeeding | 56 | 10.0 |
| (b) Keeping the baby warm | 31 | 5.5 |
| (c) Family planning | 96 | 17.1 |
| (d) Need for Institutional Delivery | 96 | 17.1 |

*Source:* Field survey.

It may be observed from Table 6.4 that the basic maternal health examination such as abdominalcheck-up's, body weight and blood pressure measures were the most commonly reported in 82 per cent and above cases while other tests such as blood test, ultra sound, urine test etc. which incurred an extra expenditure were reported infew cases at 20 per cent and below. The expected date of delivery and nutrition advice were also the most common pre-natal information given in 66.7 per cent and 54 per cent women. Contradicting to post-natal care where advice were expected to be given on breast-feeding, keeping the baby warm, family planning and the need for institutional delivery, very few women reported receiving such advice.

Overall it may be noted that among the 294 mothers who attended regular ANC visits only 25 per cent reported unsatisfactory results that the medical check-up was hurriedly done; while a sizeable 28 per cent and 47 per cent reported that the medical attendants had satisfactory and somewhat enough time to perform their duty in the ANC. Interestingly, 62.6 per cent of the mothers reported that the motivation for the antenatal check-up was 'self-motivated' while 32 per cent reported that they were motivated by a family member, 3.7 per cent by the ASHA and 1.7 per cent by others.

Thus, it may be concluded that the 55 per cent of the mothers in the present study does show that they are quite aware and does take a serious concern when it comes to taking care of themselves during their childbearing years. Included in this group are those mothers who have attained a slightly higher level of education influencing their decision-making processes and initiatives.

**Table 6.5:** Pre-natal Services Availed by Mothers

| | *No. of mothers (n=534)* | *Per cent* |
|---|---|---|
| **IFA tablets/bottles** | | |
| Received | 164 | 30.7 |
| Purchase | 40 | 7.5 |
| No | 330 | 61.8 |
| **Doses of Iron taken during the last pregnancy (n = 204)** | | |
| Taken | 133 | 65.2 |
| Can't take | 13 | 6.4 |
| No | 58 | 28.4 |
| **TT injection (n=534)** | | |
| Yes | 467 | 87.5 |
| No | 67 | 12.5 |
| **No. of times for TT injection (n = 467)** | | |
| 1 | 74 | 15.8 |
| 2 | 196 | 42.0 |
| 3+ | 197 | 42.2 |

*Source:* Field Survey.

Table 6.5 shows the access and availability of those who receive the iron and folic acid tablets (IFA), where it is found that only about 30.7 per cent received the IFA, 7.5 per cent could afford to purchase and the remaining 61.8 per cent of the mothers never availed the IFA tablets. It was reported that IFA is taken more seriously towards the last trimester period of pregnancy only among the133 women which is 24.9 per cent out of the 534 mothers. Very few mothers (n=204) responded to the question whether doses of iron was taken during last pregnancy of which 133 mothers replied in the positive and 58 mothers replied in the negative while 13 mothers responded that they could not take the iron tablets due to reasons of health complaints. With reference to the Tetanus Toxoid (TT) injection for immunisation of both mother and child, 87.5 per cent responded 'Yes' and 12.5 per cent did not take the injections. A considerable number of mothers withdraw themselves to getting only a one time or one shot injection (15.8%), twice and more than three times injection shots were also reported from 42 per cent of the mothers. This decline in the number of mothers using the TT injection was primarily due to the unavailability of injections as a free supply in the health centre, the unaffordable and lack of knowledge about the benefits of these injections.

**Table 6.6:** Childbirth and Delivery as Reported from 519 Mothers

| | *No. of mothers (n = 519)* | *Per cent* |
|---|---|---|
| **Place of Child Delivery** | | |
| Home | 451 | 86.9 |
| Hospital | 68 | 13.1 |
| **Assistance during child birth** | | |
| Hospital staff | 68 | 13.1 |
| Dais | 432 | 83.2 |
| Nurse | 13 | 2.5 |
| Others | 6 | 1.2 |
| **Last delivery conducted** | | |
| Normal | 495 | 95.4 |
| Caesarean | 24 | 46 |
| **Check-up within 48 hours after delivery** | | |
| Yes | 66 | 12.7 |
| No | 453 | 87.3 |

*Source:* Field Survey.

Table 6.6 shows the childbirth and delivery among the Thadou-Kuki mothers in the present study in which it was found that 86.9 per cent child delivery cases take place at home and only 13 per cent are at hospital (CHC or PHC). Also the fact that 83.2 per cent of all deliveries are assisted by the local Dais or midwives who in most cases are self-taught with no formal training except their hands-on experience in childbirth deliveries in the area. As the location of the study area is in rural setting it was reported that the number of trained nurse is relatively lower and most of the assistance during childbirth had taken place with the help of the local midwife or dais. For those admitted to hospital childbirth delivery was attended by hospital staff (13%), trained nurse or auxiliary midwife (2.5%) and others (1.2%). It may be noted that

population in idyllic rural setting in north east India which could be representing any hill tribal population of this region.

### *C. Health Outcome*

Health outcome will be discussed with reference to demographic characteristics of child mortality and the related causes of child deaths which reflects strong traditional beliefs and practices in spirits '*Kaose*' with indications of non-medical causes far outweighs the medical causes for a childhood disease. Also in consonance with total number of live-birth in comparison with total number of child deaths recorded in the present study.

Infant and child mortality are often the domineering contemporary socio-demographic issue which have been frequently associated with poverty, low level of education and a deficient health system. As a developing nation India is no exception being in the league of having one of the highest infant and child mortality rates in the world. On more similar grounds the infant and child mortality reported in the present study (Table 6.7) is moderately high but most severe in cases of neo-natal deaths (occurring within 0-7 days post delivery) reporting at 5.83 per cent, infant deaths below 1 years of age at 2.53 per cent, child deaths below 4 years of age at 2.11 per cent and juvenile deaths in the age group 5-14 years at 0.93 per cent respectively. The overall figure of child deaths in the age ranging from newborns until the attainment of 14 years was 11.40 per cent with more deaths occurring in males (6.34%) than the female (5.05%) children.

On closer examination about the related causes of child deaths in the present studied population as shown in Table 6.8a, the findings indicate that the child mortality among the Thadou-Kuki are related mostly with superstitious beliefs in spirits such as Kaose, unknown causes due to ignorance and lack of care by the mothers besides other health and social causes such as the Naga-Kuki conflicts in these areas of Senapati district, Manipur. Among the most common cause of death was 'cold diarrhoea' as reported by the mothers, fever, malaria, jaundice, heart/cardiac and gynaecological problem besides premature delivery.

**Medical causes**: Pre-mature delivery, Gynae problems, Diarrhoea, Cough, Cold, Fever, Tuberculosis, Chest pain, Heart problems, Jaundice, Malaria, Vomiting, Typhoid, Multiple tooth eruption, Liver problem etc.

**Table 6.7:** Child mortality which includes Neo-natal 0-7days; Infant>1yrs; Toddler 1-4yrs and Juvenile 5-14yrs mortality

| *Total No. of Mothers* | *Total No. of Live-Births* | | | *Child Mortality Rate* | | | | | | | | | | | | *Total Child Deaths* | | |
|---|---|---|---|---|---|---|---|---|---|---|---|---|---|---|---|---|---|---|
| | | | | *0–7 days* | | | *> 1 yr.* | | | *1 – 4 yrs.* | | | *5 - 14 yrs.* | | | | | |
| | *M* | *F* | *T* | *M* | *F* | *T* | *M* | *F* | *T* | *M* | *F* | *T* | *M* | *F* | *T* | *M* | *F* | *T* |
| 560 | 976 | 963 | 1939 | 61 | 52 | **113** | 30 | 19 | **49** | 21 | 20 | **41** | 11 | 7 | **18** | 123 | 98 | **221** |
| % | 50.34 | 49.66 | 50.02 | 3.15 | 2.68 | 5.83 | 1.55 | 0.98 | 2.53 | 1.08 | 1.03 | 2.11 | 0.57 | 0.36 | 0.93 | 6.34 | 5.05 | 11.40 |

*Source:* Field survey.

**Table 6.8(a):** Child Mortality and Related Causes of Child Deaths among the Present Studied Population of Thadou-Kuki

| *Age/Days* | *No. of Child-ren* | *M* | *F* | *Causes of Death* |
|---|---|---|---|---|
| 0 – 7 days | 113 | 61 | 52 | Don't know/Not known, lack of care during delivery, kaose, Premature delivery, Gynae problem, hard work etc. |
| 8 – 28 days | 3 | 1 | 2 | Don't know, kaose |
| 29 days – 1 year | 45 | 28 | 17 | Cold diarrhoea, Not known, lack of care, kaose, abnormal, fever etc. |
| 1 – 4 year | 41 | 21 | 20 | Cold diarrhoea, Not known, malaria, kaose, fever, jaundice, heartcase etc. |
| 5 – 14 year | 18 | 11 | 7 | Not known, Diarrhoea, Typhoid, Fever, Drown in water, Naga Kuki conflicts, Multiple tooth eruption etc. |
| **Total** | **220** | **122** | **98** | |

*Source:* Field survey.

**Table 6.8(b):** Nature and Causes of Deaths Reported

| | *Nature and Causes of Child Deaths* | | | |
|---|---|---|---|---|
| *Age Group* | *Medical* | *Non-Medical* | *Total* | *%* |
| 0–7 days | 10 | 103 | 113 | 5.83 |
| (%) | (8.85) | (91.15) | | |
| less than 1 month | — | 3 | 3 | 1.36 |
| (%) | | (100) | | |
| Below 1 yr. | 22 | 23 | 45 | 2.53 |
| (%) | (48.89) | (51.11) | | |
| 1–4 | 29 | 13 | 42 | 2.11 |
| (%) | (69.05) | (30.95) | | |
| 5–14 | 11 | 6 | 17 | 0.93 |
| (%) | (64.71) | (35.29) | | |
| **Total** | **72** | **148** | **220** | **11.40** |
| **(%)** | **(32.73)** | **(67.27)** | | |

*Source:* Field survey.

**Non-Medical causes:** Not known, Kaose, lack of care, hard work, displacement during Naga-Kuki conflict etc.

Figure 6.2 shows the comparison between the total number of live-births that is an incident count occurring with particular recordings of death prevalence in those specific age groups namely

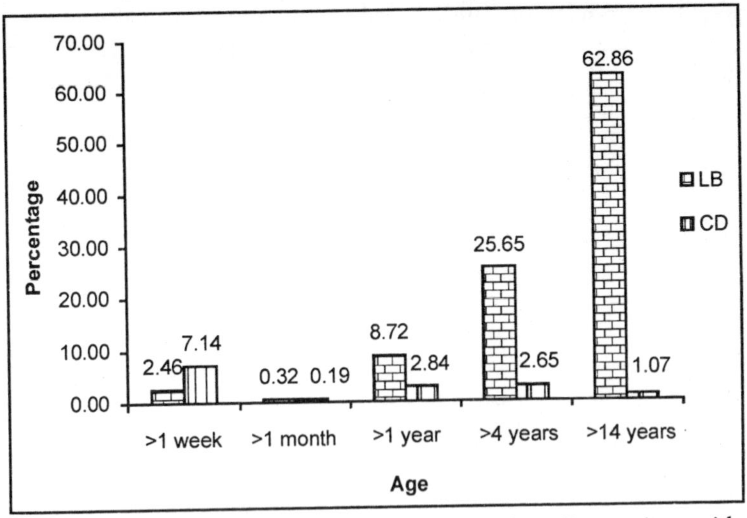


**Fig. 6.2:** Showing the Total Number of Live-Birth in Comparison with Total Number of Child Deaths Recorded in the Present Study

*Source:* Field survey.

– neo-natal (less than 1 week after birth); less than 1 month after birth, below 1 year, 4 years and 14 years respectively.

From Fig. 6.2 above, it is interesting to note the contrasting effects of mortality and survival rate which is observed at greater number in neonatal mortality which in other words mean higher child deaths occurrence during the first week after delivery (7.14%) as compared to higher live-birth incidence (62.86%) and lower death (1.07%) occurrence for children in the higher age groups of 5-14 years. In other words the rate of a surviving newborn is comparatively 9 times more in cases of live-births than neo-natal deaths. The nature and causes of child deaths in the present study for children below 14 years of age is shown in Tables 6.7 and 6.8(a).

A further sub-categorization on the causes of child deaths into a medically reported symptom *versus* a non-medical cause is shown in Table 6.8(b). It is found that non-medical causes were highly reported (67.27%) in Not known/Do not know cases which was mostly linked to a cultural belief in unnatural causes of death. Noticeably among the Thadou-Kuki the belief in 'Kaose' – an evil spirit–seems to be universally occurring phenomena resulting in death especially in children below the age of 4 years. Medical causes relating to symptoms of diarrhoea, typhoid, malarial fever, jaundice, and other medically known causes was reported at 32.73 per cent.

## Summary and Conclusion

Thus, summarising the findings from the present study we may conclude that determinants of utilisation along with the maternal health services provided in this rural population from Manipur seems to indicate that perhaps poverty and lack of access to basic health needs may not always be the hindrance or causal factor for distress in health outcomes. But demonstrations of power that culture has to shape people's perception and actions in decision making about their health in the most vulnerable state in one's life is equally important. Being self-motivated and adapting to the social environment that unequivocally provides a space for women to have a choice in availing the limited maternal health services in a gender sensitive society needs to be appreciated. The binding force that 'social networks' in this social group of women and their maternal needs especially the reciprocity of being given vital and correct information with reference to the adoption of family planning measures or the female bonded assistance provided at childbirth are examples of "make do of what you have" in the mutuality of being of what might be called as 'kinship' in a cultural phenomena.

No doubt education has a vital role to play in a woman's life, which is reflected in health outcomes on not only herself, but on her offspring(s), family and society at large. Education on Planned Parenthood or guides to parental education, maternal and child health services through outreach programmes on awareness, prevention and cautionary measures on health issues have always been taken on a positive outcome even in the remotest local village administration. These should be encouraged in right earnest to help cater to the needs of those not receiving the formal school education in the villages. Education albeit formal or informal ways of learning plays an important role in dissemination of knowledge with a conscience for better discretionary 'decision making' processes for one self and the society in which we live.

## Awareness and Constraints in Studying Poverty in NEI

At first glance it might seem that 'poverty' is a simple concept – the poor have limited monetary and material possessions – in fact poverty is complex (Dufour, 2006). For anthropologist Marshal Sahlins (2004: 37) "Poverty is not a certain small amount of goods (but) ....a relation with people......a social status.... an invidious distinction between classes...". The multifaceted nature of poverty means that we need to consider multiple dimensions to grasp poverty's effects. The material aspects of poverty such as income, possessions, education and occupation, describe only part of what it means to be poor. Many of the effects of poverty result from the interaction of material poverty with the symbolic belief system. Anthropologists have always considered that the material aspect of poverty needs to be examined in cultural context. In order to be able to appreciate the social and symbolic meanings of behaviours, relationships and material objects etc... a full bio-cultural approach is required to understand culture and all its pathways through which poverty is associated.

## Suggestions and Limitations

Improvement in communication and transport systems such as infrastructure for motorable roads and development works that are being invested in our nation or the simple communication system of understanding one another as human beings in symbolic language and dialects that bring about sharing of knowledge and goodwill is no doubt the vital link to progress and development. More importantly if it is implemented in true manner and spirit overcoming all boundaries of individualistic motives and short-term gains even among the ethnically 'small traditional societies'or the assumingly 'great tradition societies' will come a long way in bringing about change and development in this region.

## References

Bhalla, A. S. (1995). *Uneven Development in the Third World: A Study of China and India.* Basingstoke, UK: MacMillan.

*Census of India.* (2011). Provisional population totals: India.

Chandrasekhar, S., Rao, R. S., Nair, N. S., and Kutty, P. R. (1998). Socio-demographic determinants of antenatal care. *Tropical Doctors, 28(4):* 206-209.

Dufour, D. L. (2006). Biocultural approaches in human biology. *American Journal of Human Biology, 18(1):* 1-9.

Goswami, T. (1985). *Kuki Life and Lore.* Haflong, Assam: Sreeguri Press.

Haokip, E. L. (2012). Numerals in Thadou. *Language in India, 12:* 92-98.

International Institute of Population Sciences and Macro International. (2000). *National Family Health Survey,* (NFHS-II), 1998-1999, IIPS: Mumbai.

International Institute of Population Sciences and Macro International. (2007). *National Family Health Survey,* (NFHS-III), 2005-2006, IIPS, Mumbai.

Mathai, M. (2005). Patterns of routine antenatal care for low risk-pregnancy: RHL commentary. The *World Health Organisation Reproductive Health Library,* No. 8. Oxford: Update Software Ltd.

Modi, A., Moitra, M., Patel, B. H., Kapadia, P., and Kantharia, S. L. (2013). Women's Health: Profile and Practices of Anganwadi Workers. *Indian Journal of Maternal and Child Health, 15(2):* 1-11.

Sahlins, M. (2004). *Apologies to Thucydides: Understanding History as Culture and Vice-Versa.* Chicago: University of Chicago Press.

World Health Organisation. (2012). *Merck for Mothers*: WHO Issue New Maternal Mortality Data.

# 7
# Trend in Tobacco Use and Health Hazard in North-Eastern States of India
## A Time Event Analysis

*Gyan Chandra Kashyap* and *Shri Kant Singh*

## Introduction

Today India is the second largest producer of tobacco in the world and the third largest consumer. Its use and production proliferated to such an extent that, the overall 1.1 billion smokers worldwide (Bansal, John and Ling, 2005). Around 4.52 trillion cigarettes and 40.3 trillion *bidis* have been produced between 1910 and 2010, which are estimated to be responsible for nearly 100 million premature deaths in adult men of =35 years (Lal, Wilson, and Gupta, 2012) that numbers show the threat from the tobacco consumption. Tobacco addiction of a large number of adults has been initiated during the adolescence (Warren *et al.*, 2000; Patel, 1999; Gavarasana, Gorty and Allam, 1992; Sarma *et al.*,1990, Gupta 1996; Colby, 2000). Adolescents are the most vulnerable population to initiate tobacco use. More than 40 per cent of children had started the habit between 10-15 years of age (Chadda and Sengupta, 2002). Tobacco use by parents or an elder sibling increases the likelihood that a child begins smoking. Due to this, children are often introduced to such products at their very early life stages (Kapoor, Anand & Kumar, 1995; Jayant *et al.*,1991). It is now well established that most of the adult users of tobacco start tobacco use in childhood or adolescence. It is important to understand various factors that influence and encourage young teenagers to start smoking tobacco products.

Tobacco use among adolescents in India is a matter of concern. The prevalence of tobacco use in India ranged from 14 per cent among youth aged 13 – 15 years to 57 per cent among males aged 18–49 years. (Reddy and Gupta, 2004). As per the Tobacco control in India 2004, the estimated numbers of tobacco users among those aged 10 years and above were recorded as around 250 million (Reddy and Gupta, 2004). The prevalence of smoking has increased mostly in low and middle income countries, while it has declined in high income countries. Therefore, it can be understand that the vast majority of deaths will occur in low income countries (Merete, 2001). The increment in prevalence in tobacco smoking among adults and women was the highest in developing countries, which now accounts for 50 per cent of the global mortality and 56 per cent of the disease burden. At current levels of consumption, the burden from tobacco related morbidities is estimated to double by 2020 (Shibuya, Ciecierski & Guindon, 2003). Tobacco use is expected to cause approximately 8.4 million deaths, 70 per cent of which will occur in developing countries by 2020 (Enis, Brigden & Prindiville, 2000). Tobacco use, especially smoking is the largest cause of preventable death among adults in India (Lal, Wilson & Gupta, 2012). Nearly 9,00,000 people die every year in India due to diseases attributed to tobacco. Smoking has been widespread for many decades among men in India, where most adult deaths involve vascular disease, tuberculosis, or other respiratory diseases (Vendhan and Peto, 2003). The study of mortality associated with smoking in India, estimates that at least 9,30,000 adult deaths in India could be attributed to smoking, and that this would rise to over one million annually from 2010 (Jha, Jacob and Gajalakshmi, 2008). The existing trends in mortality, about 500 million people alive today will die prematurely as a result of tobacco use, with 1 billion deaths from tobacco expected during this century (Jha, Chaloupka & Corrao, 2006). The situation of tobacco consumption is grave In India where thirty per cent of the population aged 15 years and above, 47 per cent among men and 14 per cent among women either smoke or chew tobacco.

The existing prevalence transforms to almost 195 million people in India, 154 million men and 41 million women consuming tobacco. However, this study also highlights that tobacco consumption is significantly higher among socially deprived and economically marginalized groups, especially the poor, the less educated, Scheduled Castes and Scheduled Tribe populations having lesser potential to use modern health care facilities. Around 15-18 per cent of total deaths in India are preventable in nature as a large number of these deaths are due to tobacco related morbidity and lifestyle based diseases. Tobacco is also part of the socio-cultural setting in various societies, especially in the Eastern, Northern, and North-Eastern parts of the country. The prevalence of smoking and use of smokeless tobacco also vary widely across different states and had a strong association with an individual's socio-cultural characteristics (Rani, Bonu & Jha, 2003).

Continuation of tobacco consumption increases the risk of cardiovascular disease and other morbidities. In a present situation in India people start tobacco use at teenage and adulthood in all the settings. That is the danger indication of burden of disease in future from the tobacco consumption. This study is focusing on age at initiation and duration of tobacco consumption, which are the important indicator to assess its harm for the health in India. This study attempts to find the pattern and correlates of tobacco use and quitting tobacco among smokers as well as users of smokeless tobacco.

## Material and Methods

### *Ethics Statement*

The Global Adult Tobacco Survey was conducted in 2009-10. The Ministry of Health and Family Welfare (MoHFW), Government of India, designated the International Institute for Population Sciences (IIPS), Mumbai, as the nodal agency for conducting GATS in India. A formal written consent was obtained and ethical issues were taken care of before interviewing the respondent in the survey. Moreover, this study is based on anonymous public use data set with no identifiable information on the survey participants. Survey data are available upon the request on the official website of the institute at http://www.iipsindia.org.

### *Data Source*

This study is based on the data from the Global Adult Tobacco

Survey, India (GATS India). GATS India was conducted in 2009-10 as a household survey of persons in the age group 15 and above.

This study used comprehensive study design for urban and rural separately. In urban areas, three-stage sampling was adopted for the selection of households. The primary sampling units (PSU) were the city wards selected using probability proportional to size (PPS) sampling from urban sampling frame. For the secondary sampling units (SSU) were census enumeration blocks (CEB) was selected by probability proportional to size (PPS) from each selected urban ward. At the third stage tertiary sampling units (TSU) were households formed the sampling frame from which a sample of required number of households was selected. In rural areas, two-stage sampling was adopted for the selection of households. The primary sampling units (PSUs) were villages and secondary sampling units (SSUs) were households. All the villages are first stratified into different strata by using geographical regions, and further stratified by village size, proportion of Scheduled Caste, Scheduled Tribe population and female literacy. At the first stage, the list of all the villages in a state/UT formed the sampling frame. The required number of villages, i.e. (PSUs), was selected according to the probability proportional to size (PPS) sampling, within each stratum. At the second stage, a list of all the residential households in each selected village formed the sampling frame from which a sample of required number of households was selected.

The data of Global Adult Tobacco Survey India (GATS India) is the global standard for systematically monitoring adult's tobacco use (smoking and smokeless) and tracking key tobacco control indicators. A national probability survey was used to provide national and regional estimates by residence and gender and state estimate by gender. Global Adult Tobacco Survey India was carried out in all 29 states of the country and the two union territories of Chandigarh and Pondicherry, covering about 99.9 per cent of the total population of the country. The distribution of the total sampled households (79,690) was 47,959 rural and 31,731 urban. Of the total sampled households, the interview was completed in all respects in 76,069 of them, leading to an overall household response rate of 96.8 per cent. A total of 46,141 rural and 29,928 urban households successfully completed their interviews, giving a rural and urban response rate of 97.4 per cent and 96.0 per cent respectively. A total of 69,296 interviews were completed among which 33,767 and 35,529 were of males and females respectively (GATS, 2009-10).

### *Methods*

GATS survey has collected detailed information about the tobacco consumption in any form. Tobacco smoking includes manufactured cigarettes, rolled tobacco, *bidis*, cigars, cheroots, *hukkah* and smokeless tobacco includes betel quid with tobacco, *khaini* or tobacco lime mixture, *gutkha* or tobacco lime, areca nut mixture, oral tobacco, pan masala and betel quid without tobacco, nasal use of snuff. We have utilized the information on the age at initiation, current use, past use, period of use and age at quitting for both tobacco smokers as well as users of smokeless tobacco. The dependent variables used in this study are current tobacco users, current tobacco smokers, current smokeless tobacco users, time variable for the duration of tobacco use and duration of use of smokeless tobacco. Independent variables used in this study are age of respondent, sex, place of residence, education, occupation, standard of living index, region, states.

### *Statistical Analysis*

First, cross-tabulation has been used to see the state-wise prevalence of current tobacco users, current tobacco smokers and current users of smokeless tobacco. Time variables were calculated from the age at initiation and age of quitting tobacco for smokers as well as users of smokeless tobacco from the reference period of time of survey. Subsequently, those who were continuing tobacco use were considered as censored cases for this study. Cox's proportional hazards model was used to estimate the hazard ratio and their 95 per cent confidence interval for quitting tobacco. We have used the predictor variables sex, place of residence, education, occupation and region in this model. There are several reasons for choosing Cox's proportional hazards modelling to explain the effect of covariates on time until the occurrence of event where the event is quitting tobacco. Survival analysis typically examines the relationship of the survival distribution to covariates (Hosmer, Lemeshow & May, 1999). Kaplan-Meier survival analysis was graphed by sex, place of residence, education and region for smokers as well as users of smokeless tobacco. We evaluated the effect of age at initiation a time since quitting tobacco among the smokers and users of smokeless tobacco. An attempt has been made to find the progression of use of tobacco in all the regions of India by using the Kaplan-Meier Survival Analysis and Cox's Proportional Hazards Regression (Brenda, 2006; John, 2008).

Three level multilevel logistic regressions models are used to carry out the pattern and correlates of tobacco use. The state level and PSU level intercept variance in model 1 and model 2. The model expressed as intra-class correlation coefficients, these variances indicate that the variability in smoking and use of smokeless tobacco is associated with between-PSU (level 2) and between state (level 3) differences. As usually the case, between-individual differences are far more important. Model 2 incorporates all explanatory variables, i.e. individual, PSU and state level, into the model. We have utilized the variables age of respondent, sex, place of resident, education, occupation, standard of living index and different region of the country. All the analyses were done with the STATA 12.0 (Stata Corp LP, Texas 77845 USA).

## Results

### *Prevalence of Tobacco Use*

Figure 7.1(a) portrays the prevalence of the overall use of tobacco in India and its different states. The prevalence of tobacco use is the highest in Mizoram (63%) followed by four other states from the North-Eastern region, that is, Nagaland (57%), Tripura (56%), Meghalaya (55%) and Manipur (54%). The prevalence is high in Bihar (54%), Chhattisgarh (53%), and Jharkhand (50%). On the other hand, the lowest prevalence of tobacco is reported in Goa (9%), Punjab (12%), Chandigarh (14%), Puducherry (15%) and Tamil Nadu (16%). Figure 7.1(b) presents the percentage distribution of tobacco smokers according to states and UTs. The highest prevalence of tobacco smoking is reported in Mizoram (40%), followed by Meghalaya (36%), Nagaland (32%), and Arunachal Pradesh (29%). In contrast, the lowest prevalence of tobacco smoking is reported in Goa (5%), Maharashtra (7%), Punjab (7%), and Tamil Nadu (10%), whereas the national prevalence of tobacco smoking stands at 14 per cent. Figure 7.1(c) presents the

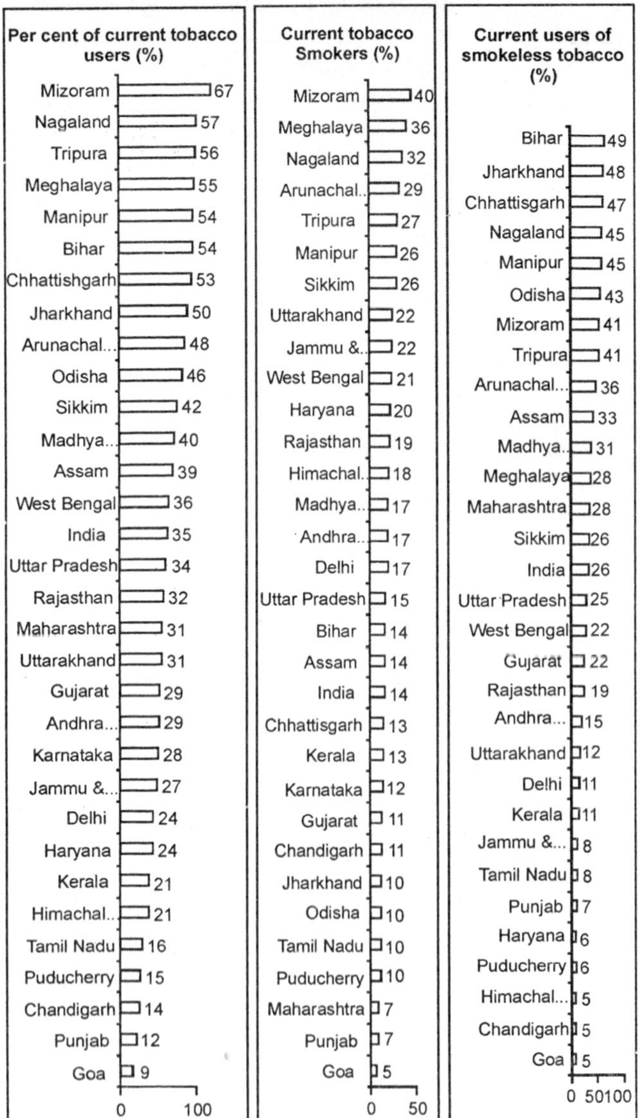


Fig. 7(*a*) Fig. 7(*b*) Fig. 7(*c*)

**Fig. 7.1(*a*):** Prevalence of Tobacco in Users India (GATS 2009-10). **Fig. 7.1(*b*):** Prevalence of Tobacco Smoking in India (GATS 2009-10). **Fig. 7.1(*c*):** Prevalence of Users of Smokeless Tobacco in India (GATS 2009-10).

*Source:* GATS, 2009-10.

percentage distribution of users of smokeless tobacco according to states and UTs in India. It is evident that there is a large variation in the prevalence of use of smokeless tobacco across different states/UTs. The highest prevalence of the use of smokeless tobacco is reported in some EAG states like Bihar (49%), Jharkhand (48%), Chhattisgarh (47%) and in the North-Eastern states of Nagaland (45%) and Manipur (45%), while the lowest prevalence is reported by the states of Himachal Pradesh, Goa, Chandigarh (5% in each) and Puducherry and Haryana (6% in each), which is significantly lower than the national level prevalence of use of smokeless tobacco, that is 26 per cent.

### *Correlates of Quitting Tobacco*

Results from Table 7.1, Cox proportional hazard model reveal that the hazard probability of quitting tobacco among females was 1.35 times ($p<.01$) higher compared to that among males. Urban people compared with their rural counterparts, had lower hazard probability of quitting tobacco (hazard ratio=0.90). As expected, the hazard of quitting tobacco increases with the level of education. Compared to uneducated persons, those with secondary education and above had 2.42 times higher hazard probability of quitting tobacco. The probability of quitting tobacco was found to be more among self-employed and retired or unemployed people than with Governmental or Non-Governmental employees. As compared to Governmental or Non-governmental employees, students as well as homemakers, were 9.2 per cent ($p<.01$) and 10.6 per cent ($p<.01$), respectively, less prone to quitting tobacco. The regional variation shows that the probability of quitting tobacco was higher in the southern and central regions (hazard ratio = 1.27), followed by the eastern regions (hazard ratio = 1.17) and western regions (hazard ratio = 1.07) compared to the north. The probability of quitting tobacco was found to be 37.6 per cent less among people from the North East compared to people from the north.

The study documented the sex of the person as a significant determinant of quitting smokeless tobacco. The hazard of quitting smokeless tobacco was high among women compared to men (hazard ratio = 1.02, $p<.01$). People living in urban areas had 1.21 times higher chances of quitting smokeless tobacco compared to their rural counterparts. Education shows a significant positive

**Table 7.1:** Cox proportional hazard ratio of quitting tobacco among smokers and users of smokeless tobacco by selected background characteristics in India, 2009-10

| *Background characteristics* | *Hazard ratio of smokers* | *Standard error* | *Hazard ratio of Users of Smokeless* | *Standard error* |
|---|---|---|---|---|
| **Sex** | | | | |
| Male® | | | | |
| Female | 1.35*** | 0.001 | 1.02*** | 0.001 |
| **Residence** | | | | |
| Rural® | | | | |
| Urban | 0.91*** | 0.000 | 1.21*** | 0.001 |
| **Education** | | | | |
| No formal schooling® | | | | |
| Less than primary | 1.01*** | 0.000 | 1.07*** | 0.001 |
| Primary but less than Secondary | 2.02*** | 0.001 | 1.59*** | 0.001 |
| Secondary and above | 2.43*** | 0.002 | 1.70*** | 0.002 |
| **Occupation** | | | | |
| Govt. and Non-Govt. employee ® | | | | |
| Self-employed | 1.12*** | 0.000 | 1.18*** | 0.001 |
| Student | 0.91*** | 0.000 | 2.50*** | 0.007 |
| Homemaker | 0.89*** | 0.001 | 1.34*** | 0.001 |
| Retired or unemployed | 1.44*** | 0.001 | 1.25*** | 0.001 |
| **Region** | | | | |
| North ® | | | | |
| Central | 1.24*** | 0.002 | 1.37*** | 0.005 |
| East | 1.17*** | 0.002 | 0.94*** | 0.003 |
| North-East | 0.62*** | 0.002 | 0.48*** | 0.002 |
| West | 1.07*** | 0.002 | 0.98*** | 0.003 |
| South | 1.27*** | 0.002 | 1.46*** | 0.005 |

*Note:* ® Reference category, ***P<0.01.
*Source:* GATS India, 2009-10.

**Table 7.2:** Log-rank Test for Equality of Survivor Functions among the Groups of Smokers

| | *Chi-square* | *d.f.* | *P-value* |
|---|---|---|---|
| Sex | 3046.14 | 1 | 0.00 |
| Residence | 29301.24 | 1 | 0.00 |
| Education | 1362857.5 | 3 | 0.00 |
| Occupation | 211780.85 | 4 | 0.00 |
| Region | 85552.70 | 5 | 0.00 |

*Source:* GATS India, 2009-10.

**Table 7.3:** Log-rank Test for Equality of Survivor Functions Among the Groups of Users of Smokeless

| | *Chi-square* | *d.f.* | *P-value* |
|---|---|---|---|
| Sex | 8814.37 | 1 | 0.00 |
| Residence | 106402.48 | 1 | 0.00 |
| Education | 374469.13 | 3 | 0.00 |
| Occupation | 165547.69 | 4 | 0.00 |
| Region | 244328.12 | 5 | 0.00 |

*Sources:* GATS India, 2009-10.

association with quitting smokeless tobacco. Compare to uneducated persons, those with secondary education and above were 1.69 times (p<.01) and those with primary, but less than secondary education 1.59 times (p<.01) more prone to quit smokeless tobacco. Compared with Governmental and Non-Governmental employees, the probability of quitting smokeless tobacco was higher among students (hazard ratio = 2.45) followed by homemakers (hazard ratio = 1.34), the retired or unemployed (hazard ratio = 1.25) and the self-employed (hazard ratic = 1.18). Again, region emerged as a significant factor affecting the chances of quitting smokeless tobacco. People from the south were 1.46 times more likely to quit smokeless tobacco followed by the central region (hazard ratio = 1.37) and the north. However, the chances of quitting smokeless tobacco were less in the North East (hazard ratio = 0.48), followed by the central (hazard ratio = 0.94) and western regions (hazard ratio = 0.98) compared with people from the northern part of the country.

### *Pattern of Tobacco Use*

Results from Table 7.4, three level multilevel logistic regressions models were used to carry out the pattern and correlates of tobacco use. The state level and PSU level Intercept variance in model 1 was 0.34 and 0.20 and in model 2 it was 0.24 and 0.36 both were statistically significant. Expressed as intra-class correlation coefficients, these variances indicate that 14 per cent and around 9 per cent of the variability in smoking is associated with between-PSU (level 2) and between state (level 3) differences. As usually the case, between-individual differences are far more important. Model 2 incorporates all explanatory variables i.e. individual, PSU

**Table 7.4:** Multilevel Odds Ratio of Smoking and Use of Smokeless Tobacco Status in India, 2009-10

| *Variables* | *Tobacco Smokers* | | *Users of Smokeless Tobacco* | |
|---|---|---|---|---|
| | *Model 1* | *Model 2* | *Model 1* | *Model 2* |
| **Intercept (coefficient)** | –1.68*** | –.65*** | –1.47*** | –2.02*** |
| **Age of respondent** | | | | |
| 15–24® | | | | |
| 25–44 | | 2.30*** | | 1.70*** |
| 45–64 | | 3.31*** | | 1.69*** |
| 65+ | | 2.86*** | | 1.77*** |
| **Sex** | | | | |
| Male® | | | | |
| Female | | 0.06*** | | 0.48*** |
| **Residence** | | | | |
| Rural® | | | | |
| Urban | | 0.87*** | | 0.48*** |
| **Education** | | | | |
| No formal schooling® | | | | |
| Less than primary | | 0.78*** | | 1.02 |
| Primary but less than secondary | | 0.51*** | | 0.84*** |
| Secondary and above | | 0.33*** | | 0.51*** |
| **Occupation** | | | | |
| Govt. and Non-Govt. employee ® | | | | |
| Self-employed | | 0.91*** | | 0.89*** |
| Student | | 0.35*** | | 0.33*** |
| Homemaker | | 0.71*** | | 0.66*** |
| Retired or unemployed | | 0.79*** | | 0.76*** |
| **Standard of Living Index** | | | | |
| Low® | | | | |
| Medium | | 0.99 | | 0.96 |
| High | | 0.85*** | | 0.70*** |
| **Region** | | | | |
| North ® | | | | |
| Central | | 0.75 | | 5.20*** |
| East | | 0.54** | | 8.18*** |
| North-East | | 2.29*** | | 8.75*** |
| West | | 0.31*** | | 2.49*** |
| South | | 0.62** | | 1.42 |
| **Random Part** | | | | |
| State variance | 0.34** | 0.24** | 1.11** | 0.22** |
| PSU variance | 0.20** | 0.36** | 0.43** | 0.40** |

*Note:* *, ** and *** indicate that the coefficient is significant at 10, 5 and 1 per cent level of significance.

*Sources:* GATS India, 2009-10.

and state level, into the model. The odds of smoking was three times higher in 45-64 (OR = 3.31***) age group compared to age group 15-24. Results highlight the positive significant impact of level of education, as education increases tobacco smoking decreases and it was the lowest at the secondary and higher level (OR = 0.33***) in comparison with no formal schooling. The prevalence of tobacco use was the highest in North East region (OR = 2.29***) in comparison of northern region. Among the users of smokeless tobacco the state level and PSU level intercept variance in model 1 was 1.11 and 0.43 and in model 2 it was 0.22 and 0.40 both were statistically significant. The variable age of respondent had the fewer variation in use of smokeless tobacco among the age group 25–44, 45–64 and 65+ in comparison to age group 15–24 (OR=1.7****) that confirmed the consistent use of smokeless tobacco after the 24 years. Females from urban area were 51 per cent less likely to use smokeless tobacco. Regional variation pointed out North-eastern (OR = 8.75***), Eastern (OR = 8.18***), Central region (OR = 5.11***), Western (OR = 2.49***) and Southern region (OR = 1.42***) are more likely to use of smokeless tobacco in comparison of Northern region. This analysis highlight that the factors like educational attainment, standard of living and regions are strongly associated with smoking and as well as use of smokeless tobacco (*see* Figs. 7.2 and 7.3).

## Discussion

The current appearance of epidemiological transition in India lies in the shift from communicable diseases to non-communicable and lifestyle based diseases accounting for the major disease burden. Recent estimates portray that deaths due to non-communicable diseases constitute about 42 per cent of all the deaths in India compared to 38 per cent of deaths due to communicable disease. Tobacco smoking and use of smokeless tobacco have been widespread for many decades among men in India, and have been responsible for most adult deaths involving cardiovascular disease, hypertension, and stroke, different forms of cancer, tuberculosis, other respiratory diseases and diseases related to the liver (Vendhan and Peto, 2003). The findings from our study show that the highest percentage of young people currently using tobacco product in the North-eastern states of India. The prevalence of

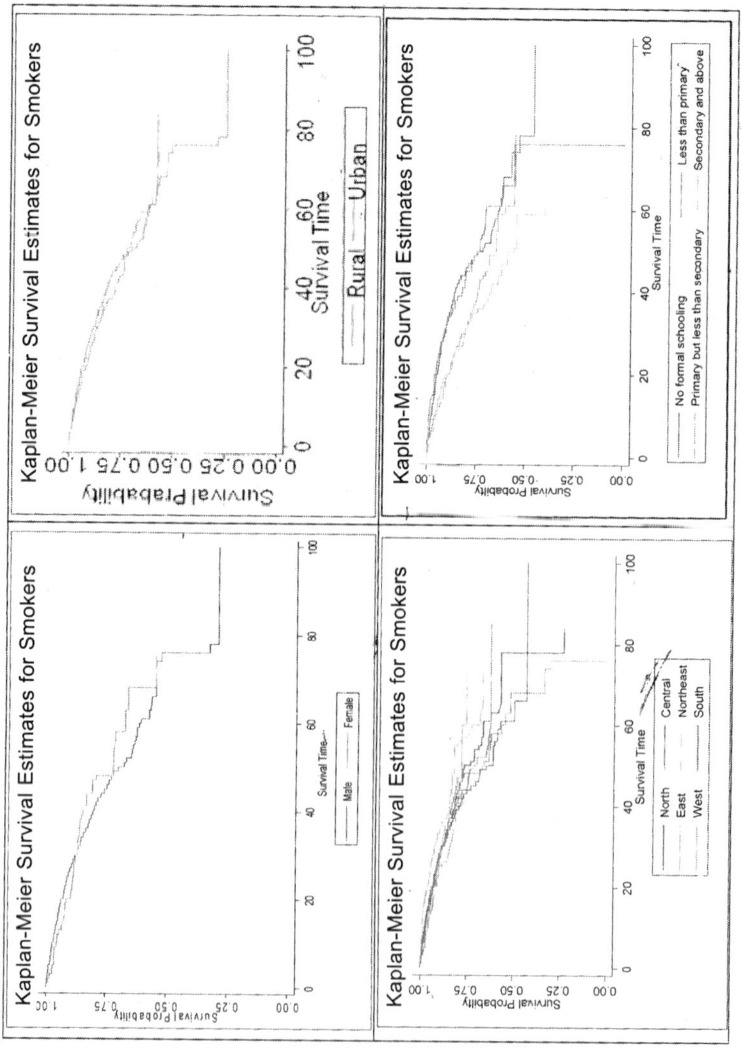


**Fig. 7.2:** Kaplan Meier Survival Estimates for Smokers by Selected Background Characteristics
*Source:* Author's Study.

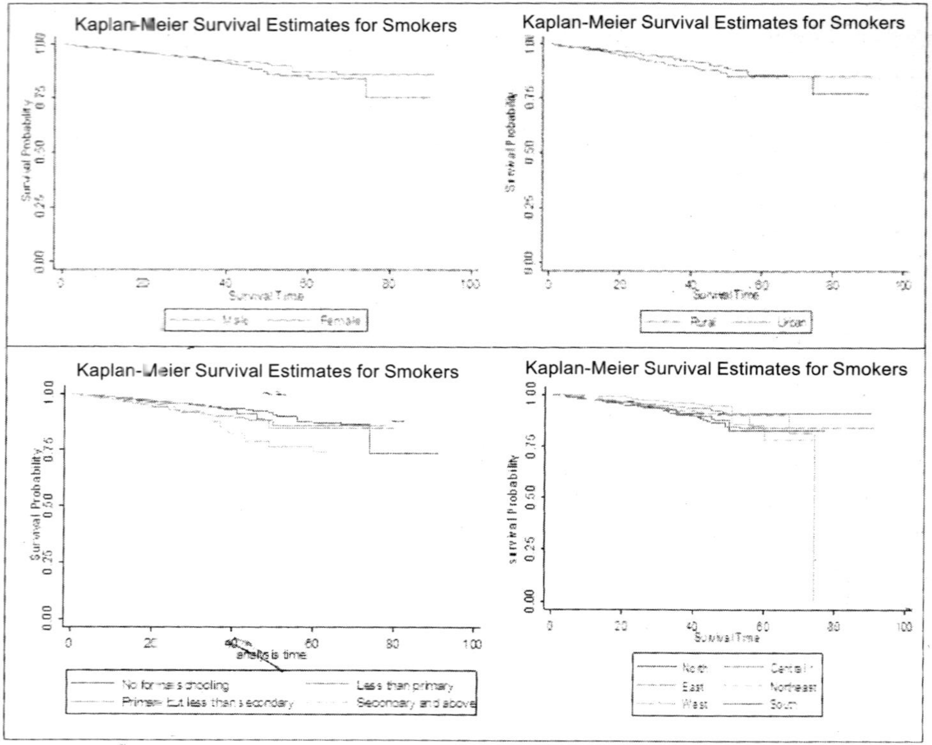


**Fig. 7.3:** Kaplan Meier Survival Estimates for Users for Smokeless by Selected Background Characteristics
*Source:* Author's Study.

tobacco use is the highest in Mizoram (63%) followed by four other states from the North-Eastern region, that is, Nagaland (57%), Tripura (56%), Meghalaya (55%) and Manipur (54%). Our concern is that, since the childhood age the children start using tobacco, and the more likely are they to become addicted, and tobacco consumption become the important things in any one's life in North-east, possible reasons may be cultural issues, living environment, parental use of tobacco. The need is more common among cigarette smokers and users of smokeless tobacco. This shows that children were already developing dependency on tobacco; they start consuming tobacco products at very young age. Many other factors may be working that showed strong association with tobacco use: parental and closest friends' tobacco use; lack of knowledge on harmful effects of tobacco; positive attitude towards tobacco use by others; and viewing of tobacco advertisements. Apart from the above states, the other three states from the North-Eastern region also rank very high in the chronology and thus all the seven sister states from the region portray the highest tobacco smoking in the country. Of course, there are many other states where tobacco smoking is higher than the national average. The highest prevalence of the use of smokeless tobacco is reported in some EAG states like Bihar (49%), Jharkhand (48%), Chhattisgarh (47%) and in the North-Eastern states of Nagaland (45%) and Manipur (45%), while the lowest prevalence is reported by the states of Himachal Pradesh, Goa, Chandigarh (5% in each).

The results from the Kaplan Meier Survival estimates pointed out that the probability of quitting is higher among women than among men and that it is relatively higher in urban areas as compared to rural areas, both for smokers as well as users of smokeless tobacco. There has been profound regional variation, where the probability of quitting is the highest in the southern states both among smokers as well as users of smokeless tobacco. Further, the Cox proportion hazard ratio, which portrays the cumulative probability of quitting tobacco use, has been computed for major socio-economic groups relevant for planning and intervention of tobacco control programmes. Three level multilevel logistic regressions models portray the pattern and correlates of tobacco use. The odds of Smoking higher in 45–64 age groups compare to age group 15–24. The variable age of respondent had the fewer variations in use of smokeless tobacco among the age group 25–44, 45–64 and 65+ in contrast to age group 15–24 that confirmed the consistent use of smokeless tobacco after the 24 years. Female belongs to urban area were 51 per cent less likely to use smokeless tobacco. This study concluded that the factors like educational attainment, standard of living and regions were associated with smoking and as well as use of smokeless tobacco.

## Conclusion

Tobacco use is growing fastest in the low-income countries due to steady population growth coupled with tobacco industry targeting and ensuring that millions of people become fatally addicted each year. As results portrays about the prevalence of tobacco smoking is the highest in North-eastern state and smokeless user were the highest in EAG states of India. Continuation of tobacco consumption up to older ages reduces the age of tobacco users, due to initiation in early age, that maximises duration of tobacco consumption. So for initiation in early ages also a danger signs for the health of teen agers and youngsters. At the same time, the chances of quitting tobacco are very low in any setting in Indian. So, that enormous consumption of tobacco use leads to disease asthma, tuberculosis, cancer etc. Auspiciously, life expectancy of male and female in India has increased but people are living their lives with diseases and disability that can be linked with tobacco consumption. Tobacco consumption should be minimized by the explaining the facts about the health risks from smoking as well as use of smokeless tobacco, ban on smoking in public places and workplaces, comprehensive bans on advertising and promotion. Although, increasing tobacco prices may be the single most effective way to reduce tobacco consumption in India.

## Recommendation

In view of the disproportionally high rate of smoking and use of smokeless tobacco in the North-Eastern states along with the progression of the tobacco epidemic, there is an urgent need of innovative strategies to strengthen cessation efforts in North-Eastern states of India. Print as well as electronic media have to play a proactive role in creating awareness among the most vulnerable groups, especially among youth and women, so that they can be convinced to quit and the tobacco related disease burden can be minimized. In view of the existing epidemiology transition and significant link between tobacco use and health hazard, the Government should effectively strengthen programmes and interventions targeting young people need to expand their focus to include both preventing initiation as well as offering youth cessation programmes.

**Authors Contribution**

Conceived and designed the experiments: SKS GCK. Performed the experiments: SKS GCK. Analysed the data: SKS GCK. Contributed reagents/materials/analysis tools: SKS GCK. Wrote the paper: SKS GCK.

**Acknowledgements**

Authors are thankful to International Institute for the Population Sciences (IIPS), Govandi Station Road, Deonar, Mumbai for providing us a GATS India (2009-10) data for this research work.

## References

Bansal, R., John, S., and Ling, P.M. (2005). Cigarette advertising in Mumbai, India: targeting different socio-economic groups, women, and youth. *Tobacco Control,* 14:201-206. doi: 10.1136/tc.2004.010173.

Brenda, G. (2006). Checking Assumptions in the Cox Proportional Hazards Regression Model. Centre for Statistical Consultation and Research, University of Michigan.

Chadda, R.K., Sengupta, S.N. (2002). Tobacco use by Indian adolescents. *Tobacco Induced Diseases,* Vol. 1, No. 2: 111–119.

Colby, S.M., Tiffany, S.T., Shiffman, S., and Niaura, R.S. (2000). Are adolescent smokers dependent on nicotine? A review of the evidence. *Drug and Alcohol Dependence,* 59: S83-S95.

Enis, B., Brigden, L.W., and Prindiville, J. (2000). Research priorities for tobacco control in developing countries: a regional approach to a global consultative process. *Tobacco Control,* 9(2): 217-223. Ottawa, Ontario, Canada.

GATS. Global Adult Tobacco Survey (2009-10) International Institute for Population Sciences (IIPS), Mumbai, India. *The Ministry of Health and Family Welfare (MOHFW),* Government of India.

Gavarasana, S., Gorty, P.V., and Allam, A. (1992). Illiteracy, ignorance and willingness to quit smoking among villagers in India. *Japanese Journal of Cancer Research*, 83: 340-343.

Gupta, P.C. (1996). Survey of socio-demographic characteristics of tobacco use among 99598 individuals in Bombay, India using handheld computers. *Tobacco Control, 5*: 114-120.

Hosmer, D.W., Lemeshow, S., and May, S. (1999). *Applied Survival Analysis.* Wiley, New York.

Jayant, K., Notani, P.N., Gulati, S.S., and Gadre, V.V. (1991). Tobacco use in school children in Bombay, India. A study of knowledge, attitude and practice. *Indian Journal of Cancer,* 28: 139-147.

Jha, P., Jacob, B., Gajalakshmi, V. (2008). A nationally representative case-control study of smoking and death in India. *N. Engl. J. Med.,* 358, 1137–1147.

Jha, P., Chaloupka, F.J., and Corrao, M. (2006). Reducing the burden of smoking world-wide: effectiveness of Interventions and their Coverage. *Drug and Alcohol Review,* 25: 597-609.

John, F. (2008). Cox Proportional-Hazards Regression for Survival Data. Appendix to an R and S-PLUS Companion to Applied Regression.

Kapoor, S.K., Anand, K., and Kumar, G. (1995). Prevalence of tobacco use among school and college going adolescents of Haryana. *Indian Journal of Paediatrics,* 62: 461-466.

Lal, P.G., Wilson, N.C., and Gupta P.C. (2012). Attributable deaths from smoking in the last 100 years in India. *Research Communications, Current Science,* 103(9): 1085-1090.

Lal, P.G., Wilson, N.C., and Gupta, P.C. (2012) Attributable deaths from smoking in the last 100 years in India. (2012). *Research Communications, Current Science,* 103(9).

Mamatha, M., and Rao, V.N. (2014). Use of Tobacco in India and the Influencing Factors: An Analysis on National Family and Health Survey Data (NFHS-III). *International Journal of Computer Science and Information Technologies,* 5(2): 1664-1667.

Merete, O. (2001). Revives. *British Medical Journal,* April 7, 322(7290): 869.

Patel, D.R. (1999). Smoking and children. *Indian Journal of Paediatrics,* 66: 817-24.

Rani, M., Bonu, S., and Jha, P. (2003). Tobacco use in India: prevalence and predictors of smoking and chewing in a national cross-sectional household survey. *Tobacco Control.* 12.e4, downloaded from http://www.tobaccocontrol.com/cgi/content/full/12/4/e4, accessed 12 May, 2015.

Reddy, S.K., Gupta, P.C. (2004). Report on Tobacco Control in India. *Ministry of Health and Family Welfare (MOHFW),* Government of India, New Delhi.

Sarma, P.V., Dhand, R., Malhotra, A., Malhotra, S., and Sharma, B.K. (1990). Pattern of smoking in north Indian adults. *Indian Journal of Chest Diseases and Allied Sciences.* 32: 83-93.

Shibuya, K., Ciecierski, C., and Guindon, E. (2003). WHO Framework Convention on Tobacco Control: development of an evidence based global public health treaty. Volume 327, *British Medical Journal,* 327: 154–157.

Vendhan, G. and Peto, R. (2003). Smoking and mortality from Tuberculosis and other diseases in India. *The Lancet,* Vol. 362, August 16: 507–15.

Warren, C.W., Riley, L., Asma, S., Eriksen, M.P., Green, L., Blanton, C., Loo, C., Batchelor, S., Yach, D. (2000). Tobacco use in youth: a surveillance report from the Global Youth Tobacco Survey Project. *Bulletin of World Health Organization,* 78: 868-876.

# 8
# Healthcare Challenges in India
## Why Healthcare Innovation Matters Today

*Laiamonriti P. Soh*

## Introduction

Indian healthcare industry is poised to double from $60 billion to $120 billion by 2015, growing at a 15 per cent CAGR (Rao, 2012). According to Fitch, the Indian healthcare sector is expected to reach US$ 100 billion by 2015 from the current US$ 65 billion, growing at around 20 per cent a year (Dutt, 2012). According to McKinsey Global Institute (2007), health care spending in India is expected to touch 13 per cent of average household income by 2025 from 7 per cent in 2005. Health service delivery in India is characterized by a three-tier system. At the lowest level are the sub-centres (each covering a population of about 5,000). Only paramedical staff is available in these sub-centres. The first points of contact with a doctor are the primary health centres (each covering about 30,000 people). Community health centres provide secondary care and are organized at the block levels. The sub-divisional hospitals and district level hospitals constitute the higher tiers. In principle, the sub-centres, primary health centres (PHCs), and community health centres (CHCs) are required to handle the preventative aspects of health care, institutionalize deliveries, treat minor diseases, and act as referral centres. The subdivision and district level hospitals would then treat major ailments as referral hospitals (Rao & Choudhury, 2012). According to Ministry of Health and Family Welfare-Government of India, there are 1,48,124 Sub-Centres, 23,887 PHCs and 4,809 CHCs functioning in the country as on March 2011.

India's the public sector accounts for only around 20 per cent of the total healthcare expenditure, representing around 1 per cent of the GDP which is among the lowest in the world with China 38.8 per cent, Thailand 63.9 per cent, Japan 82.2 per cent and US 45.1 per cent (WHO, 2008; Kothandaraman & Mookerjee, 2008). According to the WHO (2008), it was found that India's public healthcare is under-funded and small in size to meet the current health needs of the country. Items like public health, hospitals, sanitation etc. fall under the State Government, while items having wider implication at the national level like food and drugs, family planning, medical education, and vital statistics fall under the Central Government. It is mostly through national health programmes that the Central Government spent around 15 per cent of the total funds in the healthcare sector. The contribution of private sector in healthcare expenditure in India is around 80 per cent and is one of the highest in the world (Baru, 1999; Chanda, 2002). Almost 94 per cent of this amount comprises of out-of-pocket expenditure on health. The remaining 6 per cent is the expenditure on provision, which accounts for the private sector contribution to 60 per cent of all in-patient care and 78 per cent of total number of visits in outpatient care in India (Kinsey Global Institute 2007; KPMG, 2011; Narayana & Lalitha, 2013). In addition the private sector today provides 58 per cent of the hospitals and 81 per cent of the doctors in India (Kinsey Global Institute, 2007; MoHFW, 2008). Adding to the challenge is also the changing demographics and lifestyles of the people. Dealing with these challenges requires the resources and expertise of public and private sector combined.

## Challenges in the Indian Healthcare Sector

The health delivery system is an important measure that affects country's health status. Moreover, these are increasing evidence of the association between health and socio-economic status from the studies conducted throughout the world.The healthcare service delivery system is the mode to combine inputs, allow the delivery of a series of interventions or serviced actions in order to improve the health condition of the people (Bhattacharyya, McGahan, Dunne, Singer & Daar, 2008; Schneider & Barron, 2008). In many countries, reducing inequalities in health has been identified as key target of health delivery system. According to Chanda (2002) and Kinsey Global Institute (2007), the healthcare sector is one of the fastest growing sectors in the world economy in recent years with over 8 per cent growth in terms of GDP and is expected to be the third largest economy by 2050. Healthcare services which are critical to the growth in economy have seen vast improvements over the past few years in India. Yet, India's total expenditure in healthcare as a percentage of GDP is still one of the lowest in the world. Though the public health services infrastructure is widespread, starting with sub-centres, primary health centres, community health centres, secondary level district hospitals, up to medical colleges, the quality of these are not uniform and subject to regional disparities.

Although, the health sector in developing countries are facing so many challenges, these challenges are improving access, affordability and quality health, huge health status gap between urban and rural areas, low level of health awareness of the population, lack of sanitary and hygienic condition, high cost of healthcare, scarcity of specialty care and low infrastructure (Bhattacharyya, McGahan, Dunne, Singer & Daar, 2008). In recent years, these health sector problems are become more serious and higher priority has been given to delivering health service and meeting the needs of the poor (Parry & Judge, 2005; Pingali, 2010). It is recognized to strengthening health delivery system as a priority for a nation to be able to meet the basic health needs of its people, especially for poor and vulnerable populations. A challenge in a developing country like India is to find out ways that enable to address this basic health needs more effectively ( WHO, 2008; David, Sameh, Banafsheh, Katja & Marko, 2009). In this regard, innovation in health delivery system act as driving force of transforming available health resources and technology to make accessible, affordable and quality health services.

In spite of rapid economic growth, India is ranked 136 out of 185 countries in the Human Development Index. India has great social and economic inequalities. There are marked disparities among different geographical regions, between social groups, among different income level, between the sexes and demographic transition which reflects both quantitative as well as qualitative changes in the population profile (Monteiro, Moura, Conde & Popkin, 2004; KPMG, 2011). This has led to the burden of communicable, non-communicable diseases and newer diseases.

The country continues to combat against communicable diseases such as malaria, along with tuberculosis (TB), cholera, and plague, HIV, V cholera 139, hepatitis C virus. Non-communicable diseases are doubling in their incidence as well as prevalence in the country. Coronary artery disease, diabetes, renal failures, stroke and cancer are on a rise due to factors such as hypertension, metabolic syndrome and stress. In addition to this, new disease threats have emerged in the form of avian influenza, H1N1 etc. (Karl & Purnima, 2009; Gupta, 2013). Over the next 15 years, non-communicable diseases are likely to constitute nearly half of the distribution of the total disease burden, thus posing a serious future threat to the health of the Indian population. With respect to primary healthcare in the past in India, the life expectancy and mortality ratios have improved over the years though there is a need for improvement when compared with other countries of the world (KPMG, 2011; Gupta, 2013). As per the data maintained by UNDP, India's Under Five Mortality Rate (U5MR) declined from 125 per 1,000 live births in 1990 to 74.6 per 1,000 live births in 2005-06. U5MR is expected to further decline to 70 per 1,000 live births by 2015. This means India would still fall short of the target of 42 per 1,000 live births by 2015. In view of these statistics, child survival in India needs sharper focus (KPMG, 2011; Pingali, 2010). This need better managing neonatal and childhood illnesses and improving child survival, particularly among vulnerable communities. Survival risk remains a key challenge for the disadvantaged who have little access to reproductive and child health services. From a Maternal Mortality Rate (MMR) of 437 per 1,00,000 live births in 1990-91, India is required to reduce MMR to 109 per 1,00,000 live births by 2015. Between 1990 and 2006, there has been some improvement in the MMR which has declined to 254 per 1,00,000. Some of the largest states like Madhya Pradesh (62), Orissa (61), Uttar Pradesh (61), Assam (58), Meghalaya (55), Rajasthan (55), Chhattisgarh (51), Bihar (48) and Haryana (48) still have infant mortality rate (IMR) above the national estimates. India will reach maternal mortality rate (MMR) of 139 per 100,000 live births by 2015, falling short by 30 percentage points (MoHFW, 2011; KPMG, 2011).

India has a rural population of about 69 per cent, but majority of the healthcare facilities are available at urban areas. There are considerable gaps between the rural and urban areas of India, with respect to disease morbidity as well as mortality. Urban areas today have four times more health workers per 1,000 people than their rural counterparts. Moreover, 42 per cent of health workers in the rural areas identifying themselves as allopathic doctors actually, have no medical training as compared to 15 per cent in the urban areas. Compounding these disparities is an urban bias in healthcare financing. For example, almost 30 per cent of public health expenditure (both from the centre as well as states) is allocated to urban allopathic services while rural centres receive less than 12 per cent of this share (KPMF, 2011; Rao & Choudhuri, 2012).

Moreover, health expenditure in India is largely driven by private spending, namely, the out-of-pocket (OOP) expenditure, with public funds constituting an insufficient share of the total health expenditure. Despite several government initiatives in social protection, such as the Employees' State Insurance Scheme (ESIS) and the Central Government Health Scheme (CGHS), only around one-fourth of the population is covered by some form of public health insurance (Pingali, 2010; Singh & Biswas, 2012). Though several efforts, such as the NRHM, the Janani Suraksha Yojana, and the Rashtriya Swasthya Bima Yojana, have been initiated over the past few years in order to provide equitable healthcare to Indians, such programmes alone cannot accomplish the goal of universal health coverage (MoHFW, 2008, 2011). The percentage of out of pocket health expenditure in India is higher when compared to other developing countries. Approximately 29 per cent of the Indian population (almost 300 million people) live below the poverty line and depend on free health services from the public sector. The inequities in the health system are further aggravated by the fact that public spending on health has remained stagnant at around one per cent of GDP (0.9%) compared to the global average of 5.5 per cent (Kinsey Global Institute, 2007; KPGM, 2011). Yet it is found that even the public subsidy on health does not automatically benefit the poor. The poorest quintile of the population uses only one-tenth of the public (state) subsidies on health care while the richest quintile accesses 34 per cent of the subsidies (Selvaraju and Annigeri, 2001; Mahal *et al.*, 2001).

Another challenge is the shortage of skilled talent is the single biggest bottleneck affecting the growth of the sector as well as the creation of healthcare access in India. The last decade saw an increase in physicians from 0.55 per 1,000 people to a mere 0.65 per 1,000 people. This puts India behind China which has 1.3 beds per 1,000 people as per the WHO benchmark of 2.5 per 1,000 people (WHO, 2011). Despite the scarcity of medical personnel, the problem of under-utilisation persists within the system. Also, around 50 per cent of the existing medical workforce does not practise within the formal healthcare structural system. Paucity in talent can also be attributed to the uneven distribution of medical colleges in India. Presently, the southern region of India has the largest concentration of medical colleges, followed by west India. The eastern part of India on the other hand, has the least number of medical colleges (Kothandaraman & Mookerjee, 2008; Karl & Purnima, 2009).

Despite the existence of primary, secondary and tertiary health centres and public hospitals for many decades, India has one of the most fragmented and commercialized healthcare systems in the world. It was found that the national average absence rate for PHC and CHC medical providers is over 39 per cent. The absence rate for doctors exceeded 43 per cent. Such high absence rate is a clear indicator of low quality health care available at many of the PHCs and CHCs in India, making consumers seek alternate service providers mostly in the private sector (WHO, 2011; KPGM, 2011).

The cost of healthcare at private hospitals is not affordable to lower middle class and lower class consumers. In the government hospitals, there is under investment and under management. District hospitals, primary health centres (PHCs) and community health centres (CHCs) are understaffed and overworked. The KPMG study (2011) highlighted the lack of health care infrastructure in the country and noted that maternity was the second most common reason for hospitalization in India, next only to acute infection. The quality of ante-natal care and the number of institutional deliveries in the country were also found to be quite low. Importantly, the utilization of services from Non-Governmental medical care institutions was found to be expanding at the rate of 30 per cent annually.

But in the North-eastern part of India the healthcare sector is yet to garner enough steam, due to the lack of healthcare infrastructural facilities and an acute scarcity of trained medical professionals. Other than the states of Assam and Manipur, the remaining states are yet to institute a single medical college to its credibility (MoHFW, 2011; KPMG, 2011). It has been observed that the condition of all the north-eastern states, except for Assam and

Meghalaya, is better than the national average, in both the rural and urban areas alike. The states of Manipur, Nagaland and Sikkim are way ahead of the national average as well as the other north-eastern states. However, for the rural areas, their condition is below the national average as well as the other North-eastern states.

Rural healthcare infrastructure, primarily run by SCs, PHCs and CHCs, has also witnessed a couple of developments. Between 2005 and 2011, for this region as a whole, the number of SCs has declined from 7,755 to 7,259 between 2005 and 2011 (MoHFW, 2008, 2011). This is mainly due to the significant decline in the SCs in Assam and Arunachal Pradesh, whereas the number of SCs has increased in Tripura. Also, the decline in SCs in the region can be attributed to the fact that many have been upgraded to PHCs, evident from the fact that, the number of PHCs in the region have increased from 1,109 to 1,510 between 2005 and 2011 (KPMG, 2011).

The number of CHCs has increased from 215 to 244 for the entire region during 2005-2011. Apart from significant progress made by Assam, Nagaland and Arunachal Pradesh in the avenue of PCHs and by Tripura in SCs, the remaining states in the region have not taken many initiatives with respect to the establishment of health centres, even after the implementation of the NRHM in 2005. Alongside the progress in health centres, facilities available in these centres constitute a critical aspect. In this regard, the condition of the north-eastern region has been deplorable (MoHFW, 2011).

As far as the availability of trained medical professionals are concerned, it has been observed that the states of Assam, Manipur, Sikkim and Tripura have a surplus of doctors in PHCs, while other states have been experiencing acute shortages. Similarly, Assam, Manipur, Meghalaya and Tripura have a surplus of pharmacists in PHCs and CHCs, whereas the remaining states, except for Arunachal Pradesh and Sikkim enjoy a surplus in nursing staff in PHCs and CHCs (KMPG, 2011). The entire region faces an acute shortage of specialists and radiographers in CHCs. In addition to this, more than 75 per cent of PHCs in Meghalaya and Mizoram and 69 per cent of PHCs in Nagaland have been functioning with only doctor, while for the other states the percentage of PHCs with only one doctor is less than the national average (62.18%). The states of Manipur, Tripura and Assam are in a better position, with more than three doctors operating out of PHCs as compared to the rest of the country (6.89%) (KPMG, 2011).

## Why Innovation in Healthcare Matters Today?

Innovation is a key driver of success not only in the industrial sector, but also the service sector like healthcare. Drucker (1985) discussed innovation as the power to redefine the industry or the effort to create purposeful focused change in an enterprise's economic or social potential. Innovation in health delivery system are new ways of delivering services through new technology and management concept and from the patient point of view, it is the improved quality healthcare services provided at right time (Faulkner & Kent, 2001; Nobuo, Michel & Fred, 2005). When it comes to service design, clarity is a must to initiate innovations in services in healthcare or in other words service innovation in healthcare. Service design encompasses a number of elements namely customers, service concept, service encounters, and service delivery system. Service design acts as an integrator of these components. The purpose of service design is to have processes that consistently deliver high quality services to drive customer satisfaction and retention, while at the same time maintaining process efficiency (Oslo Manual, 2008; Tidd & Bessant, 2009). Innovation is driven by strategic implementation and absorption of information technology and information systems. Studies on innovation have indicated that success and survival of the health care industry depend on the effectiveness and efficiency of IT/ IS uses or implementation (Liaw, 2002; Walker, 2006). Effective and easy use of technology should enable innovation in the health care industry. Moreover, an organization would be open to adopting an innovative idea if they anticipate that the adoption of an innovative idea would give them a relative competitive advantage. Studies indicate that besides relative advantage, perceived complexity and compatibility of the new technology also influence its adoption decision. For example, although electronic medical records (EMRs) have been around since the early 1960s, until recently, they were not adopted extensively by the majority of healthcare management organizations because of the complexity of maintaining the electronic medical records of the patients (Walker, 2006; Prada, 2008).

India's healthcare challenges can be addressed only through innovative approaches. India has a low cost base and a large talent pool of scientists and engineers (Shaw, 2014). India is now driving a new model of innovation that focuses on quality and affordability. Affordable innovations will ensure better healthcare for all especially the poor. Innovation is the application of new ideas to solve problems, which are sometimes specific to a region or a context, with resultant benefits to different stakeholders (Krishnan, 2013). Healthcare sectors are looking for ways to improve services to customers as now-a-days, they are not only for treating patients, but also support healthcare provision by offering health-check programmes, pre-diagnosis testing, as well as following up with the customers after treatment. The service innovations of the hospital are complicated by many factors. For example, hospital personnel reflect various skills and specialism, such as doctors, nurses, technicians, radiologists, pharmacists, marketing officers, IT officers, and service officers. Innovation in healthcare are new services and new working methods and technologies which offer benefits to patients that include healthier lives and less suffering from illness at affordable cost (Lansisalmi *et al.*, 2006; Salge & Vera, 2009). From the point of view of hospitals, novel ideas include new products including medicines, medical technology, and IT systems. Novel services are clinical treatment regulations, supporting services such as conference services and new processes such as treatment strategies, patient practice concepts, or new organization structures (Lansiaslmi *et al.*, 2006; Salge & Vera, 2009).

## Public-Private-Partnership (PPP) as an Innovation in Healthcare

Public-Private-Partnership refers to forms of cooperation between public authorities and the world of business, which aim to ensure the funding, construction, renovation, management or maintenance of an infrastructure or the provision of a service (European Commission, 2012). Public-Private-Partnerships (PPPs) are defined as a variety of co-operative arrangements between the government and the private sector in delivering goods or services to the citizens. PPPs provide a vehicle for coordinating with Non-Governmental sectors to undertake integrated, comprehensive efforts to meet community needs. They aim to take advantage of the expertise of each partner, so that resources, risks and rewards can be allocated in a way that best meets clearly defined public needs. (WHO, 2000; Ajith, 2014) A public-private-partnership (PPP) in the healthcare sector is an approach to address public health problems through the combined efforts of public, private, and development organizations. It can encourage innovation in service delivery, better institutional integration throughout the life cycle of the facility, accessibility and quality healthcare at affordable cost. Thus, PPP can be seen as procurement of innovation (EU Commission, 2012).

Poor performance in the healthcare public sectors in India is well documented. The inability of the public health sector has forced poor and underprivileged section of the population to seek health services from the private sector. Evidence indicates that, in many parts of India, the private sector provides a large volume of health services, but with little or no regulation (Singh & Biswas, 2012; Ajith, 2014). The private sector is not only India's most unregulated sector but also its most potent and untapped sector. To address the inefficiency and inequity in the health system, many State Governments have undertaken innovative health sector reforms. One of these reforms has been collaboration with the private sector through Public-Private-Partnership (PPP). State Governments in India are experimenting with partnerships with the private sector to reach the poor and underserved sections of the population (Singh & Biswas, 2012; Ajith, 2014).

Partnership with the private sector has emerged as a new avenue of reforms, in part due to resource constraints in the public sector of governments across the world (Mitchell, Weaver & Manning, 1992). There is growing recognition that, given their respective strengths and weaknesses, neither the public sector nor the private sector alone can operate in the best interest of the health system. There is also a growing belief that public and private sectors in healthcare can potentially gain from one another (ADBI, 2000; Wang, 2000; Agha, Karim, Balal & Sossler, 2003). Involvement of the private sector is linked to the wider belief that public sector bureaucracies are inefficient and unresponsive and that market mechanisms will promote efficiency and ensure cost effective, good quality services (WHO, 2001). Another perspective on this debate is linked to the notion that the public sector must reorient its dual role of financing and provision of services because of its increasing inability on both fronts (Mitchell, Weaver & Manning, 1992). Under partnerships, public and private sectors can play innovative roles in financing and providing health care services.

This is evident from the successful implementation of PPP in healthcare in the States of Gujarat, Tamil Nadu and Meghalaya. Gujarat is one of the industrially developed states in India. As per the term and condition of the partnership; the private providers have to provide affordable health service to BPL women and children State Government reimburse the service charge to the private provider as per the tariff (MoHFW, 2008, 2011; KPMG, 2011). The success of the PPP model can be to address the larger issue of reducing maternal and deaths. Tamil Nadu has encouraging public partnerships to provide health care access in tribal areas. It has collaboration with Private sector and NGOs for ambulance services, facility maintenance, medical equipment, blood banks and provision of training and support for community health workers in remote areas. It is found that this approach has helped to reduce maternal mortality and infant mortality rate in Tamil Nadu (MoHFW, 2011; KPMG, 2011). Meghalaya, a hilly tribal state in North East India, has adopted Public-Private-Partnership (PPP) approach involves the management and operations of poorly performing health centres located in remote areas. The use of management tools, intensive use of installed capacity, novel medical reimbursement models help to increasing patient turnover and reduce average cost per patient (MoHFW, 2011; Singh *et al.*, 2012). PPP model can bring about innovation in healthcare delivery system through better financial innovation which helps in minimizing operational cost and cross subsidization; marketing innovation through social marketing and tailoring of services franchising; technological innovation like m-health, Health information system and telemedicine; and effective operational innovation which utilise maximum human resourse, process reengineering and increasing its outreach to the needy. All these innovation ultimately lead to accessible and affordable quality healthcare services (Singh and Biswas, 2012).

### Innovative Service Delivery System and Innovative Health Service Providers in India

In the effort to improve health system, India face the challenge of integrating traditional government health resources with a large and growing private health sector, where many poor people seek care. Below are some of the most innovate healthcare services available in India.

**Emergency Management and Research Institute (EMRI)** programme is a centralized emergency response service addressing the challenge of poor of non-existence access to emergency support across India as it was found that many states lack transportation and have weak referral systems, which pose significant challenges to poor communities' ability to access health facilities when in need of urgent medical care. It was initially launch in 2005 in the state of Andhra Pradesh and it has expanded to eight other states of Assam, Goa, Gujarat, Karnataka, Meghalaya, Rajasthan, Tamil Nadu and Uttarakhand. EMRI is expected to spread to other part of the country (MoHFW, 2008, 2011). EMRI's operation which is over 95 per cent cost are funded by the National Rural Health Mission, Government of India. Its goal is to respond to 30 billion emergencies and save 1 million lives using an innovative delivery model of emergency response services under PPP structure that provides emergency and pre-hospital care free of charge to the patient through a mix of private and government funding. In addition to a supportive government, the key to EMRI's well functioning system is an integrated emergency management infrastructure that includes a toll-free number accessible from landlines and mobile phones, a geographic information system to locate emergencies, a fleet of ambulances for quality care, trained personnel for pre-hospital care, and detailed maps and information about public and private healthcare facility locations and capacities (MoHFW, 2008, 2011).

**Health Management and Research Institute (HMRI)** is an easily accessible digital health platform integrating a medical advice hotline, a mobile medical outreach component, and telemedicine solutions. It was established in 2007 and it HMRI serves 80 million people in rural Andhra Pradesh and it plans to scale up medical advice services nationally as more than 72.2 per cent of Indians live in rural and semi-urban areas and face the challenges of poor or non-existent access to healthcare services (MoHFW, 2011). Mobile medical services cover approximately 3.9 million people a month, focusing on rural areas. HMRI's operations are financed by the Government of Andhra Pradesh, which covers over 90 per cent of costs with the support of the National Rural

Health Mission, Government of India. The HMRI programme is built around two core components technology and public education, which effectively leveraged to create citizen-centered health services at no cost to the consumer. HMRI's 24/7 call centre averages 50,000 calls a day, with most originating in small villages with no permanent medical facilities or staff. All calls are routed to the appropriate medical personnel (doctor, nurse practitioner, or psychologist) or in case of an emergency, linked to the EMRI emergency service (MoHFW, 2011).

**World Health Partners (WHP)** is an international collaboration working to bring healthcare and family planning services to rural areas by harnessing the existing private sector and incentivizing it to create viable health networks addressing communities' health needs. It was launched in 2008 in three districts of Uttar Pradesh, whose population is 185 million, servicing an estimated 4 million people. Uttar Pradesh has some of the worst social and demographic indicators in India (Dimovska, Sealy, Bergkwist & Pernefeldt, 2009). Basic amenities of developed countries are sparse: 57 per cent of households have no electricity, 90 per cent lack water, and 67 per cent do not have a toilet. Despite the intense poverty, the population is growing, further straining limited resources. Unmet need for family planning is 21.9 per cent, but in rural areas, where three-fourths of the population lives, it is 23.8 per cent. WHP envisions expanding in India and replicating the model across developing countries. Funding WHP is funded by a large, anonymous U.S.-based donor. WHP is an innovative programme that aspires to bring healthcare and family planning access to the most underserved parts of developing countries by organizing existing resources and creating viable health networks, training village providers, and encouraging broader community social development in addition to medical access (Dimovska, Sealy, Bergkwist & Pernefeldt, 2009). WHP organizes health network providers into sub-networks that are the units of operation for product supply and distribution as well as medical referrals. Each village practitioner that WHP works with belongs to the village health network, which provides the access to four tiers of healthcare products and services: village shops, basic rural village health providers, centrally located telemedicine centres, and medical clinics in a nearby town (Dimovska, Sealy, Bergkwist & Pernefeldt, 2009).

**Life-Spring Hospitals Private Limited (LHPL)** is a for-profit, high-volume, low-cost hospital providing quality and affordable healthcare to women and children from lower income households across India, as India has very high levels of maternal mortality—more than 1,00,000 women die every year from pregnancy-related causes and an equal number suffer moderate to severe complications LHPL was established in 2005 and it operates six hospitals serving 23,000 patients, with plans to scale up to 140 hospitals in 2014 in the states of Andhra Pradesh, Karnataka, and Maharashtra. LHPL is jointly operated by Hindustan Latex Limited and the Acumen Fund (Dimovska, Sealy, Bergkwist & Pernefeldt, 2009; Ajith, 2014). Life Spring is a for-profit hospital operated as a 50/50 equity partnership between the Acumen Fund and Hindustan Latex Limited. Life Spring's prices are 30 to 50 per cent lower than market rates. A tiered pricing model helps its commercial viability. Women, for instance, can choose to give birth in a general ward, semi-private room or private room. Rates will rise accordingly. Life Spring's focus on a particular niche—maternal and child care—cuts down on the need for many specialist doctors and also on the range of equipment needed (Dimovska, Sealy, Bergkwis & Pernefeldt, 2009; Ajith, 2014). Specialising in inpatient gynaecology and obstetrics leads to easy standardization. It has over 90 standard procedures, including standardized surgery kits and clinical protocols.

**Janani** is a non-profit organization that uses a network of private health practitioners and health facilities to provide safe and low-cost options for family planning, health, and reproductive health services in rural areas through social marketing, a clinic based service delivery programme, and a social franchising programme. It was launched in 1995. Janani covers Bihar and Jharkhand, two of India's poorest states comprising 118 million people, and 10 districts of Madhya Pradesh. It has further included expansion to Assam, Chhattisgarh, Orissa, Rajasthan, Uttar Pradesh, Uttarakhand, and West Bengal, raising the target population to almost 600 million people. Janani implements the social franchise through a network of partner health facilities. It is supported by the Government of India, the David and Lucille Packard Foundation, and a large, anonymous donor (Dimovska, Sealy, Bergkwis & Pernefeldt, 2009; MoHFW, 2008). Janani started a social marketing and social franchise programme that uses India's large private health sector and its existing service delivery resources to provide family planning and reproductive healthcare services. The social franchise has a network of rural health practitioners who work in partnership with a female family partner. She serves as the conduit between the clinics and rural communities. After receiving Janani training, rural practitioners are franchised as *Titli* (Butterfly) Centres, and they sell non-clinical products and over-the-counter tests. Under the private-public-partnership of the National Rural Health Mission, the government has accredited 15 of Janani's Surya Clinics as authorized sterilization centres, which the government reimburses $35 per sterilization. More than 40,000 trained networked rural providers are monitored by project field teams set up by entrepreneurs, and the 620 franchisee medical clinics are supervised by Janani (Dimovska, Sealy, Bergkwis & Pernefeldt, 2009; MoHFW, 2011).

**Byrraju Foundation Health Programme** is a not-for-profit organization, which implements holistic programmes for sustainable rural transformation, including self-reliant, local healthcare infrastructure. It was launched in 2001 and is currently works in 200 villages in six districts of Andhra Pradesh covering nearly 3 million people. The Byrraju Foundation Health organization works in partnership with rural communities and several public and private organizations. Its operations are supported through a mix of donor and partner funding, contributions from trustees and individual user fees (Dimovska, Sealy, Bergkwis & Pernefeldt, 2009). The Foundation considers quality health services at all levels of care to be a vital component of building progressive self-reliant rural communities. To improve the availability and quality of healthcare in underserved areas, the Foundation capitalizes on all available resources by relying on local resources, harnessing village volunteer time, building partnerships with public and private providers in the area and using knowledge and technology innovations as tracking multiple metrics, telecardiology, comprehensive health worker training, research in morbidity trends, and so on. The foundation sets up a small primary health centre in which neighbouring villages can also access (Dimovska, Sealy, Bergkwis & Pernefeldt, 2009).

**NICE Foundation** is a registered charitable trust based in Hyderabad, designs and implements all health programmes in partnership with State Governments, the private sector, and civil societies. It provides a wide range of targeted medical services to the most vulnerable segments of society through innovative service delivery and risk pooling. It was launched in 2002 and operates its programmes in Andhra Pradesh and Rajasthan, with plans to expand to other states (Dimovska, Sealy, Bergkwis & Pernefeldt, 2009). NICE Foundation's programmes are financed through public funding sources including State Governments and the Central Government and through private donations from individuals and grant-making organizations. It runs two health programmes in Andhra Pradesh—the Schoolchild Healthcare Plan and the Tribal Reproductive Child Health—and operates the Institute for the Newborn in Hyderabad, which provides neonatal care and conducts training and research. The Schoolchild Healthcare Plan has been replicated in three districts of Rajasthan, and further rollout is planned in the state (Dimovska, Sealy, Bergkwis & Pernefeldt, 2009).

**Smile-on-Wheels Programme** is a national mobile hospital programme catering to underprivileged children and women in remote rural areas and urban slums using primarily volunteer physicians and nurses. It was launched in 2006 and operates in several locations across India in the states Chhattisgarh, Delhi, Maharashtra, Orissa, Tamil Nadu, and Uttarakhand reaching nearly 7,50,000 people in 249 villages and slums. Three more units are being added in Ahmadabad, Hyderabad, and Lucknow. Smile-on-Wheels is implemented by the Smile Foundation, a not-for profit organization working in education and healthcare for underprivileged children across India (Dimovska, Sealy, Bergkwis & Pernefeldt, 2009). The Smile Foundation partners with local organizations in each state to run Smile-on-Wheels, including: Ambuja Cement Foundation (Roorkee, Uttarakhand), Berojgar Mahila Sewa Samiti (Bhilai, Chhattisgarh), Operation Blessing India (Delhi), Orissa Institute of Medical Research and Health Services (Cuttack, Orissa), and Sevadham Trust (Pune, Maharashtra). The Foundation receives funding from several domestic and international partner organizations. Focusing on women and children, Smile-on-Wheels is a national multi centric mobile hospital programme that provides medical care to rural and semi-rural areas and urban slums where governmental healthcare facilities are scarce, non-existent, or non-functional. Under this programme five vans travel through 25 kilo metres of rural areas every day, visiting two to three villages on a rotating basis to deliver healthcare at a nominal cost to the community (Dimovska, Sealy, Bergkwis & Pernefeldt, 2009).

**Rashtriya Swasthya Bima Yojana (RSBY)** literally "National Health Insurance Programme" is a state-managed national health insurance programme designed to improve access to quality medical care for informal workers living below the poverty line. The scheme starts enrolling on 1st April, 2008 and has been implemented in 25 states in India. A total of 36 million families are enrolled in the scheme as of February, 2014 (Dimovska, Sealy, Bergkwis & Pernefeldt, 2009; MoHFW, 2011). RSBY is a Central Government Scheme, launched by the Ministry of Labour and Employment. Now, it has been transferred to the Ministry of Health and Family Welfare (Government of India) from 1st April, 2015. The insurance scheme is being implemented by State Governments with the participation of both public and private insurance companies. RSBY receives 75 per cent of its funding (90% in the North-eastern states and Jammu & Kashmir) from the Central Government and the remainder from State Governments. The scheme target informal sector workers living below the poverty line. Beneficiaries pay only Rs. 30 per family per year to register (Dimovska, Sealy, Bergkwis & Pernefeldt, 2009; MoHFW, 2011). Through competitive bidding State Governments select a public or private insurance company to administer the scheme. This engages local intermediaries such as Non-Governmental Organizations (NGOs) and micro-finance institutions to provide grassroots outreach and assist members in using services after enrolment. Healthcare services are delivered by a network of empanelled public and private hospitals, and payment is made using a cashless smart card. Enrolments entitle beneficiaries to most medical and surgical procedures that can be performed for Rs. 30,000 rupees or less. For 725 in-patient surgical procedures, the government has predefined package rates that include all hospital charges, including food. Pre-existing diseases are covered from day one, and beginning in 2009/10 maternity and newborn care will also be included. The unit of enrolment in RSBY is a household, which includes up to five members. The smart card technology and key management system are unique features of the scheme; they make fraud very difficult while building accountability for different stakeholders ((Dimovska, Sealy, Bergkwis & Pernefeldt, 2009; MoHFW, 2011).

## Conclusion

The health system of India is facing so many challenges includes huge health status gap between urban and rural areas, low level of health awareness, lack of sanitary and hygienic condition, cost of healthcare, scarcity of specialty care and under-resourced infrastructure. Moreover, there health system is unable to deliver health service in an effective and efficient manner because of resource constrain, lack of managerial practices and technology. In this situation, the innovation acts as supportive tool to overcome from all these challenge of health system as it helps people to have greater choices in diagnostics and treatment. At the same time, the use of technology depends on many factors, including the skills of service personnel, service processes, technology, tools, equipment, and safety factors. The different innovation concepts give positive impact on the performance of health delivery system and improve health outcome. Therefore, there is need to implement innovation base health delivery system enable to provide accessible, affordable and quality health services to all individual. This is possible through the adoption of PPP model in healthcare. This calls for a holistic approach to health development, supported by relevant human resource capacities, convergence, integration, and public-private partnerships. PPP will provides an opportunity for promoting equity, serving the under privileged, and empowering communities in a sustainable manner. India is striving to achieve the Millennium Development Goals, and the expectations to attain various targets are variable. Policy pronouncements by government alone are not sufficient for PPP to succeed. Visionary leadership, social entrepreneurship and relationships based on trust between the stakeholders are equally important for successful partnerships.

## References

ADBI. (2000). Public-Private-Partnerships in Health. Executive Summary Series No. S34/01. Executive Summary of Proceedings (30 October–3 November), Ayutthaya, Thailand. Tokyo: Asian Development Bank Institute.

Agha, S., Karim, A. M., Balal, A. A. and Sossler, S. (2003). A Quasi Experimental Study to Assess the Performance of a Reproductive

Health Franchise in Nepal. Commercial Market Strategies (CMS). Country Research Series Paper No.14. Washington DC.

Ajith, P. (2014). Affordable healthcare service innovation from India. *Pacific Business Review, 6*, 87-94.

Baru, R. (1999). *Private Health Care in India: Social Characteristics and Trends.* New Delhi: National Council for Applied Economic Research. Delhi: National Institute of Public Finance and Policy. Background paper for the Commission on Macro-Economics and Health (India). Delhi: Sage Publications, *Development 26*(4): 45-67.

Bhattacharyya, O., McGahan, A., Dunne, D., Singer P.A., and Daar A. (2008). *Innovative Health Service Delivery Models for Low and Middle Income Countries,* The Rockefeller Foundation, Washington.

Chanda, R. (2002). Trade in health services, *Bull World Health Organzation,* 80(2): 158–163.

David, H.P., Sameh E., Banafsheh S., Katja J., and Marko V. (2009). Improving Health Service Delivery in Developing Countries, The World Bank, Washington, DC, 978: 8213-7888.

Dimovska, D., Sealy, S., Bergkwist, S., and Pernefeldt, H. (2009). *Innovative Pro-poor Health Financing and Delivery Models*. Rockefller Foundation, Washington DC.

Drucker, P. (1985). *Innovation and Entrepreneurship: Practice and Principles.* 1st ed. New York, NY: Harper & Row.

Dutt, S. (2012). Making India an evolved healthcare market. Retrieved from http:// www.financialexpress.com/news/making-india-an-evolvedhealthcare- market/976447

European Commission (2012). *Health and Economic Analysis for an Evaluation of the Public-Private Partnerships in Health Care Delivery across Europe*. B-1049, Brussels.

Faulkner, A. and Kent, J. (2001). Innovation and regulation in human implant technologies: developing comparative approaches. *Social Science and Medicine, 53*: 895-913.

Gupta, A. (2013). International Business Environment: Challenges and Changes, *Research Journal of Management Sciences,* 2(11): 34-38.

Karl, K. and Purnima M. (2009). Leveraging human capital to reduce maternal mortality in India, enhanced public health system or public-private-partnership? *Human Resources for Health,* 7-18.

Kinsey Global Institute (2007). The bird of gold: The rise of India's consumer market from http://www.mckinsey.com/locations/india/mckinseyonindia/pdf/India_Consumer_Market.pdf.

Kothandaraman, P., and Mookerjee, S. (2008). Healthcare for All: Narayana Hrudayalaya, Bangalore, United Nations Development Programme, New York:, *GIM Case Study.*

KPMG. (2011). Emerging trends in healthcare. Retrieved, from http:// www.kpmg.com/IN/en/IssuesAndInsights/ThoughtLeadership/Emreging_trends_in_healthcare.pdf.

Krishnan, R.T. (2013). Does India need innovation? Retrieved from http://www.thehindubusinessline.com/features/newmanager/does-india-need-innovation/article5322323.ece.

Lansisalmi, H., Kivimaki, M., Aalto, P., and Ruoranen, R. (2006). Innovation in Healthcare: A Systematic Review of Recent Research. *Nursing Science Quarterly*, 19: 66-72.

Liaw, S. S. (2002). Understanding user perceptions of world-wide web environments. *Journal of Computer Assisting and Learning, 18*(2): 137-48.

Mahal, A.; Singh, J.; Afridi, F.; Lamba, V.; Gumber, A. and Selvaraju, V. (2001). *Who Benefits from Public Sector Health Spending in India.* National Council of Applied Economic Research Working Paper 56371, New Delhi.

Michell-Weaver, C., and Manning, B. (1992). Public-Private-Partnerships in Third World Development: A Conceptual Overview, *Studies in Comparative International Development*, 26(4): 45.

Ministry of Health and Family Welfare, Government of India. (2008). Report by the Task Force on Medical Education constituted. Retrieved from www.health.report-mohfw@nic.in

Ministry of Health and Family Welfare, Government of India. (2011). Annual Report retrieved from www.health.report-mohfw@nic.in

Nobuo T., Michel, G., and Fred G. (2005). *The Measurement of Scientific and Technological Activities.* UNESCO Institute for Statistics, Oslow Manual, 3rd edition.

Oslo Manual. (2008). *The Measurement of Scientific and Technological Activities.* OECD.

Parry, J., and Judge K. (2005). Tackling the wider determinants of health disparities in England: a model for evaluating New Deal for Communities regeneration initiative. *American Journal of Public Health, 95*(4): 626-628.

Pingali, P. (2010). Affordable, high quality core maternal healthcare for low-income women in India. Retrieved from http://www.changemakers.com/browse/human-rights-peace/gender-equity?page=8.

Prada, G. (2008). Exploring technological innovation in health systems: in Canada measuring up? *Journal of Management Marketing, 1*(4): 362-74.

Rao, M. G. and Choudhury, M. (2012). Health care financing reforms in India (Working Paper No: 2012-100).

Salge, T. O. and Vera, A. (2009). Hospital innovativeness and organizational performance: Evidence from English pubic acute care. *Health Care Management Review, 34*: 54-67.

Schneider, H. and Barron P. (2008). *Achieving the Millennium Development Goals in South Africa through the revitalization of primary health care and a strengthened District health system,* University of Cape Town.

# 9
# Services Quality in Government Health Organization
## Case Study of Porto Velho City, Brazil

*Natália Talita Araújo Nascimento, José Delcias Moura dos Santos, Anderson Emanuel Cantanhêde, Flávio de São Pedro Filho,* and *Jayashree Patil-Dake*

## Introduction

The chapter focuses on the public service delivery, provided by a government health sector of Porto Velho City, Rondonia, Brazil. The methodology and procedure of case study analysis is implemented to understand the innovative actions and ways of compliance in the institution are studied. The purpose is to seek the quality improve in the current service provided to the public. The question to be answered here is: What is a contribution of innovation processes to the quality of service delivery in organizations of public health?

The present work aims to study the influences of innovative actions in the quality of public service delivery by health organizations. And to meet this general objective, specific objectives were proposed: (1) to analyze the current conditions of service to the public in the research institution; (2) to conduct theoretical and conceptual confrontation with the data obtained in research; and (3) to introdûce measures suitability for the quality of service.

## Theoretic and Conceptual Reviews

The theoretical constitutions of Administration developed by questioning the concepts, seeking adjustments in the weaknesses and inconsistencies in existing approaches; geared to the best management practices of organizations. While evaluating different effective models of organizational structure from Classical Theory, the Contingency Theory is described as the exposure of the existence of a functional relationship between environmental conditions and appropriate administrative techniques for the effective range of the organization's objectives, which directs its concepts for flexibility and agility, determining that there is no absolutism in organizations (Chiavenato, 2003).

Chiavenato (2003) describes the organization as a "social entity composed of people and resources, deliberately structured and oriented to achieve a common goal." Overlooking the issue to direct the attendance in a base theory, Chiavenato (2003) also describes the organization as a "social entity composed of people and resources, deliberately structured and oriented to achieve a common goal." Overlooking the issue to direct the delivery of services in our base theory, we found the support of Contingency Theory applies better to the correlation between human resources and organizational effectiveness.

### *Analysis of Public Services Delivery in Government Institutions*

In this item and it is sub items the theoretical insights that involve the service delivery to the public as the innovation approach are presented, relating the legal descriptions, bureaucratic and of delivery in the context of the public sphere.

#### *Morality and Efficiency Principles*

Madeira (2008) sets that the moral can be conceived as a set of shared values among members of the community at determined epoch. Thus, it is perceived the role of the morality in the social context, when defines the values that guide the action of the individual, establishing duties for himself through his own consciousness. He also states that the role of the administrator, to do not configure violation of the administrative morality, should therefore; always concentrate himself at the end desired by the public Administration, which is the common good.

The principles of morality and efficiency were introduced in the Brazilian Constitution by the Constitutional Amendment No. 19, of June 5, 1998. It preaches the duty of the Public Administration as a ruler being in order to manage resources, inputs, people and materials, as well as finance with proper optimization. Thus, it is necessary to use these means to meet the purposes of public interest. Madeira (2008) deals of this principle, discussing that in theory, the efficiency would be neither beginning, but the result of an administrative activity. Efficiency in Public Administration relates to the ability to generate benefits to society with the resources originated from it; thus demonstrates the citizen taxpayer the due respect, as if to give him back the counterparts of these "inputs" or inputs provided by all citizens. Thus, it seeks to avoid waste in the execution of activities, while prioritizes lower costs through the better execution method of the public functions.

### *The Bureaucracy in Public Organizations*

Weber, creator of bureaucratic concepts based himself on the rationality to develop his ideas in response to the inconsistencies between Classical Theory and Human Relations, with the goal of creating a model of organization that would involve all the variables. Chiavenato (2003) states that the bureaucracy is a form of human organization based on rationality, in other words, the adequation of the goals (ends) intended and Matias-Pereira (2010) defines that in the bureaucratic context, rationality means the quest for efficiency. For Weber (cited Matias-Pereira, 2010), the bureaucracy may be understood as a group of regulations, laws and standards that the employee, supervised by his supervisor, shall fulfil, always respecting the hierarchical structure, which he must obey faithfully and worthily.

Matias-Pereira (2010) discusses two main causes of the distortion of the concept of bureaucracy, the first relates to the centralization and the verticalization of the decision process, resulting in the slowness of the procedural steps in the hierarchical structure in upward direction and the second is about the lack of flexibility, in other words, obsessive preoccupation to follow rules, with no place to modification. On the other hand, the bureaucratic advantages are guided by the rationality in relation to the achievement of objectives, definition of positions, operations and duties, rapidity in decision process and channels through which the information about orders, rules and procedure are transmitted. Under these conditions, cites Matias-Pereira (2010) that the work is professionalized, nepotism is avoided and working conditions favour the economic morality and difficult the corruption. Matias-Pereira (2010) also argues that the fairness of bureaucratic rules, almost always based on universal standards of fairness and equal treatment, has the virtue of ensuring cooperation, since, the people comply rules mainly because the ends achieved by the entire structure are highly valued. In the studies of Weber, the author also identified dilemmas faced by the bureaucracy that undergoes constant external pressures to force the organization develop different ideas of the rules employed. Accordingly, as describes Matias-Pereira (2010), the organization to be effective, requires a special kind of legitimacy, rationality, discipline and range limitation, which remits to an evaluation of the methods as applied to measuring its effectiveness in meeting the proposed objectives.

*Innovation in Public Management: Organization and Processes*

In face of this impasse described by Weber when dealing with bureaucratic dilemmas, is noticeable to identify the relationship of innovation as one of the factors driving the changes of the rules committed by this administration model. Adair (2010) states that innovation means creating or presenting something new in particular. He combines two main processes that overlap themselves, namely, (1) have new ideas and (2) implement them. Druker (1985 cited Bessant, Pavitt and Tidd, 2005) expressly says that innovation is the specific tool of entrepreneurs, through which they exploit the change as an opportunity for different business or services. It is liable of being presented as a discipline, liable of being learned, liable of being practiced. So, the public organization may develop actions for a innovatory learning process, using the inputs available, such these values, that should be incorporated by the structure as a whole, involving the various employees that comprise the public mechanism.

The importance of changes in organizational processes happens mainly in response by the adaptation to environmental conditions that surround business organisms. Bessant, Pavitt and Tidd (2005) believe that innovation is an essential process, concerned to renew that the company offers, noting that, in non-profit organizations the development of innovative actions can be directed to reducing costs and improving quality. Adair (2010) states that organize something is to impose on this element a sequential and/or spatial manner and Bessant, Pavitt and Tidd (2005) complement that understand the innovation as a process is to clarify that the knowledge originated by this process creates the manner how this process is managed and experienced.

As instruments for the execution of administrative processes were established the routines of organizational behaviour, according to Levitt and March (quoted in Bessant, Pavitt and Tidd, 2005) are *ipse literis*, procedures that involve established sequences of actions to perform tasks in a mixture of technologies, procedures or formal and informal strategies, and, conventions or informal habits. These tasks are related to the central competencies of planning, management and evaluation, where the routines of behaviour must be integrated in order to constitute the capacity of manageability in the innovation processes. In the relationship of modifications caused by the innovation of the process, we emphasize the difficulties conceived by the presence of routines rooted in government institutions, which entails a blockade to the realization of innovative actions aiming at the improving of the quality of the processes. On this blockade, Bessant, Pavitt and Tidd (2005) state that it is essential from the point of view of the innovation management, not just the building of routines, but also recognize when and how to destroy them and allow to create new ones. The authors add that the effective management of innovation is basically resulting from the design and development of effective routines and learn to do them depends on recognizing and understanding such routines and facilitate its emergence inside the corporation.

### *Attendance (Delivery) in Public Organizations*

The definition of attendance provided by public organizations is presented as a service of social nature and necessary to respond to the community demand. The Brazilian Service of Support for Micro- and Small Enterprises [SEBRAE] is a benchmark in the country to conceptualize the attendance, for it provides support to several companies since the very beginning stage and acts as the assistance organ to improvement of the quality of the processes of these organizations. According SEBRAE (2013), attendance service refers to our judgement value as a whole. To serve is much more than treat. Treat is essential and basic. Serve is to exceed expectations, to surprise the customer. Débora Martins, an expert in the management of the relationship between company and customer and auditor by the National Service for Industrial Apprenticeship in São Paulo [Senai/SP] NBR 9001:2008 that specifies requirements for a Quality Management System, states that attendance is related to any liability that the company places on its employees to meet the client properly, on the right time and satisfactorily.

The issue of attendance in Brazil, especially in the services provided by public organizations, has a notorious shortage related to the processes of excellence and quality. Dantas (2004) argues that poor customer service is not an issue of who execute the attendance, but a management issue, that passes through the training aspect of the service personnel and adequacy of the environment and ends on the ongoing assessment of quality. So, it is clear that broach the attendance service in a individualized manner and of responsibility of the one who executes it, is actually delimit itself to identify only one of the agents involved in the process. According Bandeira de Melo (apud Matias-Pereira, 2007), public administration is the offering by the State or its designee, of utility or community aimed at satisfaction of the community, under the regime of public law and in accordance with the public interests. In this respect, it becomes even more noticeable the complexity of the attendance service in these conditions, because of the diversity found in the public to which the service is directed.

### *Theoretical and Conceptual Elements in Confrontation with the Techniques of Attendance Service*

The development of an organization, especially in the public context, is related to the ability to identify failures and inadequacies within the process, seeking the application of preventive measures and mitigatory (resolving) in the face of the adequacy of the institution to the processes of management quality. Assess the necessity for change requires, as cited by

George and Jones (2011), the recognition that there is a problem and the identification of its cause. In this respect, the theoretical elements presented orient and expand the knowledge levels of the public administrator, who can use tools, previously tested by scientists and experts, to prove the efficiency of the method in order to improve the quality.

### *Measures of Innovation Adequacy in Public Service Organizations*

Innovation is a process that integrates the entire organization and, therefore, it is necessary that exists the integration and the work together in order to reach the goals that seek quality and the improvement of services. Abreu, Coral and Ogliari (2008) state that the first step to implement a process of management of innovation in the company is to establish an appropriate organizational structure. Thus, it becomes necessary to make a diagnosis of the organization to assess the main variables that make up the innovative process, as well as determine the resources applied to the process of innovation. Lewin (cited in Cameron, 2009) presents a model of the organizational changing process in three steps: unfreeze the current state, then go to a new state through participation and involvement and refreeze and stabilize the new state by establishing new policies and standards and recognition of the success of the process. Organizational change involves the development of a restructuring process that as cited by Cameron (2009) aims to align the organization to perform its best strategy.

## Methodology

The methodology can be defined as the set of methods used to perform a search. Siena (2007) describes that method can be understood as the form and the pathway of the manner of think. It is the way to approach the level of abstraction of phenomena. Is the group of processes or mental operations employed in the study? Severino (1941) complements this concept when broaches that science forms itself applying techniques by following and relying on epistemological grounds. In this context, we present the methods used in research as follows.

### *Methods and Procedures of the Research*

The methodology applied in this research has a qualitative nature, according to the recommendations suggested by Flick (2004). We adopted the method of case study as indicated in Yin (2005). For validation of the results it was decided by the support of the group of focus as has been recommended in Pedro Filho (2012), of the Master's Programme in Administration from the Foundation of the Federal University of Rondônia.

The questionnaire method was formulated as a procedure for data collection as on the website Survey Monkey. The questions were multiple choices, so as to allow the measurement of data, analysis and critique of the causal relationship. Since the public (respondents) focused of this present study did not have access to email or a internet tools to receive the file *via* internet, the facts recorded in research were investigated by inference of the matters contained in the printed document. The data obtained from the questioning of the actors surveyed were inserted into the platform of the website Survey Monkey by manual feeding of information, strictly observing the data insertion in identical reference to the written record made by individuals who responded to the questionnaire. With the data tabulation it was possible to obtain the graphics and the tables of information to compare the margins of asymmetry and concordance between the responses of individuals in the context of the items investigated.

A further methodological procedure was adopted *in loco* the location of observation, which allowed us to assess the performance of the actors involved in institutional attendance (delivery) of service with the registry about the local phenomena measured in conformity with the conceptual and theoretical confrontation. We seek for our study the measure recommended by Severino (2007); on the "layout" and other factors that compose the environment of the location of the research, the field observations, considering the theoretical bases built in order to perform the comparison between the practices found in the public organism (organization) and the scientific recommendations raised by theoretical and conceptual research. The data (respondent) group is obtained by methodology that allows the comparative analysis of causal relationship. And inferences about research scenario are drawn in order to identify the proposals for improvements, adaptations and adjustments. The recommendations proposed are followed by the social scientists and are supported by the theoretical and conceptual fundamentals of this case study. As from the data group obtained by means of methodological procedures presented, the comparative analysis of the causal relationship was performed.

### *Group of Focus*

The Group of focus is an instrumental procedure for collection, data capture and information that assist the researcher in the processing, analysis and description of the facts related to the object that is being investigated. Morgan and Freitas (quoted Vergara, 2006) emphasize that the group of focus can be a simultaneous providence (available) to the (research) search procedures when it seeks to stimulate or interact in face of the collection of opinions of the social actors involved in any way with the subject researched. For the purposes of this study the group of focus (respondents) consists of 15 participants, where seven individuals were appointed from among the employees related to the attendance (delivery) of service of the health system under study, and eight are customers (patients) randomly selected; in both cases we seek to obey the protocol of ethics of the Social Research, through informed consent, free acceptance and interest in collaborating with the results of the survey as recommended in Pedro Filho (2012).

## Case Studies on Innovation in Service Attendance (Delivery) in Government Health Organization

Here the results obtained are presented by means of methodological procedures applied in research that seeks to meet the specific objectives initially proposed in this study. The research was conducted in a health care facility that serves as a centre of medical specialties, organ of the prefecture of the city of Porto Velho, state of Rondônia. The government institution was opened in March 2012; the investments made by the government with the management of resources of social compensations arising from the construction of Hydroelectric Jirau located on the Madeira River in Rondônia state. The goal of creating an exclusive unit for concentration of the attendance (delivery of) services in some areas of medical specialties emerged as a mitigatory (mitigation) measure to improve the quality of the services provided to the population (people), which also serves to a fundamental right that guarantees individuals' access to health. The research developed in this work was directed to the subdivision of medical and statistical files who manages the administrative and (delivery) attendance issues, which include the reception, instruction and guidance of patients referred by health service stations and from different locations of the city, in addition of other (province) counties in the state. Among the individuals that constituted the group of focus of this research, in Table 9.1 are described the characteristics of the group of actors questioned.

**Table 9.1:** Socio-Economic Profile of the Respondents

| *Characteristic* | *Socio-economic Profile* |
|---|---|
| Gender | 73% Male 27% Female |
| Age | 40% – 18 a 27 years 26% – 28 a 37 years<br>20% – 38 a 47 years 14% – 48 a 57 years |
| Scholarity | 6% basic education 33% High school 61% College |
| Naturality | 80% Northern Region 13% South Region 7% North-east Region |
| Occupation | 46% civil servants 26% Students 15% merchants 13% Independent workers |

*Source:* Formulated by the Authors Based on the Research (2013).

## *Analysis of Public Attendance Services in the Research Institution*

In order to perform the study on the influence of innovative actions in the public attendance (delivery of) service provided by health organizations, the data obtained in research is compared with the theoretical and conceptual bases and presented.

### *Legal Principles of Morality and Efficiency*

The social actors involved in the process of attendance (delivery of) service of the researched organization are investigated through the facts. When asked about the principles of morality and efficiency in order to obtain the opinion of these individuals about the performance of the public administration to serve and apply them appropriately in the attendance service process following results were obtain and the results as shown in Fig 9.1:

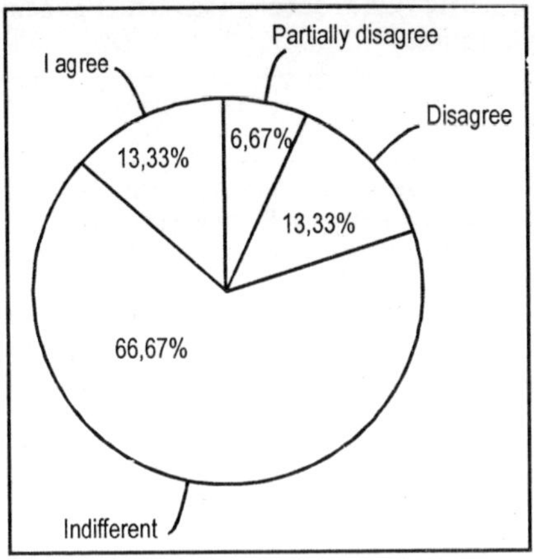


**Fig. 9.1:** Fulfillment of the Principles of Morality and Efficiency
*Source:* Survey by the authors for present study (2013).

According to the opinion of the respondents the most part was indifferent to determine whether there is fulfillment and applicability of the principles of morality and effectiveness by the Public Administration. This issue may be related to the ignorance of the principles, that although they were informed at the meeting of the group of focus, they were identified as new elements to the individuals consulted. It is Important to consider the low level of the involvement of citizenship as well as their inability of perception about relevant issues that should be incorporated to the routine of the public employees.

*The Bureaucracy in Public Organizations*

The factors obtained in this research aimed to identify characteristics of bureaucracy in the organizational environment and obtain the opinion from the users and employees on the role of bureaucracy in the process of attendance service provided by the organization where it was developed the case study for this activity. In relation to the characteristics related to the bureaucracy, are presented in Fig. 9.2 are the practices identified by the respondents.

**Table 9.2:** Bureaucratic Characteristics in Processes of Public Administration

| *Process of administration* | *Description* |
|---|---|
| Planning | Presents rules, policies and regulations; Detailed and in long term; |
| Organization | Centralized in authority; Formal and with specific responsibilities; |
| Direction | Directed to the supervision of the tasks performed; Supervision closed; |
| Control | Directed to ensure the compliance of the procedures. |

*Source:* Findings of the research conducted by authors for present study (2013).

When asked about the role of bureaucracy in the processes of attendance delivery of service, there was unanimity in the responses, where respondents stated that bureaucratic activity has a negative effect on the process of attendance service, creating obstacles and clutter in the process. The analysis of this question enabled us to identify the association that the respondents create between the bureaucracy and the malfunctions existing in a system or task, where individuals claim that bureaucratic operations generate disorders and damage the provision of the attendance service.

*Innovation in Public Management: Organization and Processes*

In this topic we sought to infer about the perception of the respondents regarding to the innovative actions in the environment where the attendance service is conducted to the public. On this question the data were collected, as illustrated in Fig. 9.1. At this question none of the individuals questioned consider the environment in which the attendance delivery of service is performed in the organization investigated as an environment innovative and creative, which emphasizes and affirms again the association of the provider institution of this public service as an organization where bureaucratic dysfunctions prevail, since, respondents in this study used the term bureaucracy as a nomenclature of flaws and inadequacies observed and existing service process. In Face of this challenge, most of the individuals studied showed indifference to express their opinion on the level of satisfaction that the attendance service provided to the public provides, demonstrating, therefore, that there is an identification of dysfunction. However, the social actor does not express nor has a method to evaluate and present measures for a quality attendance service, according to data gathered in the meeting of the group of focus.

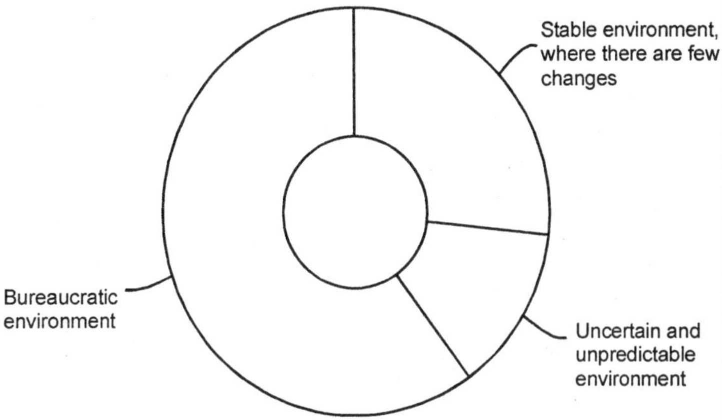


| Reply Options | Reply | |
|---|---|---|
| Stable environment, where there are few changes | 26.67% | 4 |
| Innovative and creative environment | 0% | 0 |
| Uncertain and unpredictable environment | 13.33% | 2 |
| Bureaucratic environment | 60% | 9 |
| **TOTAL** | | **15** |

**Fig. 9.2:** Characteristics of the Environment where Occurs the Attendance Service to the Public.

*Source:* Findings of the research conducted by authors for present study (2013).

*Attendance Service in Public Organizations*

In the applied study on the attendance service in the organization focus of this research, we identified the following observations as shown in Fig. 9.3, which shows the level of satisfaction of users and employees with public attendance service; Table 9.1

of these elements is responsible for the excellence in attendance service providing.

With the study and the conclusion of the analysis it was possible to identify weaknesses and threats that compromise the quality of attendance service provided by public unit and propose improvements and adaptation measures for seizing opportunities and invigorate the strengths found. The theoretical and conceptual confrontation on this research allowed the comparison of the recommendations of experts, scientists and researchers with the practices developed by the organization in its routine. These factors were addressed by the methods initially proposed and thus here the suggestions and considerations of research are presented.

### *Proposals for Adequacy Measures for the Attendance Service of Public Organizations*

According to the facts raised in loco, coordination of the group of focus and application of research methods were considered proposals for improvements and adjustments, shown in Table 9.4.

## Conclusion

In face of the data collected, research and analysis performed it was possible to identify the relationship of the individual in public context and the practices of the attendance service provided by health institutions. In this context when responding to the problematic about what is the contribution of innovation processes to the quality of the attendance services in organizations of public health, it was possible to ascertain that innovation generates benefits in applying the Organizational Learning through the use of available resources in a creative and dynamic manner aiming to improve the performance of processes. Thus, innovative actions can be implemented in the public organizations by the practice of everyday activities with the use of the "inputs" arranged in the organization, which include the development of the human element as a motivator of innovative initiatives. The organization surveyed showed ability to the fulfillment of its activities in relation to the structure, staffing and organization, however, are raised points which were suggested improvement proposals that aim to make the creative work environment and dynamic, since the

**Table 9.4:** Proposals for Improvements and Adjustments to the Process of Attendance Service

| | *Indicative raised* | | *Description of the measures of adequacy* |
|---|---|---|---|
| 1 | Inadequation in organizational processes | 1.1 | Analyse the routines and seek, within the public context, simplify the possible processes; |
| | | 1.2 | Disclose the procedures and standards to all employees in order to disseminate the purpose of the organization; |
| 2 | Failure in the centralization of the organization | 2.1 | Inform staff about the organization's hierarchy, clarifying who are the managers or employees responsible for each task; |
| 3 | Deficiency by the direction with focus on the task | 3.1 | Evaluation of the performance of the employees; perception about the motivators of the improvement of the quality of the work. |
| 4 | Inadequacy in control | 4.1 | More formal control of the unit, definition of tasks and deadlines; |
| 5 | Rigid environment, inflexible | 5.1 | Work the actions of Organizational Learning (OL) to utilize the available resources in view of the better performance, encouraging an innovative and creative environment; |
| 6 | Lack of maintenance in work environment | 6.1 | Conservation of the cleaning, care, organization, concern for the public served; |
| 7 | Lack of participation of social actors in the process | 7.1 | Involvement of citizens in the public process, in order to criticize the dysfunctions, but also to contribute to the resolution of these. |

*Source:* Formulated by the authors based on the present case study research (2013).

emphasis of the respondents was pointed to the bureaucratic dysfunctions.

It is presented also that the participation of social actors in the process, exists in order to identify failures and inadequacies, however, the training and the experience with the public sphere to intervene in these relationships in order to modify them, appeared as factor underexplored and developed by the individuals questioned, a situation in which is suggested as a new research topic that could have as a target the study about the citizen participation in collective organism. In short, the realization of the conceptual and theoretical confrontation with the practices developed by the organization allowed beyond the study of the subject proposed; visualize the concepts of users and employees of the public attendance service process, allowing a reflection on the performance of the organization and of the citizen within the scenario researched.

## References


Abreu Aline Coral, Elisa Ogliari André (2008). *Gestão integrada da inovação.* São Paulo: Atlas.

Adair John (2010). Liderança para a inovação: como estimular e organizar a criatividade para sua equipe de trabalho produzir ideias inovadoras. São Paulo: Clio.

Bessamt John Pavitt, Keith Tidd Joe (2005). *Gestão para a inovação.* Porto Alegre: Bookman.

Cameron Esther (2009). Gerenciamento de mudanças: guia completo, com modelos, ferramentas e técnicas, para entender e implementar as mudanças nas organizações. São Paulo: Clio.

Chiavenato Idalberto (2003). Introdução à teoria geral da Administração: uma visão abrangente da moderna administração das organizações. Rio de Janeiro: Elsevier.

Dantas Edmundo Brandão (2004). Atendimento ao público nas organizações: quando o marketing de serviços mostra a cara. Brasília: Editora SENAC.

Flick Uwe (2004). *Uma introdução à pesquisa qualitativa.* Porto Alegre: Bookman.

George JM and Jones GR (2011). *Fundamentos da Administração Contemporânea* (4a ed.) Porto Alegre: Bookman.

Madeira José Maria Pinheiro (2008). *Administração Pública,* Rio de Janeiro: Elsevier.

Matias-Pererira José (2010). *Curso de Administração Pública: foco nas instituições e ações governamentais.* São Paulo: Atlas.

Pedro Filho, Flávio de São (2012). *Apostila de Administração da Produção I.* Federal University of Rondônia. Porto Velho, UNIR.

Serverino Antônio Joaquim (2007). *Metodologia do trabalho científico.* São Paulo: Cortez.

Siena, O. (2007). Metodologia da pesquisa científica: elementos para elaboração e apresentação de trabalhos acadêmicos. Porto Velho: UNIR.

Vergara Sylvia Constant (2006). *Métodos de pesquisa em Administração.* São Paulo: Atlas.

Yin, R.K. (2005). *Estudo de caso: planejamento e métodos.* Porto Alegre: Bookman.

# 10
# Look Before You Leap
## Access to Basic Health Infrastructure in the North East India

*Atanu Sengupta* and *Ganesh Naskar*

### Introduction

Preventive health is often less expensive and less demanding on human body and soul. From the economic point it is important that curative health causes financial burdens and curds the productive capacity of an individual even if the diseases is curable. For a poor man it often becomes a luxury to bear the burden of curative costs through prevention. It is the lack of awareness of some simple life habits that can prevent or at least mitigate some of the costs of curative burden.

This focuses on the basic health facilities and health infrastructure. They are often a backbone of the preventive health care machine. We are tò see how and to what extent even this basic health facilities are unequally divided among the groups and locations across the length and breadth of our country. The chapter is here to merely chart the contour of inequality that has plagued our health infrastructural amenities like sanitation, drinking water and drainage or even the use of less health hazardous the cooking fuels. These are the basics from which the health mapping of India should start. Too much emphasis on the curative aspects and neglect of the preventive aspects may bar the dream of a healthy India.

The chapter is presented as follows—Section 2 gives a brief profile of the existing studies on the various types of exclusions and the access to basic health infrastructure. In section 3 we chart out the data used and the methodology that we have designed to fashion our index of basic health infrastructure. Section 4 gives the basic contour of iniquitous distribution for a number of various aspects that we deemed important to the study. Section 5 describes the data with the indices that we have developed. In the empirical analysis we have categories or data according to various social groups (*Dalits* and General), economic classes (Poor and Non-Poor) geographical locations (Rural and Urban) with an interspersing of each other. The myriad of picture that emanates from the discussion is concluded in section 6.

## Health and Social Exclusion

There has been a long debate in the health literature regarding the relationship between health outcome facilities and its socio-economic origin. Historically, the idea was first developed by the British economist William Petty and French economist Louis-Rene Villerme. Petty tried to show the influence of societal resources on wealth status. Villerme was a resident in the suburbs of Paris. His work was more elaborate. He considered various attributes of health (such as stunting, illness, and deformities) and linked them with panorama of factors—social, cultural, economic and anthropological as well as natural. He found the mortality patterns were strongly correlated with incidence of poverty. Fradirch Engels found that the health of destitute workers and their children were worst affected by extreme adverse living and working conditions (Nayar & Oliver, 2006).

All these studies are international in nature. In the case of India the problem of health is accentuated by the coexistence of poverty and caste. The Indian Constitution has specifically identified three categories of most deprived classes—Schedule Tribe (ST), Schedule Caste (SC) and Other Backward Caste (OBC). In the common typology he may categories former two under *Dalits*. However the category is not homogeneous. Among the *Dalit*, the "Untouchable" are the most deprived. It was Professor Amartya Sen who first considered the social exclusion in a rigorous way. He pointed out the various dimension of social exclusion. Firstly, he distinguishes between 'Unfavourable exclusion' and 'Unfavourable inclusion'. In the later case, people are included (even forcefully included) at a greatly unfavourable term. The result is almost same as "unfavourable exclusion". Unfavourable exclusion is a situation where people are excluded from some functioning or opportunities that are important. It may be contrasted with favourable exclusion such as containment of patients suffering from infectious diseases in a secluded place. He also differentiated between active and passive exclusion. Active exclusion is involving the deliberate act of exclusion (such as untouchable). Passive exclusion involves exclusion not deliberately but in effects. Sometimes low caste children are excluded from some schools from the logic of low merit.

Thirdly some differentiate between constitutive exclusion and instrumentive exclusion. Constitutive exclusion refers to exclusion of those which result in a loss of livelihood or social impoverishment. Cost of the exclusion in health is of this type. If a person of low caste is not properly treated, or if a tribal folk is not allowed to enter a doctor's chamber, the result is fatal. Many a time this exclusion may take the form of passive exclusion. Language problem, lack of communicative skill, inabilities to locate the scientific terminologies involved in the understanding and the healing of illness are all building up walls between the medical care providers (doctors, nurses and technicians) and the low caste poor patients. Similar logic can be applied to the provision of preventive health facilities (Drinking water, Sanitation, Drainage etc.).

Another related exclusion is instrumental. In this case the direct consequence of exclusion is not so fatal but end effect is basically the same. An example from health is the case of vaccination. Non-vaccination guarantees illness and increases manifold risks.

## Data and Methodology

The fabric of Indian social milieu is orchestrated into a divisive world. In this study, we have considered only three dimensions of such social divisions. They are locational, social and economic. Locationally rural people face a lot of constraints that are often encountered in an urban existence. For example the long journey of ailing persons through a topsy-turvy potted road is often a daily scene for a country folk, though even a poor person in a city may not have to encounter such an unbelievably nightmarish journey.

Thus the rural-urban division is the basic problem in accessing to health infrastructural facilities. The next component is the social division that is uniquely Indian. We have clubbed the Schedule Tribe (ST), Schedule Caste (SC), and Other Backward Castes (OBCs) in the *Dalit* categories. They face a lot of incompleteness in a society that is socially biased. Often the health infrastructural facilities have been cornered by the socially powerful groups. Very often the *Dalit* are denied access to such facilities. The *Dalit* themselves are often powerless and fail to register their rights. The last devised pattern that we have considered is the economic one. We have taken the monthly per capita expenditures of families with the official poverty level-mark. Those who fail to meet this official figure are deemed as poor while others as relatively rich. There is lot of controversy regarding the official lines. However, the official line may be regarded as a bare minimum level of existence. Thus, the 'Poor' in our exercise are the worst possible among the economically deprived. It is to be seen how this economic deprivation is reflected in accessing to basic health facilities and infrastructural amenities.

To establish the relation between the rural and urban scenario we need data. Therefore, the objectives cannot be completed without the availability of relevant information. The data used in this study have been collected from the 60th round (January-June 2004) of NSSO (National Sample Survey Organization) published by the Ministry of Statistics and Programme Implementation, Government of India. This round covered a wide range of Indian healthcare infrastructural facilities and consumer health expenditure that focused basically on the enquiry on the "Morbidity and Healthcare". This round of unit level data also emphasis on the curative aspects of the general healthcare system of India, utilization of health care services provided by the public, private system and the consumer health expenditures while availing these services. The published NSSO report provides detailed information regarding rural urban distinction in case of using healthcare facilities at the state level. At aggregative level, we get detailed information covering 8 states of North-East India of both at urban and rural level.

In the next section we have calculated the inter-state disparity using Principal Component Analysis. Before running PCA, we convert the raw data into a normalized form. This is done to make the raw data unit free as well as to get the relative position of each state in respect of health infrastructure. First the actual and minimum values in a particular infrastructural indicator are identified. In case of all indicators, the highest value is treated as the best value and the lowest as the worst value. Once the maximum and minimum values are identified, the following formula is used to obtain normalized values: (Observe-Minimum)/(Maximum- Minimum).Therefore, the normalized values always lie between 0 and 1. Once the normalized values are obtained for all the health infrastructural variables across the states, next step is to assign factor loadings and weights. The PCA is used to compute the factor loadings and weights of these infrastructural indicators. Using this loadings and weights we arrive at the health infrastructure indices for the 8 major states of North-East India. In our exercise, we have considered three variables to construct the infrastructural index— (i) percentage of water treated before drinking, (ii) percentage of latrine and (iii) percentage of drainage.

## Some Socio-Economic Features of a Socially Fragmented Economy

Our intellectual journey begins with the study of a set of variables that are deemed important from the point of view of health infrastructural facilities. These factors are studied through the lens of divisiveness that marsh our societies. For each variable we consider three dimensions—locational, social and economic. In fact they are interrelated parts. We consider the social and economic categorization under both rural and urban distinction.

Our first variable is the condition of housing. NSSO categorises houses as '*kuchcha*' (serviceable, non-serviceable and without structure) and '*pucca*'. The worst category appears to be the people who live in houses with no structure. They are the homeless people. Unfortunately, however, the data is scanty or unreliable. Thus, we consider the category serviceable-*kuchcha* and unserviceable-*kuchcha* as low quality housing. Now, we consider the state-wise distribution of poor quality housing across the social, economic and locational terrains. First consider the rural-urban break-up. For all the North East states, the preponderance of low quality housing is higher in the rural sector than in urban area. However, the rural-urban gap is larger for some North East states than others.

For example, in Arunachal Pradesh the intensity of low quality housing in urban area (36.39%) is half of that of the rural (78.82%). Situation is more or less similar in Mizoram. In Assam the situation is worse (41.21% in rural, 7.76% in urban). When we go to Manipur and Meghalaya, this difference is wider. In fact the wide rural-urban gap is seen in the 3 states—Arunachal Pradesh, Assam, and Sikkim. It is really disheartening.

Next we consider the *Dalit* housing. Again there is the rural urban gap and states where the gap is frightening are Arunachal Pradesh, Assam, and Manipur. In many states the rural-urban division is reflected even in the *Dalit* categorization. A rural *Dalit* is thus doubly inflected—he belongs to a socially deprived class as well as to a locationally deprived position.

The next dimension is economic. Here also the rural-urban division is multifaceted with domination of urban population. Again the disparity is alarming for states Assam and Nagaland. May be, in the urban area, the poor get some facilities from the public authorities and from their rich neighbours. Also credit facilities may be easily available in the urban area. Our general conclusion for the housing condition is simple. The locational condition becomes an important factor.

A similar asymmetry may be found in all the other variables considered by us—namely drainage condition, major source of drinking water as well as source of cooking energy. The proportion of disadvantaged families is high for the rural Dalits and the Poor people. They have the highest percentage of inadequate drainage; use of unsafe and untreated drinking water and have to cope up with health-risky traditional sources of cooking. However the rural-urban inequality is multifaceted in both the social and economic groupings. All the other categories, social or economic, get subdued under this simple, but important factor. Living in a village is still living in a gloomy night. This adds to the woes generated otherwise.

## Indexation of Health Access and Facilities in Socially Fragmented Economy

We now come to the profile according to the infrastructural index constructed by us. We have shown the result in a concrete form in Tables 10.1, 10.2 and 10.3. Our result indicates a clear profile across the rural, urban and aggregative North East state of India. There are states, which show good performance for all the categories as well as for all the groups. In rural North East India, Manipur, Sikkim, Tripura and Nagaland are such states. However, we have small data in case of the Nagaland. There are states which remain permanently at the bottom. They are Assam, Meghalaya and Mizoram.

**Table 10.1:** High and Low Health Infrastructure (Rural)

| | *Dalit* | *Poor People* | *All Groups* |
|---|---|---|---|
| High Health Infrastructure | Nagaland | Nagaland | Nagaland |
| | Manipur | Meghalaya | Manipur |
| | Sikkim | Sikkim | Sikkim |
| | Mizoram | Manipur | Tripura |
| | Tripura | Assam | Mizoram |
| Low Health Infrastructure | **India** | Tripura | **India** |
| | Arunachal Pradesh | Arunachal Pradesh | Arunachal Pradesh |
| | Assam | **India** | Meghalaya |
| | Meghalaya | Mizoram | Assam |

*Source:* National Sample Survey Organization 60th Round.

States such as Arunachal Pradesh changes their position for the Poor People. Meghalaya is well placed, but for the category of *Dalit* people they are the below the average.

**Table 10.2:** High and Low Health Infrastructure (Urban)

| | *Dalit* | *Poor People* | *All Groups* |
|---|---|---|---|
| High Health Infrastructure | Nagaland | Manipur | Nagaland |
| | Sikkim | Nagaland | Manipur |
| | Manipur | Assam | Meghalaya |
| | Arunachal Pradesh | Arunachal Pradesh | Sikkim |
| | Meghalaya | Mizoram | Assam |
| Low Health Infrastructure | **India** | Sikkim | **India** |
| | Mizoram | **India** | Mizoram |
| | Assam | Meghalaya | Arunachal Pradesh |
| | Tripura | Tripura | Tripura |

*Source:* National Sample Survey Organization, 60th Round.

More or less similar picture emanates for urban North-East India. However states Assam lies above average for Poor People while Arunachal Pradesh for *Dalit*. The proportion of bad states is lower for Poor People as compared to the average in rural North

East India. For urban North-East India however, the proportion of bad states are slightly lower for *Dalit* and Poor as compared to all North East India.

**Table 10.3:** High and Low Health Infrastructure (All North East)

| | *Dalit* | *Poor People* | *All Groups* |
|---|---|---|---|
| High Health Infrastructure | Nagaland<br>Manipur<br>Sikkim<br>Mizoram | Nagaland<br>Manipur<br>Sikkim<br>Meghalaya | Nagaland<br>Manipur<br>Sikkim<br>Meghalaya |
| Low Health Infrastructure | Arunachal Pradesh<br>**India**<br>Tripura<br>Assam<br>Meghalaya | **India**<br>Tripura<br>Assam<br>Arunachal Pradesh<br>Mizoram | **India**<br>Tripura<br>Assam<br>Arunachal Pradesh<br>Mizoram |

*Source:* National Sample Survey Organization, 60th Round.

## Conclusion

Our study is a discourse on a less trodden terrain. The issue of preventive health infrastructure is looking through the prism of social and economical exclusion. Economically, we have considered the families who are below the official poverty level. Socially, we have considered the category called '*Dalits*' including Schedule Caste, Schedule Tribe and Other Backward Castes. We have also considered the locational dimension—living in an urban or rural environment. All these factors are assumed to have effect on the spread and availability of basic healthcare infrastructure. This exercise was a tapestry of facts and figures culled from the NSSO unit level (2004) survey data. Our analysis shows that there are wide socio-economic implications for bad healthcare in both rural and urban North East states of India. The picture that emanates from our analysis is a mixture of social and economic exclusion with its impacts on the supply of healthcare. Proper policy prescription is needed to surmount the barriers of asymmetry.

# Appendices

**Table A1:** Housing Condition of the North East States—Socio-Economic Groupings

| North East States | All Groups | | | | Dalits | | | | Poor People | | | |
|---|---|---|---|---|---|---|---|---|---|---|---|---|
| | Rural | | Urban | | Rural | | Urban | | Rural | | Urban | |
| | % of Pucca | % of low Quality Housing | % of Pucca | % of low Quality Housing | % of Pucca | % of low Quality Housing | % of Pucca | % of low Quality Housing | % of Pucca | % of low Quality Housing | % of Pucca | % of low Quality Housing |
| Arunachal Pradesh | 4.40 | 78.82 | 38.92 | 36.39 | 4.39 | 78.55 | 41.38 | 31.18 | 1.18 | 84.02 | 19.18 | 64.38 |
| Assam | 15.52 | 41.21 | 63.94 | 7.76 | 13.55 | 41.33 | 49.37 | 8.86 | 15.52 | 41.21 | 63.94 | 7.76 |
| Manipur | 5.70 | 39.07 | 19.81 | 9.23 | 5.68 | 39.17 | 19.02 | 10.07 | 3.70 | 59.26 | 6.45 | 29.03 |
| Meghalaya | 37.50 | 19.22 | 78.66 | 4.60 | 38.70 | 18.08 | 82.68 | 4.47 | 19.35 | 22.58 | 60.00 | 20.00 |
| Mizoram | 52.03 | 9.64 | 76.55 | 3.17 | 51.79 | 9.69 | 76.67 | 3.02 | 0.00 | 33.33 | 61.90 | 4.76 |
| Nagaland | 40.83 | 2.92 | 69.17 | 2.50 | 40.83 | 2.92 | 69.72 | 1.83 | 0.00 | 0.00 | 50.00 | 50.00 |
| Sikkim | 61.14 | 11.13 | 91.25 | 1.25 | 60.33 | 11.27 | 91.53 | 1.69 | 33.33 | 15.69 | 66.67 | 0.00 |
| Tripura | 5.00 | 20.00 | 35.42 | 16.23 | 4.70 | 21.74 | 29.75 | 1.65 | 0.44 | 32.44 | 16.42 | 4.48 |

*Source:* NSSO 60th Round Unit level Data, Calculation is done by the authors.

**Table A1.1:** Ratio of Urban to Rural Proportion for the Housing Condition

| *North East States* | *All Groups* | | *Dalits* | | *Poor People* | |
|---|---|---|---|---|---|---|
| | *Ratio* | | *Ratio* | | *Ratio* | |
| | *% of Pucca* | *% of low Quality Housing* | *% of Pucca* | *% of low Quality Housing* | *% of Pucca* | *% of low Quality Housing* |
| Arunachal Pradesh | 8.85 | 0.46 | 9.43 | 0.40 | 16.25 | 0.77 |
| Assam | 4.12 | 0.19 | 3.64 | 0.21 | 4.12 | 0.19 |
| Manipur | 3.48 | 0.24 | 3.35 | 0.26 | 1.74 | 0.49 |
| Meghalaya | 2.10 | 0.24 | 2.14 | 0.25 | 3.10 | 0.89 |
| Mizoram | 1.47 | 0.33 | 1.48 | 0.31 | 0.00 | 0.14 |
| Nagaland | 1.69 | 0.86 | 1.71 | 0.63 | 0.00 | 0.00 |
| Sikkim | 1.49 | 0.11 | 1.52 | 0.15 | 2.00 | 0.00 |
| Tripura | 7.08 | 0.81 | 6.33 | 0.08 | 37.32 | 0.14 |

*Source:* NSSO 60th Round Unit level Data, Calculation is done by the authors.

**Table A2:** Sanitation Condition of the North-East States-Socio Economic Groupings

| *North East States* | *All Groups* | | | | *Dalits* | | | | *Poor People* | | | |
|---|---|---|---|---|---|---|---|---|---|---|---|---|
| | *Rural* | | *Urban* | | *Rural* | | *Urban* | | *Rural* | | *Urban* | |
| | *% of latrine with septic tank* | *% of no. latrine* | *% of latrine with septic tank* | *% of no. latrine* | *% of latrine with septic tank* | *% of no. latrine* | *% of latrine with septic tank* | *% of no. latrine* | *% of latrine with septic tank* | *% of no. latrine* | *% of latrine with septic tank* | *% of no. latrine* |
| Arunachal Pradesh | 7.57 | 11.97 | 42.41 | 0.63 | 5.91 | 10.81 | 41.95 | 1.15 | 1.78 | 22.49 | 30.14 | 0.00 |
| Assam | 13.71 | 13.71 | 71.49 | 0.63 | 11.62 | 15.30 | 63.29 | 1.27 | 13.71 | 13.71 | 71.49 | 0.63 |
| Manipur | 23.93 | 1.12 | 45.38 | 0.19 | 23.94 | 1.14 | 46.09 | 0.22 | 7.41 | 22.22 | 56.45 | 0.00 |
| Meghalaya | 4.10 | 39.55 | 76.15 | 1.26 | 3.93 | 41.26 | 74.86 | 1.68 | 3.23 | 16.13 | 20.00 | 10.00 |
| Mizoram | 12.94 | 10.91 | 54.20 | 0.32 | 12.76 | 10.97 | 54.29 | 0.16 | 0.00 | 60.00 | 33.33 | 0.00 |
| Nagaland | 22.92 | 0.00 | 69.17 | 0.00 | 22.92 | 0.00 | 69.72 | 0.00 | 0.00 | 0.00 | 50.00 | 0.00 |
| Sikkim | 41.82 | 3.64 | 91.25 | 3.75 | 41.55 | 3.76 | 91.53 | 3.39 | 19.61 | 3.92 | 66.67 | 33.33 |
| Tripura | 10.73 | 4.63 | 40.00 | 2.08 | 8.70 | 5.22 | 38.02 | 4.13 | 12.44 | 8.00 | 22.39 | 5.97 |

*Source:* NSSO 60th Round Unit level Data, Calculation is done by the authors.

**Table A3.1:** Ratio of Urban to Rural Proportion for the Drainage Condition

| North East States | All Groups | | Dalits | | Poor People | |
|---|---|---|---|---|---|---|
| | Ratio | | Ratio | | Ratio | |
| | % of under ground | % of no. drainage | % of under ground | % of no. drainage | % of under ground | % of no. drainage |
| Arunachal Pradesh | 0.23 | 0.27 | 0.34 | 0.17 | 0.00 | 0.45 |
| Assam | 3.23 | 0.31 | 6.68 | 0.50 | 3.23 | 0.31 |
| Manipur | 0.65 | 0.46 | 0.75 | 0.35 | 0.00 | 0.34 |
| Meghalaya | 2.21 | 0.14 | 2.80 | 0.13 | 0.00 | 0.66 |
| Mizoram | 1.28 | 0.52 | 0.62 | 0.52 | 0.71 | 0.55 |
| Nagaland | 0.00 | 0.10 | 0.00 | 0.08 | 0.00 | 0.00 |
| Sikkim | 0.00 | 0.10 | 0.00 | 0.09 | 0.00 | 0.57 |
| Tripura | 0.00 | 0.68 | 0.00 | 0.75 | 0.00 | 0.81 |

*Source:* NSSO 60th Round Unit level Data, Calculation is done by the authors.

**Table A4:** Major source of Drinking Water of the North East States-Socio Economic Groupings

| North East States | *All Groups* | | | | *Dalits* | | | | *Poor People* | | | |
|---|---|---|---|---|---|---|---|---|---|---|---|---|
| | *Rural* | | *Urban* | | *Rural* | | *Urban* | | *Rural* | | *Urban* | |
| | % of safe drinking water as source | % of treated water before drinking | % of safe drinking water as source | % of treated water before drinking | % of safe drinking water as source | % of treated water before drinking | % of safe drinking water as source | % of treated water before drinking | % of safe drinking water as source | % of treated water before drinking | % of safe drinking water as source | % of treated water before drinking |
| Arunachal Pradesh | 83.49 | 19.67 | 96.20 | 46.52 | 84.12 | 21.28 | 93.68 | 53.45 | 71.01 | 13.61 | 94.52 | 42.47 |
| Assam | 67.32 | 23.17 | 82.81 | 57.65 | 65.25 | 24.20 | 84.18 | 56.96 | 67.32 | 23.17 | 82.81 | 57.65 |
| Manipur | 42.80 | 58.79 | 76.54 | 60.77 | 42.19 | 59.41 | 74.27 | 59.96 | 29.63 | 66.7 | 77.4 | 67.74 |
| Meghalaya | 43.10 | 39.37 | 92.47 | 65.69 | 41.45 | 39.49 | 90.50 | 72.07 | 51.61 | 61.29 | 100.0 | 40.00 |
| Mizoram | 20.05 | 41.37 | 56.58 | 55.63 | 19.90 | 41.07 | 56.67 | 55.71 | 0.00 | 0.00 | 61.90 | 47.62 |
| Nagaland | 34.17 | 98.75 | 60.00 | 98.33 | 34.17 | 98.75 | 57.80 | 99.08 | 0.00 | 0.00 | 100.0 | 50.00 |
| Sikkim | 34.77 | 51.36 | 98.75 | 95.00 | 34.04 | 51.41 | 98.31 | 96.61 | 23.53 | 47.06 | 100.0 | 100.0 |
| Tripura | 70.49 | 47.32 | 96.25 | 70.00 | 66.78 | 45.04 | 96.69 | 61.98 | 61.78 | 34.67 | 97.01 | 50.75 |

*Source:* NSSO 60th Round Unit level Data, Calculation is done by the authors.

**Table A4.1:** Ratio of Urban to Rural Proportion for the Source of Drinking Water

| *North East States* | *All Groups* | | *Dalits* | | *Poor People* | |
|---|---|---|---|---|---|---|
| | *Ratio* | | *Ratio* | | *Ratio* | |
| | *% of Safe Drinking Water as Source* | *% of Treated Water Before Drinking* | *% of Safe Drinking Water as Source* | *% of Treated Water Before Drinking* | *% of Safe Drinking Water as Source* | *% of Treated Water Before Drinking* |
| Arunachal Pradesh | 1.15 | 2.37 | 1.11 | 2.51 | 1.33 | 3.12 |
| Assam | 1.23 | 2.49 | 1.29 | 2.35 | 1.23 | 2.49 |
| Manipur | 1.79 | 1.03 | 1.76 | 1.01 | 2.61 | 1.02 |
| Meghalaya | 2.15 | 1.67 | 2.18 | 1.83 | 1.94 | 0.65 |
| Mizoram | 2.82 | 1.34 | 2.85 | 1.36 | 0.00 | 0.00 |
| Nagaland | 1.76 | 1.00 | 1.69 | 1.00 | 0.00 | 0.00 |
| Sikkim | 2.84 | 1.85 | 2.89 | 1.88 | 4.25 | 2.12 |
| Tripura | 1.37 | 1.48 | 1.45 | 1.38 | 1.57 | 1.46 |

*Source:* NSSO 60th Round Unit Level Data, Calculation is done by the authors.

**Table A5:** Source of Cooking Energy of the North East States—Socio-Economic Groupings

| North East States | All Groups | | | | Dalits | | | | Poor People | | | |
|---|---|---|---|---|---|---|---|---|---|---|---|---|
| | Rural | | Urban | | Rural | | Urban | | Rural | | Urban | |
| | % of traditional source | % of modern source | % of traditional source | % of modern source | % of traditional source | % of modern source | % of traditional source | % of modern source | % of traditional source | % of modern source | % of traditional source | % of modern source |
| Arunachal Pradesh | 90.65 | 9.08 | 35.44 | 25.39 | 92.40 | 7.09 | 34.48 | 64.94 | 97.64 | 2.37 | 49.32 | 50.68 |
| Assam | 94.17 | 5.78 | 24.11 | 75.05 | 94.82 | 4.84 | 32.91 | 67.09 | 94.17 | 5.78 | 24.11 | 75.05 |
| Manipur | 79.53 | 20.47 | 35.58 | 64.42 | 79.84 | 20.15 | 37.36 | 62.64 | 85.19 | 14.81 | 69.35 | 30.65 |
| Meghalaya | 97.76 | 2.24 | 43.10 | 55.64 | 98.04 | 1.97 | 49.16 | 49.16 | 96.77 | 3.23 | 80.00 | 20.00 |
| Mizoram | 68.02 | 31.98 | 13.15 | 86.21 | 68.37 | 31.63 | 13.49 | 86.35 | 100.0 | 0.00 | 90.48 | 4.76 |
| Nagaland | 70.41 | 29.58 | 4.16 | 94.17 | 70.41 | 29.58 | 4.59 | 93.58 | 0.00 | 0.00 | 0.00 | 50.00 |
| Sikkim | 77.95 | 20.91 | 7.50 | 85.00 | 78.64 | 20.42 | 6.78 | 86.44 | 96.08 | 3.92 | 66.67 | 33.33 |
| Tripura | 94.75 | 5.00 | 52.08 | 47.92 | 95.48 | 4.17 | 64.46 | 35.54 | 99.11 | 0.44 | 98.51 | 10.45 |

*Source:* NSSO 60th Round Unit level Data, Calculation is done by the authors.

**Table A5.1:** Ratio of Urban to Rural Proportion for the Source of Cooking Energy

| North East States | All Groups | | Dalits | | Poor People | |
|---|---|---|---|---|---|---|
| | Ratio | | Ratio | | Ratio | |
| | % of Traditional Source | % of Modern Source | % of Traditional Source | % of Modern Source | % of Traditional Source | % of Modern Source |
| Arunachal Pradesh | 0.39 | 2.85 | 0.37 | 9.16 | 0.51 | 21.38 |
| Assam | 0.26 | 12.98 | 0.35 | 13.86 | 0.26 | 12.98 |
| Manipur | 0.45 | 3.15 | 0.47 | 3.11 | 0.81 | 2.07 |
| Meghalaya | 0.44 | 24.84 | 0.50 | 24.95 | 0.83 | 6.19 |
| Mizoram | 0.19 | 2.70 | 0.20 | 2.73 | 0.90 | 0.00 |
| Nagaland | 0.06 | 3.18 | 0.07 | 3.16 | 0.00 | 0.00 |
| Sikkim | 0.10 | 4.07 | 0.09 | 4.23 | 0.69 | 8.50 |
| Tripura | 0.55 | 9.58 | 0.68 | 8.52 | 0.99 | 23.75 |

*Source:* NSSO 60th Round Unit level Data, Calculation is done by the authors.

**Table B1:** Health Infrastructure Index—Socio-Economic Groupings

| North East States | All Groups | | Dalits | | Poor People | |
|---|---|---|---|---|---|---|
| | Rural | Urban | Rural | Urban | Rural | Urban |
| Arunachal Pradesh | 0.2354 | 0.5007 | 0.2507 | 0.5167 | 0.4129 | 0.5485 |
| Assam | 0.2185 | 0.5576 | 0.2212 | 0.3730 | 0.4897 | 0.6609 |
| Manipur | 0.6532 | 0.6396 | 0.6564 | 0.6114 | 0.5992 | 0.7281 |
| Meghalaya | 0.2201 | 0.6058 | 0.2144 | 0.4920 | 0.7018 | 0.4119 |
| Mizoram | 0.3866 | 0.5177 | 0.3844 | 0.4305 | 0.0345 | 0.5267 |
| Nagaland | 1.0000 | 1.0000 | 1.0000 | 1.0000 | 0.7546 | 0.6803 |
| Sikkim | 0.5776 | 0.6052 | 0.5711 | 0.9456 | 0.6745 | 0.5124 |
| Tripura | 0.4083 | 0.3407 | 0.3834 | 0.2827 | 0.4603 | 0.3895 |

*Source:* NSSO 60th Round Unit level Data, Calculation is done by the authors.

**Table B2:** Health Infrastructure Index—Socio-Economic Groupings (All North East)

| North Eastern States | All Groups | Dalits | Poor People |
|---|---|---|---|
| Arunachal Pradesh | 0.2728 | 0.4466 | 0.2577 |
| Assam | 0.2191 | 0.3050 | 0.3513 |
| Manipur | 0.6381 | 0.7516 | 0.7845 |
| Meghalaya | 0.2506 | 0.2940 | 0.5719 |
| Mizoram | 0.4898 | 0.5854 | 0.1371 |
| Nagaland | 1.0000 | 1.0000 | 0.8666 |
| Sikkim | 0.5961 | 0.6843 | 0.5929 |
| Tripura | 0.1230 | 0.3500 | 0.3595 |

*Source:* NSSO 60th Round Unit level Data, Calculation is done by the authors.

## References

National Sample Survey Organization, NSS 60th Round 2004. *Morbidity, Healthcare and the Condition of the Aged*. NSSO New Delhi and its unit level household data.

World Development Indicators 2012, Washington, DC: The World Bank.

Nayar, K. R. and Razum, O. (2006). Millennium Development Goals and Health: Another selective development? *International Studies*, 43: 317-22.

Qadeer, I. (1985). Health services system in India: an expression of socio-economic inequalities, *Social Action*, 35: 199-222.

Raychaudhuri, A., and Haldar, S.K. (2009). An Investigation into the Inter-District Disparity in West Bengal, 1991-2005. *Economic and Political Weekly*, June 27, XLIV (26 and 27): 258-263.

Sen, A., and Dreze, J. (2013). *An Uncertain Glory: India and its Contradictions*. New Delhi: Allen Lane, Penguin Group Publications.

Sen, A.K. (2015). Universal healthcare: the affordable dream, Health Long read, 6th January, 2015, *The Guardian*, online. Available at http://www.theguardian.com.

Thorat, S. (2007). *Human Poverty and Socially Disadvantage Groups in India*, Discussion Paper Series-18, UNDP India.

# 11
# Public Health Expenditure in India with Special Reference to North Eastern States

*Sonam Gupta* and *Prahlad Kumar*

## Introduction

> "Growth in national income by itself is not enough, if the benefits do not manifest themselves in the form of more food, better access to health and education." —*A.K. Sen*

The health condition of the people of a nation largely depends on an effective and well developed healthcare system, which can easily be affordable and accessible for the people, but to make accessible the healthcare facilities to all, we need healthcare infrastructure and for this we need not only large volume of investment in this sector, but its utilization is also necessary. However, even after six and half decades of planned development process initiated in India, its healthcare sector is quite unsatisfactory. India has the lowest health spending as a proportion of gross domestic product (GDP), with the overall number looking a little better due to the contribution by the private sector. According the data in the **Economic Survey 2014-15,** General government (Central and State) spends around 1.3 per cent of GDP on health in 2008-09 and it almost constant over the last 5 years with the marginal increase. In 2014-15 government spend only 1.2 per cent of GDP, which is 4 per cent of total government expenditure, while China and Russia that are among the low spenders among the 11 countries identified in the government document, spending at least a percentage point more. Only Indonesia has a poorer allocation (2.6%) among the 11 countries, while Brazil and South Africa are neat the 9 per cent range. This makes India the worst performer among the BRICS group. The government has admitted to low health allocation, is the major driver for high infant and maternal mortality rates in the government document. In spite of government spending on Health care facilities, the improvement has been much uneven across regions with large scale inter-state variations. For development of health care system, government has to spend more on health sector and monitor its utilization.

## Objectives

In this context the present study tries to explore the growth of health spending in North Eastern state, the extent of utilization and the increase of health care facilities and various health indicators, towards achieving the Millennium Development Goals that is reduce child mortality and improve maternal health.

## Status of North East India

North Eastern States comprises Seven Sisters States that is (Arunachal Pradesh, Assam, Manipur, Meghalaya, Mizoram, Nagaland and Tripura). These states cover about 3.7 per cent (44.98 million) population of India's total population, according to Census 2011. It is generally considered to be a backward state of a progressive economy.

We are discussing here plan expenditure on Health in the North Eastern States. We can see from Table 11.1. In the North Eastern State, Manipur is the best performer, to increase health allocation in this five year with 239.73 per cent, where Tripura stood second best performer with 203.04 per cent. Meghalya and Assam perform third and forth respectivily. Arunanchal Pradesh is the worst performer in terms of health allocation with 4.55 per cent increase.

In the context of utilization, we can see in Fig. 11.1 all the North Eastern State perform well over the year 2007-08, and trying to improve their utilization, but in term of trend of resource utiliztion, Meghalaya present impressive growth over the year and Manipur is the worst performer, while it got highest health allocation among the North Eastern State. Higher allocation of fund to the region

**Table 11.1:** Allocation, Expenditure and the Extent of Utilisation in North Eastern States

*(Rs. in Lakh)*

| Medical and Public Health | | | | | | | | |
|---|---|---|---|---|---|---|---|---|
| *Year* | *Flow* | *Arunanchal Pradesh* | *Assam* | *Manipur* | *Meghalaya* | *Mizoram* | *Nagaland* | *Tripura* |
| 2007-08 | Allocation | 5554.95 | 18979.0 | 4402.00 | 6040.00 | 4275.00 | 2256.89 | 8452.41 |
| | Expenditure | 3014.66 | 7043.50 | 1774.19 | 6038.26 | 4181.17 | 2281.89 | 6035.19 |
| | *Utilisation* | *54.26* | *37.11* | *40.30* | *99.97* | *97.80* | *101.11* | *71.40* |
| 2008-09 | Allocation | 2036.10 | 16095.00 | 6786.66 | 6700.00 | 10612.00 | 3303.00 | 10526.34 |
| | Expenditure | 1888.11 | 16085.21 | 2002.25 | 6608.52 | 10525.52 | 3313.00 | 10503.80 |
| | *Utilisation* | *92.73* | *99.93* | *29.50* | *98.63* | *99.18* | *100.30* | *99.78* |
| 2009-10 | Allocation | 5945.28 | 42185.00 | 9457.16 | 9250.00 | 18800.00 | 4295.37 | 10902.29 |
| | Expenditure | 5945.00 | 41964.00 | 2725.36 | 9709.57 | 17493.67 | 3373.60 | 14026.48 |
| | *Utilisation* | *99.99* | *99.47* | *28.81* | *104.96* | *93.05* | *78.54* | *128.65* |
| 2010-11 | Allocation | 7698.88 | 57176.00 | 14973.56 | 10200.00 | 6140.00 | 4917.00 | 10809.54 |
| | Expenditure | 7698.88 | 56519.78 | 8992.48 | 14036.68 | 7432.82 | 4917.00 | 11281.48 |
| | *Utilisation* | *100.00* | *98.85* | *60.05* | *137.61* | *121.05* | *100.00* | *104.36* |
| 2011-12* | Allocation | 5808.00 | 47486.71 | 14955.00 | 17300.00 | 8775.00 | 3224.00 | 25615.36 |
| | Expenditure | 5808.00 | 59250.71 | 26345.00 | 16800.00 | 8726.62 | 4838.38 | 22407.33 |
| | *Utilisation* | *100.00* | *124.77* | *176.16* | *97.10* | *99.44* | *150.07* | *87.47* |
| Total 11th Plan | Allocation | 27043.21 | 181921.71 | 50574.38 | 49490.00 | 48602.0 | 17996.26 | 66305.94 |
| | Expenditure | 24354.65 | 180863.2 | 41839.28 | 53193.03 | 48359.8 | 18723.87 | 66254.28 |
| | *Utilisation* | *90.05* | *99.42* | *82.73* | *107.48* | *99.50* | *104.04* | *99.92* |

*Note:* * Anticipated Expenditure.
*Source:* Planning Commission of India.

has not been a problem in the last decade, rather the region is facing at present the problem of utilization of fund, and more so their proper utilization.

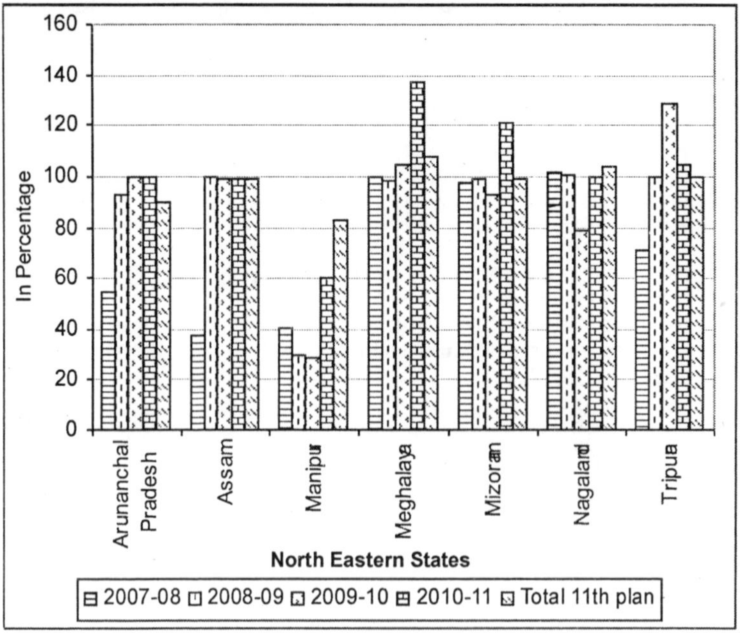


**Fig. 11.1:** Utilization of Plan Expenditure on Health
*Source:* Based on Table 11.1.

Table 11.2 shows the requirement, in position, shortfall and surplus of basic healthcare facilities of Sub-Centre, Primary Health Centres (PHCs) and Community Health Centres (CHCs) according to the prescribe norms on the basis of the rural population in NESs. We can see in Table 11.2 that Mizoram and Tripura show surplus in the availability of sub-centre according to prescribed norm that is, each sub-centre will cover 5,000 popultion. Meghalaya is the worst performing state to provide basic health infrastructure with 44 per cent shortfall amoung the NESs, Assam, Manipur and Nagaland stand respectivily.

In the context of Primary Health Centres, Arunanchal Pradesh, Assam, Manipur, Mizoram and Nagaland show surplus according

**Table 11.2:** Shortfall in Health Infrastucture as per 2011 Population in NESs ( As on 31st March, 2014)

| States | Total Population in Rural Areas | Sub-Centre | | | | PHCs | | | | CHCs | | | |
|---|---|---|---|---|---|---|---|---|---|---|---|---|---|
| | | R | P | S | % Short fall | R | P | S | % Short fall | R | P | S | % Short fall |
| Arunanchal Pradesh | 10,66,358 | 318 | 286 | 32 | 10 | 48 | 117 | * | * | 12 | 52 | * | * |
| Assam | 2,68,07,034 | 5850 | 4621 | 1229 | 21 | 954 | 1014 | * | * | 238 | 151 | 87 | 37 |
| Manipur | 20,21,640 | 509 | 421 | 88 | 17 | 80 | 85 | * | * | 20 | 17 | 3 | 15 |
| Meghalaya | 23,71,439 | 759 | 422 | 337 | 44 | 114 | 108 | 6 | 5 | 28 | 27 | 1 | 4 |
| Mizoram | 5,25,435 | 172 | 370 | * | * | 25 | 57 | * | * | 6 | 9 | * | * |
| Nagaland | 14,07,536 | 455 | 396 | 59 | 13 | 68 | 126 | * | * | 17 | 21 | * | * |
| Tripura | 27,12,464 | 691 | 972 | * | * | 109 | 84 | 25 | 23 | 27 | 18 | 9 | 33 |

*Note:* We are not considering 2011-12 data because it is anticipated data and not actual. So here, we analyse only data from 2007-08 to 2010-11.

*Source:* NRHM, R—Required, P—In Position, S—Shortfall, *—Surplus.

to the PHCs norm that is, One PHCs for every 30,000 population in plain areas. Tripura is the worst performer amoung NESs. In the respect of Community Health Centres (CHCs), Arunanchal Pradesh, Mizoram and Nagaland present surplus according to the requirement and Assam is the worst performer amoung NESs. We find that basic healthcare facilities are not uniform amoung the NESs and Mizoram is the best performing state to develop and provide basic health infrastructure (Sub-centres, PHCs, and CHCs) according to the prescribed norms amoung the NESs.

Here we examine the State Programme Implementation Plan (SPIP) approval and expenditure under Child and Maternal Health to analyse the correlation between their fund utilization and improvement in the related indicators. The State Programme Implementation Plan (SPIP) is made by the Executive Committee (EC) of the State Health Socity and approved by the State Government/ Governing Board. The EC of State Health Society implements the approved plan, with governance and oversight exercised by the governing board and the State Health Mission (Ministry of Health and Family welfare, GoI). Government allocate resources through plans, programmes and policy initiatives to achieve some target, which indicates the development process. In this study we discussed about allocation and utilisation of resources for health, so, it is important to take a close look at the some indicators related to health, in India as well as in North Eastern State (NESs). We have taken indicators related to health from the project of Millennium Development Goals (MDGs), becouse the set time for achieving these goals is near about.

**Millennium Development Goals (MDGs):** MDGs adopted by the United Nations in the year 2000. According to this project we have to achieve the MDGs goals by the year 2015. Due to limitation of the study we are focusing on only 3 goals of MDGs, which is related to health and education. These are given below:

(a) **Reduce Child Mortality:** Reduce by two thirds (2/3), between 1990 and 2015, the Percentage of One Year old Children Immunized against Measles and Infant Mortality Rate per thousand live births.

(b) **Improve Maternal Health:** Reduce by three quarters (3/4), between 1990 and 2015, the maternal mortality ratio per lakhs live births and Proportion of Deliveries attended by Skilled Health Personnel.

We can see from Table 11.3, in Assam, Meghalaya and Nagaland, there is sharp decline in the utilization pattern of the

**Table 11.3:** SPIP Approval and Expenditure under Child Health for 2011-12 to 2014-15 in North Eastern State

*(In Lakh Rs.)*

| States/ UTs | 2011-12 | | 2012-13 | | 2013-14 | | 2014-15 | |
|---|---|---|---|---|---|---|---|---|
| | SPIP Approval | Expenditure | SPIP Approval | Expenditure | SPIP Approval | Expenditure | SPIP Approval | Expenditure up to 31.12.2014 |
| Arunachal Pradesh | — | 0.4 | 212.7 | 61.87 | 137.83 | 64.8 | 126.49 | 10.94 |
| Assam | 410.04 | 414.15 | 1,474.33 | 776.09 | 2,575.66 | 1,568.67 | 3,003.88 | 990.86 |
| Manipur | 26.2 | 15.24 | 93.76 | 11.8 | 38.13 | 74.84 | 177.08 | 134.02 |
| Meghalaya | 12.12 | 13.49 | 283.01 | 34.91 | 178.22 | 12.9 | 364.5 | 38.45 |
| Mizoram | 23.81 | 1.18 | 62.5 | 17.34 | 140.1 | 78.16 | 86.45 | 6.77 |
| Nagaland | 33.86 | 38.11 | 199.34 | 63.84 | 178.9 | 46.39 | 128.97 | 9.11 |
| Tripura | 200.48 | 68.41 | 221.21 | 56.63 | 58.07 | 88.35 | 255.55 | 99.23 |
| **Grand Total** | **21,107.00** | **10,402.47** | **48,360.22** | **17,391.32** | **32,584.35** | **22,332.48** | **32,558.24** | **12,405.30** |

*Source:* SPIP—State Programme Implementation Plan.

resources allocated for providing to develop child health care facility there might be one of the reason that they have developed the sufficient healthcare facilities and some states like Mizoram, Manipur and Tripura showing an increasing pattern of utilization and there might be one of the reason that they are trying to improve their child health facility.

**Table 11.4:** Utilization of SPIP Approval and Expenditure under Child Health

(%)

| | 2011-12 | 2012-13 | 2013-14 | 2014-15 |
|---|---|---|---|---|
| Arunachal Pradesh | – | 29.09 | 47.01 | 8.65 |
| Assam | 101.00 | 52.64 | 60.90 | 32.99 |
| Manipur | 58.17 | 12.59 | 196.28 | 75.68 |
| Meghalaya | 111.30 | 12.34 | 7.24 | 10.55 |
| Mizoram | 4.96 | 27.74 | 55.79 | 7.83 |
| Nagaland | 112.55 | 32.03 | 25.93 | 7.06 |
| Tripura | 34.12 | 25.60 | 152.14 | 38.83 |

*Source:* Based on Table 11.3.

**Table 11.5:** Percentage of One Year old Children Immunized against Measles

| % of One Year old Children Immunized against Measles | | | | | | | | |
|---|---|---|---|---|---|---|---|---|
| Year | Arunanchal Pradesh | Assam | Manipur | Meghalaya | Mizoram | Nagaland | Tripura | INDIA |
| 1992-93 | 27.5 | 25.8 | 37 | 13.2 | 65.1 | 10 | 28.9 | 42.2 |
| 2005-06 | 53.5 | 37.4 | 52.8 | 43.8 | 69.5 | 27.3 | 59.9 | 58.8 |
| 2007-08 | – | 71.2 | – | 52.5 | 89.3 | – | 83.3 | 77.6 |
| 2009 | 48.2 | 80.1 | 60.3 | 74.1 | 81.1 | 52.2 | 68.8 | 74.1 |
| Likely Achievement 2015 | 91.2 | 100 | 91.6 | 100 | 82.0 | 100 | 100 | 89.1 |
| Target 2015 | 100 | 100 | 100 | 100 | 100 | 100 | 100 | 100 |

*Source:* Millennium Development Goals, India Country Report, 2015.

We can see from the table that Assam, Meghalaya, Nagaland and Tripura almost achieve the MDGs target to immunized one year old children against Measles, they all performing well, while Mizoram is the most awful performing state among the NESs with 17 percentage point improvement and it perform poor as compare to India.

**Table 11.6:** Infant Mortality Rate

| Year | Arunanchal Pradesh | Assam | Manipur | Meghalaya | Mizoram | Nagaland | Tripura | INDIA |
|---|---|---|---|---|---|---|---|---|
| 1990 | 75.3 | 76 | 29.1 | 54.3 | – | – | 46 | 80 |
| 2007 | 37 | 66 | 12 | 56 | 23 | 21 | 39 | 55 |
| 2009 | 32 | 61 | 16 | 59 | 36 | 26 | 31 | 50 |
| 2010 | 31 | 58 | 14 | 55 | 37 | 23 | 27 | 47 |
| 2011 | 32 | 55 | 11 | 52 | 34 | 21 | 29 | 44 |
| 2012 | 33 | 55 | 10 | 49 | 35 | 18 | 28 | 42 |
| 2013 | 32 | 54 | 10 | 47 | 35 | 18 | 26 | 40 |
| Likely Achievement 2015 | 27.8 | 53.21 | 9.94 | 47 | – | – | 25.61 | 39 |
| **Target 2015** | **25.10** | **25.33** | **9.70** | **18.10** | **–** | **–** | **15.33** | **26.67** |

*Source:* Millennium Development Goals, India Country Report, 2015.

The trend of IMR is similar for child mortality (Mohanty, 2009). We can see from Table 11.5 that all the NESs trying to reduce their infant mortality rate except Mizoram over the period. According to MDGs target Manipur almost achieved it, so, in this context Manipur is the best performing state toward achieving the MDGs target of IMR. Arunanchal Pradesh, Assam, Meghalaya, Nagaland, Tripura, these five states trying to improve their IMR but Mizoram is the state where IMR increases in 2013 over 2007 and show a negative trend.

**Table 11.7:** Infant Mortality by Sex (Per 1000 live Birth)

| Year | Arunanchal Pradesh | | Assam | | Manipur | | Meghalaya | | Mizoram | | Nagaland | | Tripura | | India | |
|---|---|---|---|---|---|---|---|---|---|---|---|---|---|---|---|---|
| | M | F | M | F | M | F | M | F | M | F | M | F | M | F | M | F |
| 2006 | 38 | 43 | 67 | 68 | 10 | 13 | 53 | 52 | 24 | 25 | 17 | 23 | 31 | 41 | 56 | 59 |
| 2010 | 31 | 32 | 56 | 60 | 11 | 16 | 55 | 56 | 36 | 39 | 19 | 28 | 25 | 29 | 46 | 49 |
| 2011 | 33 | 31 | 55 | 56 | 8 | 15 | 52 | 52 | 31 | 37 | 15 | 26 | 29 | 29 | 43 | 46 |
| 2012 | 32 | 35 | 54 | 57 | 10 | 11 | 48 | 50 | 33 | 37 | 15 | 22 | 26 | 29 | 41 | 44 |
| 2013 | 32 | 33 | 53 | 55 | 9 | 10 | 46 | 48 | 33 | 37 | 14 | 23 | 22 | 30 | 39 | 42 |

*Source:* Millennium Development Goals, India Country Report, 2015.

All the States performs well to reduce the infant mortality rate except Mizoram where infant mortality rate increases for both the sexes. If we see the infant mortality rate by sex in the NESs, we find that Assam is the best performing state and Mizoram perform much poor in both the sex, male and female and if we see the infant mortality rate for female as compare to male, we find that Tripura perform well to reduce the infant mortality of female as compare to male and Arunanchal Pradesh stood second best. The government on has admitted to low health allocation, which is the major driver for high infant and maternal mortality rates (Economic Survey, 2013-14).

In the sum up, we find that utilization of child healthcare approval and the improvement in the child health indicator are positively correlated. Higher growth rate and lower regional disparity in the indicator of human development can be achieved by increasing public investment in Social Sector (Ghosh, 2006).

From Table 11.7 and Fig. 11.2, it is clear that all the North Eastern States trying to improve their utilization under resource allocated for Maternal Health except Meghalaya where resource utilization continuously decreases over the time and it perform very poor while Assam is the best performing state

In term of Maternal Mortality rate, we are unable to analyse the performance of North Eastern states because the MMR data is not available, there might be one of the reason that auditing of the MMR are not going well, yet the NESs is the high focus state under the National Health Mission. We get MMR data for Assam and we find that it is the worst performing state as compare to all the state of India.

We can see from Table 11.8 that all the NESs trying to increase that more and more deliveries have been attended by skilled health personnel. Assam, Arunanchal Pradesh, Tripura and Manipur improves fast among NESs, but Nagaland and Meghalaya show slow improvement and Meghalaya is the worst performing state among NESs with only 6 point improvement over the period. We find that Assam utilize the resources under Maternal health and perform well in terms of deliveries attended by skilled health personnel and Meghalaya not utilize their resources and perform poor, in the sum up, we find that utilization of maternal health approval and the improvement in the maternal health indicator are positively correlated.

**Table 11.8:** State SPIP Approval and Expenditure under Maternal Health for F.Y. 2011-12 to 2014-15

*(In Lakh Rs.)*

| States / UTs | 2011-12 | | 2012-13 | | 2013-14 | | 2014-15 | |
|---|---|---|---|---|---|---|---|---|
| | SPIP Approval | Expenditure | SPIP Approval | Expenditure | SPIP Approval | Expenditure | SPIP Approval | Expenditure up to 31.12.2014 |
| Arunachal Pradesh | 172.9 | 138.06 | 283.09 | 180.83 | 451.95 | 301.2 | 572.63 | 35.63 |
| Assam | 11,561.35 | 9,452.87 | 14,374.31 | 13,581.92 | 16,621.84 | 13,642.00 | 22,028.59 | 4,450.53 |
| Manipur | 293.59 | 184.49 | 644.43 | 225.06 | 713.71 | 486.83 | 913.25 | 292.59 |
| Meghalaya | 175.47 | 132.95 | 822.86 | 243.66 | 685.89 | 111.24 | 1,084.11 | 302.16 |
| Mizoram | 319.39 | 134.7 | 480.22 | 207.07 | 427.59 | 347.83 | 447.14 | 44.97 |
| Nagaland | 333.24 | 203.49 | 620.79 | 364.4 | 704.33 | 514.7 | 736.71 | 24.9 |
| Tripura | 1,226.47 | 689.01 | 1,433.98 | 929.64 | 1,245.37 | 1,055.02 | 1,681.23 | 137.78 |
| **Grand Total** | **2,29,696.73** | **1,80,953.80** | **3,22,387.50** | **2,47,332.47** | **3,68,511.92** | **2,90,863.78** | **3,72,157.74** | **87,555.86** |

*Source:* SPIP—State Programme Implementation Plan.

**Table 11.9:** SPIP Approval and Expenditure under Maternal Health

| *State* | *2011-12* | *2012-13* | *2013-14* |
|---|---|---|---|
| Arunachal Pradesh | 79.85 | 63.88 | 66.64 |
| Assam | 81.76 | 94.49 | 82.07 |
| Manipur | 62.84 | 34.92 | 68.21 |
| Meghalaya | 75.77 | 29.61 | 16.22 |
| Mizoram | 42.17 | 43.12 | 81.35 |
| Nagaland | 61.06 | 58.70 | 73.08 |
| Tripura | 56.18 | 64.83 | 84.72 |

*Source:* Based on Table 11.7.

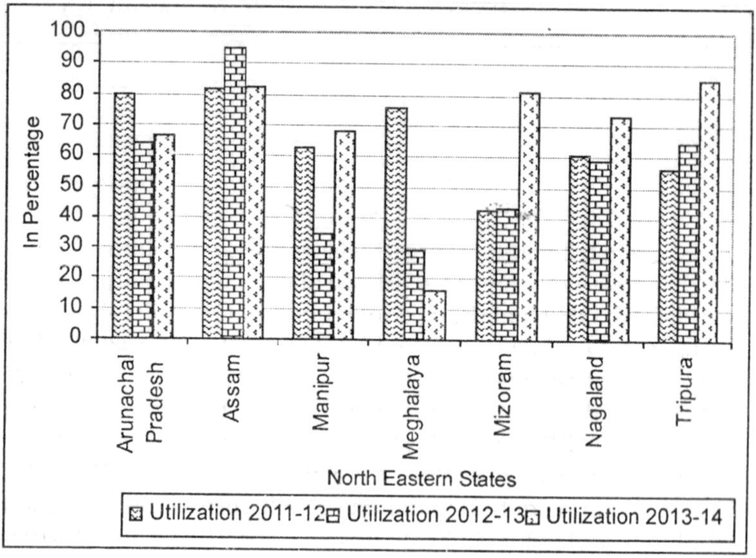


**Fig. 11.2:** Resource Utilization Allocated for Maternal Health
*Source:* Based on Table 11.7.

Considering the above variables, we can say that there is positive correlation between utilization of resources and improvement in the related indicators. Improvement in Infant Mortality Rate and Maternal mortality rate has been accelerated, but overall progress is still short of meeting the Millennium Development Goals.

**Limitations and Suggestion**

Flow of funds from Central to State has two parts, Plan Expenditure

**Table 11.8:** Deliveries Attended by Skilled Health Personnel in NESs

| | *Proportion of Deliveries attended by Skilled Health Personnel* | | | | | | | |
|---|---|---|---|---|---|---|---|---|
| *Year* | *Arunanchal Pradesh* | *Assam* | *Manipur* | *Meghalaya* | *Mizoram* | *Nagaland* | *Tripura* | *India* |
| 1992-93 | 22 | 18 | 39.9 | 37.9 | 62.2 | 18.9 | 32.2 | 33 |
| 2005-06 | 20.8 | 27.5 | 52.8 | 22.2 | 47.4 | 17.9 | 45.4 | 39 |
| 2007-08 | 48.8 | 39.9 | 55.3 | 28.9 | 63.3 | 24.7 | 47.2 | 52 |
| 2009 | 71.9 | 65.5 | 82.7 | 65.2 | 85.1 | 43.8 | 83.1 | 76.2 |
| Likely Achievement 2015 | 74.9 | 71.7 | 82.9 | 43.9 | 76.7 | 38.3 | 78.8 | 77.3 |
| Target 2015 | 100 | 100 | 100 | 100 | 100 | 100 | 100 | 100 |

*Source:* Millennium Development Goals, India Country Report, 2015.

and Non-Plan Expenditure. Here we examine only plan expenditure, but the large share of non-plan expenditure is not discussed in this chapter:

- There should be transparency in the flow of funds and its utilization.
- Take a close look on health outlay and its utilization, it is an essential area of concern because many of maternal, infant and child survival depends upon public health system.
- It should be audited that whether the fund is being used, for what purposes, it should be questioned.
- Because we have limited resources, so, we should provide basic amenities only for targeted people, not for all.
- Funds should be spent on the adornment of the city only and only when we provide at least basic amenities of vulnerable people.
- We can do adornment of the city by different angle, providing more and more amenities in public health system and education institutions.

## References

Berman, P. and Ahuja, R. (December 2010). *Government Health Financing in India: Challenges in Achieving Ambitious Goals.* Washigton DC. URL or DOI.

Economic Survey. (Various Issues). New Delhi: Ministry of Finance GOI, downloaded from http://www.researchgate.net/publication/236177139_

Ministry of Health and Family welfare, GOI URL or DOI

Mohanty, S.K. (2009). *Progress and Prospects of Millennium Development Goals in India*. Mumbai: International Institute for Population Sciences. URL or DOI.

Nayah Purusottam (2012). *Human Development in Northeastern Region of India: Issues and Challenges*. MPRA paper no. 41582.

Saikia, D. and Das, K.K. (2014). Access to Public Healthcare in the Rural North East India. *The NEHU Journal*, 12: 77-100.

Sample registration system (2013). *Maternal and Child Mortality and Total Fertility Rates*. Office of Registrar General. India.

www.nrhm.gov.in

www.planningcommisson.com

Author or Agency (2015). *Millennium Development Goals India Country Report*. New Delhi: Central Statistical Organization Ministry of Statistics and Programme Implementation GOI.

# 12
# Community Participation and Effectiveness of ICDS
## A Case Study of Kamrup District of Assam

*Nayanakhee Sarma*

### Introduction

The holistic development of women and children plays an influential role in the overall upliftment of the society. Children play a crucial role in the human resource development of a nation and are now-a-days given utmost priority in human resource development. This is because young children are the most vulnerable and also because, human development of children takes place during this period. Today all over the world investment in human development is given utmost importance as it eventually leads to economic development of the nation. There is an inter linkage among survival of children, growth and development and it requires to look at it as a holistic approach. Education, health and nutrition must have a balanced linkage among them for the development of children.

Well-functioning public services, especially in fields such as education and health, are critical in fostering participatory growth as well as in ensuring that growth leads to rapid improvement in people's living conditions. There should be systematic evaluation of the different evaluation programmes which in turn helps to increase the effectiveness of the programme. Moreover, there should be active initiation, involvement and awareness about the various government policies and programmes by the intended beneficiaries and make it more demand driven.

The Government of India launched the Integrated Child Development Services (ICDs) in 1975 in order to cater to the needs of early childhood care and also to lay the foundation of the human development in India. ICDS has today expanded all over India and at present it is the world's largest and most unique programme for the holistic development of the children. The main objectives of the programme is to provide pre-school education on one hand and to break the inter-generational cycle of malnutrition, reduction of morbidity and mortality caused by nutritional deficiencies, reduce school dropouts and to enhance the capability of the mother to look after the normal health and nutritional needs of the child through proper nutrition and health education by reaching out the children, pregnant women, lactating mothers and adolescent girls.

Focusing on some of the goals of the Millennium Development Goals (MDGs) viz. eradication of extreme poverty and hunger, reduction in child mortality and to improve maternal health; there is a need to assure nutritional and health security to every child and women. ICDS is a child development programme currently functioning in India which has the potential to achieve the MDGs in India. At this point of time when we have reached 2015, India has not been able to achieve the MDGs and the gaps still exist (Table 12.1) in the areas of nutrition, health and education of children and women which are the main aspects in the process of overall development of an individual. According to the first five-year review in 2005 by UN, it was found that the MDGs had become central to the way government, international development agencies, and Non-Governmental Organizations (NGOs) carry out their development efforts. India too worked out towards achieving the MDGs. India has its own indicators as per Indian framework for the different targets under MDGs. Table 12.1 clearly shows that India lags behind in terms of nutritional and health status of children and women, and will miss the targets of MDG 2015. So at this point there is a need of well functioning government policies and programme and improve the effectiveness of the existing programmes to bridge the gaps and achieve the MDGs.

The importance of a programme like ICDS is realised when we consider some facts regarding the child population of India. India is home to the largest child population in the world with 158 million children, constituting 15.42 per cent of the population

**Table 12.1:** Showing Gaps in achieving MDGs in India

| India | 2005-06 | 2012 | Likely achievements 2015 | Target 2015 |
|---|---|---|---|---|
| Under weight children (< 3 years) | 40.4 | NA | 32.85 | 26 |
| Under 5 mortality rate | 74.3 | 52 | 49 | 42 |
| Infant mortality rate | 57 | 42 | 40 | 27 |
| % of one year old child (12-23 months) immunised against measles | 58.8 | NA | 89.06 | 100 |
| MMR (death per 1,00,000 live birth) | 254 | 178 | 140 | 109 |

*Source:* India Country Report 2014: Ministry of Statistical and Programme Implementation (2014) Millennium Development Goals.

below 6 years as per 2011 census. A significant proportion of them lives in economic and social environment of poverty, poor environmental sanitation and drinking water facility which eventually lead to spread of disease and infection, inappropriate feeding practices and child care and also inadequate access to primary health etc. In India, approximately 60 million children are underweight. In 1998-99, 47 per cent of children under three were underweight or severely underweight, and a further 26 per cent were mildly underweight such that, in total, underweight afflicted almost three-quarters of Indian children. It is seen that even after reaching 2015 there is a huge proportion of children in India who are underweight. Economic growths alone will not reduce the existing malnutrition among children in India and meet the MDG target and bridge the gap. It can be achieved either through effective implementation of the existing programmes or implement new programmes to bridge the gaps.

The effectiveness of a public policy or a programme on child development also to a great extent depends on the role of women and local community in the overall development of children and the society. Development scholars like M.P. Todaro and S.C. Smith view that women play the central role in the process of development. Globally, women tend to be poorer than men. They are more deprived in health and education and in freedom in all forms. Moreover, women have primary responsibility for child rearing, and the resources that they are able to bring to this task will determine whether the cycle of poverty from generation to generation will be broken. Children need better health and education, and studies from around the world confirm that mothers tend to spend a significant high fraction of income under their control for the benefit of their children than their fathers do. To make the biggest impact on development, the society must empower and invest in its women (Todaro and Smith, 2012). Women's education and literacy tend to reduce the mortality rates of children. The influence works through many channels, but perhaps most immediately, it works through the importance that mothers typically attach to the welfare of the children, and the opportunity the mothers have, when their agency is respected and empowered, to influence family decisions in that direction. Moreover, active inanition of the members of the society and involvement of the community in the overall development of children and women is important at the grassroots level which helps in proper implementation and functioning of the different government development programmes.

Therefore, ICDS being a development programme for children and women in India there is a need for effective implementation of ICDS at grassroots level and reaches the target population and intended beneficiary. So, at this point to know the effectiveness of the ICDS it is important to look at the supply side indicators of ICDS, find out the gaps that exist in the field, at the same time it is necessary to look at its outcome indicators and to what extent it has been successful in reaching its goal and target population. It is also impotent to look at the involvement and participation of the community and the stakeholders in the programme and to what extent it is demand driven.

## Literature Review

As per the Planning Commission Report 2011, at the national level there have been only three evaluations of ICDS schemes – NIPCCD (1992) and (2006) and NCAER in (1998) and Das Gupta (2005).

One of the most recent studies of ICDS at nation level taken by Planning Commission in 2011 of all the states of India shows that gap exists in ICDS. Some of the outcomes of the study were: AWC surveys cover about 62 per cent of the estimated number of children. At the national level, of those recorded in the delivery register for ICDS benefits, 64 per cent received SN (may not be for all 300 days), immunisation and other benefits, 12 per cent received other benefits, but not supplementary nutrition and 24 per cent did not receive any benefits. Around 78 per cent of the women (pregnant and lactating) and 42 per cent of adolescent girls recorded in the delivery register actually received benefits under SNP (not necessary for all 300 days and as per entitlement). At the national level, 41 per cent of children, 38 per cent of women and 10 per cent adolescent girls are estimated to have received supplementary nutrition in 2008-09. Some of the good performing states in terms of frequency of delivery of Supplementary nutrition to child beneficiaries for 300 days are Haryana, Karnataka, Kerala, Maharashtra, Odisha, Tamil Nadu, West Bengal whereas low performing states are Assam, Bihar, Madhya Pradesh, Rajasthan, Uttar Pradesh and Uttarakhand. Moreover, according to the study the most important condition for successful implementation of the ICDS programme is the adequacy of infrastructure of Anganwadi Centres (AWCs).

The findings of NCAER (2001) study also shows the status and gaps that exist in ICDS, some of the findings were: Regarding infrastructure 40 per cent of AWC with *pucca* structures, 50 per cent AWC had adequate cooking space, indoor and outdoor space.Toilet facilities at AWC were dismal (nearly 17%). Seventy five per cent AWC reported having weighing scales. Finding of educational qualifications of AWWs shows 50 per cent AWWs were matriculate and above 30 per cent were educated up to middle school, 15 per cent educated up to primary level. Regarding training of AWW, in service training was quite low (less than 30%), 84 per cent of AWWs received some kind of training. Findings of coverage of SN showed that, 65 per cent of the eligible children were registered in AWC and of the registered 64 per centres availed of SNP, 67.3 per cent of AWC provided food supplements for more than 21 days during the last month of survey. Acceptability of SN showed that, about 63 per cent of AWWs reported poor quality of nutrition effecting the functioning of AWC, 42 per cent of the households perceived that the nutrition supplied by the AWC was very good. Interruption in distribution of SN 67 per cent of *Anganwadi* perceived that there was irregular supply of nutrition in their respective AWC. Regarding PSE, 60 per cent of the eligible children were enrolled for PSE. Inadequate in service training of AWWs in some of the states and inadequate availability of PSE materials were some reasons for low enrolment. 68.5 per cent of

kept the government on its toes, making it difficult, for instance, "for an *Anganwadi* to remain closed without immediate enquiry"

Moreover, women's agency also played a crucial role in this success story, in several ways. First, ICDS in Tamil Nadu is managed almost entirely by women, not only at the *Anganwadi* level, but also at higher levels. Second, women have helped to hold the system accountable. The "pressure from below", i.e. demands for the services comes largely from women—women who value the ICDS and are able to voice their demands. Third, women have also helped to make health and nutrition political issues. For instance, women's votes in Tamil Nadu matter a great deal, and this forces political leaders to respond to their aspirations, including those relating to child development.

According to another study on Community Participation in ICDS, Banarjee (2008), in North Kolkata, published in "Research on ICDS: An Overview" by NIPCCD, recommended after evaluating the findings that, there is need to have a short duration preparation phase to raise awareness of the community regarding ICDS services, and the benefits that the community could derive from the programme, the ICDS package should be made flexible to meet needs of the community and the training of project functionaries should be strengthened to impart them specific skills to elicit community participation. Therefore, there is a need for home visits by the AWW and the community health workers for greater participation of the community in the programme and make it more demand driven.

The study titled "Child Malnutrition" Ghosh (2004) published in *'Economic and Political Weekly'* showed that ICDS has to be converted into a true health, nutrition and development programme, and not limited to a food dole programme. It was found that 30 per cent of newborns have weight below 2.5 kgs, among whom mortality is higher and also 47 per cent children under 4 years of age are malnourished (NFHS-2; 1998-99), and 18 per cent are severely malnourished. Some of the main reasons are poor living conditions and lack of awareness of the young child's food requirements. Therefore, there is a need for spreading awareness about the feeding practices of children through ICDS among the members of the community.

In another study titled "Food Dole or Health, Nutrition and Development Programme" Ghosh (2006), it was found that almost a third of babies born in India are under weight, they weigh less than 2.5 kg at birth, mainly due to young age and poor nutrition of mother. According to National Family Health Survey (1998-99), 14 per cent of girls aged 15-19 years were married and 61 per cent of all women were married before 18 years. According to NFHS-2 only one third of Indian children are offered semi-solid food between 6-9 months of age. This sets the beginning of malnutrition. This is not because of lack of food in the households but because of lack of knowledge. Therefore, there is a need to create awareness among people about the nutritional needs of the children through ICDS and prevent malnutrition among children in India. The AWW must make regular home visits and meeting with the mothers to spread the knowledge about child's nutritional and health status.

To examine what India is doing for the survival, well-being and rights of children there is need to address the structural roots of child deprivation mainly mass poverty, social discrimination, lack of education and gender inequality. The first six years of life have a decisive and lasting influence on the on the child's health, well-being, aptitude and opportunities. At this point there is a need to rethink ICDS as a right based prospective and the arguments put forward by Dipa Sinha (2006) in her paper is that every mother and child has right to health and well-being and it is non-negotiable, state obligation to ensure all mothers and children have access to basic health care and nutrition and also a change in existing social norms. Therefore, ICDS should not only just be a welfare scheme but protect the rights of children and women (right to nutrition, health and education) and make it more demand driven. ICDS and the service provided at the *Anganwadi* centre is still not explicitly acknowledged as an institution created to fulfil the state's obligation towards the protecting of the rights of mother and children, and this is mainly due to absence of social norms such as gender discrimination, attitude towards women, pregnancy, nutrition and child care which have a great impact on the status of maternal and child health. Moreover, there is also a need to create new social environment because in absence of supportive environment even the best services do not reach the target groups. There is a need to mobilize entire community for health of mother and child, inclusion of gram *panchayat* and local bodies for reviewing the functions of *Anganwadi*. Therefore, unless the services of ICDS are not demand driven, ICDS cannot achieve its intended goals and the programme gaps will exist.

In a review undertaken by the DSW (District Social Welfare) of Assam in March 2012 identified several improvements as well as service gaps in ICDS. For example, while the coordination between the health sector and ICDS is better, additional effort from ICDS functionaries is needed to make it more successful and sustainable. Whereas the introduction of village health and nutrition days (VHND) caused a marked increase in health check-up of children under six years of age, referral services, a crucial component for identifying and providing timely treatment to ICDS beneficiaries, are weak and need strengthening. Overall, the State's child health and nutrition indicators are not encouraging as noted in the National Family Health Survey-III (NFHS -III, 2005-06). More than 40 per cent of children below age three years in Assam are underweight, and the weighing efficiency of children in the age group of 0-5 years in ICDS in the state is only 46.6 per cent.

According to the Annual Report of Ministry of Women and Child Development, 2009-10, in Assam only 61.7 per cent of Anganwadi Centres are operational against the sanctioned Anganwadi centre, which is the lowest compare to the other North Eastern states. Assam has spent only 75.6 per cent (which is also the lowest among North Eastern states) of money released by Government of India for making Anganwadi Centre, salary etc. other than food. Assam spent only 90.50 per cent (including state share) money on Supplementary nutrition food in the year 2008-09. The percentage of amount spent by Assam is far behind than other NE States. Other states had spent more than the sanctioned amount; in fact 5 NE states had spent more than double the sanctioned amount. In the year 2009-10, there were 219 ICDS projects in Assam, out of which 196 projects are operational.

Comparing Assam with India as per the "Evaluation Report on Integrated Child Development Services" by Programme Evaluation Organisation, Planning Commission Government of India (2011), Assam had more than 60 per cent AWC with their own building. This is better than the national average of AWC with their own buildings which is only 42.5 per cent.

Assam is ranked 14th in the State-wise performance of ICDS programme in Infrastructure facilities. The source of drinking water in AWC's in Assam is primarily hand-pump which is about 75.1 per cent and that of pipe source is only about 8.1 per cent whereas the National average for pipe sourced drinking water is 28.4 per cent and that of hand-pump source is 58.8 per cent.

Assam has about 16.2 per cent of AWC's having Flush system of Toilets which is better than the national average of 12.4 per cent. But 56.1 per cent of the AWCs of Assam does not have any facilities of toilets. This average on the national level is 61.5 per cent. 87.5 per cent of AWCs of Assam has their own Weighing Scales (Baby) whereas the national average is 68.9 per cent.

In Assam 73.9 per cent of AWW reported a regular visit of ANM and 83.7 per cent reported of receiving a medical kit whereas the national average of AWW reporting regular visit by ANM is 61.7 per cent and that of receiving medical kit is 62.4 per cent. In Assam 93.4 per cent of AWWs are trained well to conduct pre-school education which is almost similar to the national average of 93.6 per cent.About 70 per cent of community leaders on National level felt that the ICDS programme was "very beneficial" to the community and 26.5 per cent of them regarded the programme to be beneficial to "some extent". In Assam only 39 per cent of the community leaders are of the opinion that the AWC are "very beneficial" which is lowest among all the states and about 58.5 per cent felt it to be beneficial to "some extent".

Assam is one of the North Eastern states of India. Its total population is 3,12,05,576 as per 2011 census and its total rural population is 2,68,07,034, i.e. 85.90 per cent of the total population and its urban population is 43,98,542, i.e. 14.10 per cent of the total population. According to 2011 census total population of children in the age group 0-6 years in Assam is 46,38,130, i.e. 14.86 per cent of the population. It is seen here that Assam has a very high IMR, i.e. 55 per 1000 live birth in 2011 as compared to 44 at all India level. Again IMR in rural Assam is 58 per 1000 live birth and that of urban Assam is 34 in 2011. Again Assam has high under five mortality rate of 78 per 1000 live births as against 55 at all India level. On the other hand according to the NFSHS round 3 survey 2005-06 it is seen that only 26.8 per cent of the children in the age group 0-6 years received services of AWC in Assam as against 28.4 per cent at all-India level.

Now, coming to the districts of Kamrup and Kamrup Metro; are two adjourning districts and are nearest to the capital of Assam, Dispur and Dispur comes under Kamrup Metro district. The total population of Kamrup is 15,17,542 and that of Kamrup Metro is 12,53,938. The population of children in the age group 0-6 years in

Kamrup is 2,00,061, i.e. 13.18 per cent and of Kamrup Metro is 1,25,386, i.e. 10 per cent of the total population.The total rural population of Kamrup is 13,75,148, i.e. 90.62 per cent and that of Kamrup Metro is 2,16,927, i.e. 17.30 per cent. The urban population of Kamrup is 1,42,394, i.e. 9.38 per cent and that of Kamrup Metro is 10,37,001, i.e. 82.70 per cent according to 2011 census. Since there is more concentration of rural population in Kamrup for this study two rural ICDS block of Kamrup was taken, i.e. Hajo and Chayani Bordwar, and for the urban part of the study two ICDS Blocks from Kamrup Metro was taken, i.e. Dispur and Guwahati Urban Block. The following data shows that there is difference in delivery of services of ICDS in urban and rural blocks of Kamrup and Kamrup Metro.

The literature shows that gaps exist in the functioning of ICDS at national level, state level and also at the district level. It also shows that there is lack of awareness about the programme among the members of the community and there is a need for community participation in the programme to make it more effective.

## Relevance of the Topic

The study tries to see how community participation and women's involvement in ICDS can help to fulfil the gaps that exist in ICDS and make it more effective in both rural and urban areas. As far as ICDS is concerned, the main challenge is to break the vicious circle of low awareness, low expectations, weak demand and lethargic implementation. In a recent evaluation of ICDS by the Planning Commission, startling contrasts were found in women's awareness of children's food entitlements under the programme. So, there is a need for more initiative and involvements at the grassroots levels and make ICDS more demand driven.

It is also necessary to understand the difficulties faced at the *Anganwadi* centres level by the *Anganwadi* Workers. The real problem lies in its implementation of the programme, which arises out of inadequate funding, lack of convergence, accountability of those managing and implementing the programme, lack of community ownership and the general perception about this being a feeding programme and not an Early Childhood Development programme.

The study also has relevance because Assam has a significant proportion of children in the age group 0-6 years and the same time has high IMR (Infant Mortality Rate) of 55 per 1000 live births. Since ICDS aims at combating child mortality it important to understand the functioning of ICDS in Assam at the grassroots level and identifying the difficulties in functioning, community initiative and involvement in the programme, women's role and participation in ICDS both in rural and urban areas. The study between rural and urban areas may reveal how there is a difference in functioning, community participation and women's role in ICDS in rural and urban areas of Assam.

Research in this topic will bring to light the challenges and opportunities faced by various Governmental and Non-Governmental Programmes at the grassroots level and how this can vary in different context (as in rural and urban).

Purpose of taking this topic as my research is its. Moreover, it will also bring to light how ICDS has importance as a planning scheme and has greater importance towards the development of women and children in India and how through ICDS India can move forward towards the achievement of the MDGs.

## Objectives

In order to study the difference in the performance of ICDS in different blocks of rural and urban areasat first it is necessary to study the supply side indicators both from the perspectives of AWW and the mothers whose children attend AWC centre. On the other hand it is also necessary to study the demand side indicators from the perspective of mothers whose children attend AWC and also from the perspective of the AWW. At last it is also necessary to examine the level of co-operation and participation of the local community in improving the performance of ICDS since it is a community based programme.

The main research questions taken here is to see is there any difference in the performance of ICDS in urban and rural areas and dose community participation and involvement of women in ICDS programme improves its performance.

## Methodology

The study is based on both secondary and primary data. Secondary information's are collected from various published articles and published reports both at national and state level. Primary data was collected from 60 AWCs over a period of one month, 30 AWCs from urban blocks and 30 AWCs from rural blocks. Two projects each from rural and urban blocks of Kamrup Metro and Kamrup districts were randomly selected. The blocks are, Dispur Block and Guwahati Urban Block of Kamrup Metro and Hajo Block and Chayani Bordwar Block of Kamrup. The AWCs (*Anganwadi* centres) were randomly selected and fifteen (15) AWC from each block were selected and the total sample size is sixty (60).

Data was collected from the functionaries of ICDS at grassroots level, i.e. the AWWs (*Anganwadi* workers) and also from the mothers of the children who attend the AWC in the age group (3-6) years. Altogether 60 AWW from the 60 AWC visited were interviewed by interview schedule method trough close ended coded questions. 30 AWW from rural and 30 AWW from urban were interviewed. Similarly, mothers of children whose children attend AWC were interviewed in the same method and also through focus group discussion. Altogether 120 mothers have been interviewed, 60 from rural and 60 from urban.

The analysis of the data has been done in SPSS 20 version using statistical tools like cross tabulated data for comparing urban and rural outcomes of frequency and relative frequency expressed in terms of percentage. The second part of the analysis is devoted to comparing the difference between the performance of ICDS in rural and urban areas, and to know if the differences are statistically significant. Since the data collected are categorical in nature, Mann Whitney U test has been used.

The study analyses the grassroots level responses received from the AWW and the mothers, whose children attend AWC. The study looks at the supply side/input indicators, outcome indicators and the demand indicators from the perspective of the AWW at the AWC level. Further, we look at the supply side indicators (both output and input), demand and co-operation indicators along with general profile of the mothers from the prospective of the mothers whose children attend AWC.

## Findings

Responses regarding the supply side indicators, demand side

indicators and the level of co-operation has been taken from the prospective of both AWW and the mothers whose children attend AWC has been taken and analysed in two different context, i.e. rural and urban. Responses from both the givers side, i.e. AWW and the receiver's side, i.e. the mothers whose children attend AWC at grassroots level will bring to light the functioning of ICDS at grassroots level in rural and urban blocks of Assam. It will also bring to light if gap exist in the delivery of services and receiving of services by the stakeholders in scheduled period.The findings have been recorded for the responses receive from 30 AWW of rural and 30 AWW of urban in Table 12.2. And in Table 12.3 the responses from 60 mothers from rural and 60 mothers from urban.

implies 2-tailed p-value of the Mann Whitney U test is significant at 95 per cent confidence interval, if the p-value is greater than 0.05 then we accept our null hypothesis that there is no significant difference between rural and urban and if the P is less than 0.05 we reject our null hypothesis and accept our alternative hypothesis that there is significant difference between rural and urban.

## Analysis

Children in the age group 0-6 years make a significant proportion of the population of Assam (14.86%), but at the same time it has a high IMR of 55 per 1000 live births, with 58 per 1000 live birth in rural Assam and 34 in urban Assam as per 2011 census. Assam also has high under five mortality rate of 78 per 1000 live birth. So at this point it is important to study the effectiveness of ICDS comparing rural and urban centres in Assam taking Kamrup and Kamrup Metro districts because ICDS is one such programme, which one of the goals is to reduce child mortality. Again though in most of the national level studies on ICDS Assam as a whole has been include in the studies, but there has not been much research at district level comparing rural and urban. So, the study it tries to analysis that is there any difference in effectiveness of ICDS in rural and urban areas of Kamrup as whole and also see to what extent the services of ICDS are demand driven and co-operation of the community both in rural and urban Kamrup and find that does it have any effect on the effectiveness functioning of ICDS.

**Table 12.2:** Finding on the Services Received as Obtained from the Responses of AWW

| | *Response from AWW* | | | *Percentage of Positive Response* | | |
|---|---|---|---|---|---|---|
| *Supply Side Indicators* | *Broad Areas* | *Material or Service Provided* | *Variables used to study the broad areas* | *Rural %* | *Urban %* | *Test Statistic Asymp. Sign. (2-tailed)* |
| | 1. Materials Received | Infrastructure | AWC running in | | | 0.108 |
| | | | Rented House | 13.3 | 33.3 | |
| | | | Own house | 46.7 | 36.3 | |
| | | | Club House | 29 | 20 | |
| | | | Primary School | 16.7 | 10 | |
| | | | Type of house | | | 0.522 |
| | | | Pucca house | 76.7 | 83.3 | |
| | | | Kachcha house | 23.3 | 16.7 | |
| | | | Drinking water source | | | 0.109 |
| | | | Own Source | 30 | 16.7 | |
| | | | Public Well | 10 | 3.3 | |
| | | | Public Tap | 33.3 | 36.7 | |
| | | | From Nearby House | 16.7 | 30 | |
| | | | Presence of Sanitation | 63.3 | 50 | 0.301 |
| | | | Presence of weighting machines | 63.3 | 50 | 0.301 |
| | 2. Delivery of Services | Regularity of Supplementary Nutrition | Hot Cooked Meals | 100 | 100 | |
| | | | Take home ration | 96.6 | 3.3 | |
| | 3. Man Power | AWW profile | Education Qualification AWW | 43.3 (10th passed) | 40 (12th passed) | 0.139 |
| | | | Training Received by AWW | 100 | 93.3 | |
| | | How often health personals visit AWC | Once a week | 3.3 | 3.3 | 0.037 |
| | | | Once in 15 days | 43.3 | 20 | |
| | | | Once a month | 43.3 | 53.3 | |
| | | | Once every 3 month | 10 | 6.7 | |
| | | | Rare | 0 | 16.7 | |
| Demand Side Indicators | 1. Services of ICDS demanded | | | 73.3 | 24.3 | 0.019 |
| | 2. Which Service Demanded | | Supplementary nutrition | 56.7 | 46.7 | |
| | | | PSE | 96.7 | 96.7 | |
| | | | Immunization | 3.3 | 6.7 | |
| | | | Health Check up | 23.3 | 10 | |
| | | | Referral Services | 3.3 | 0 | |
| Co-operation | | | By local community and stakeholders | 100 | 93.3 | |
| | | | Local women | 60 | 43.3 | |
| | | | Mothers whose children attend AWC | 90 | 63.3 | |
| | | | Local community leader | 43.3 | 16.6 | |

*Note:* * indicates that the Test statistics is significant at 5 per cent level of significance.

*Source:* Field Survey, February 2015.

**Table 12.3:** Findings on the Services received as obtained from the Response of the Mothers whose Children attend AWC

| *Arial* | *Response of the mothers whose children attend AWC* | | | *Percentage of Positive Response* | | |
|---|---|---|---|---|---|---|
| *Supply side indicators* | *Broad Areas* | *Material or Service Provided* | *Variables used to Study the Broad Areas* | *Rural* | *Urban* | *Test Statistic Asymp Sign.(2-tailed)* |
| | 1. Materials Received | Services to pregnant mothers | Mothers registerred in AWC when pregnant. | 96.7 | 68.3 | 0.00 |
| | | | Did mothers receive anything when registered during pregnancy; | 83.3 | 61.7 | 0.008 |
| | | Services for children attending AWC | Was the child weighted by the AWW | 88.1 | 91.7 | 0.524 |
| | | | Discussion of child's nutrition and growth chart | 72.9 | 81.7 | 0.255 |
| | | | Receiving of medicines. | 54.2 | 43.3 | 0.236 |
| | 2. Delivery of services | Perception of quality of food given as SNP, | Good | 44.1 | 56.7 | 0.129 |
| | | | Acceptable | 52.5 | 43.3 | |
| | | | Bad; | 3.4 | 0 | |
| | | Perception of Quality of PSE, | Not Good | 3.4 | 1.7 | 0.200 |
| | | | Somewhat good | 61 | 51.7 | |
| | | | Good | 35.6 | 46.7 | |
| | | Regularity of opening of AWC | Regular | 98.3 | 86.7 | 0.017 |
| | | | Not Regular | 1.7 | 13.3 | |
| Demand Side Indicators | 1. What knowledge mothers have about ICDS | | Free Education | 36.3 | 33.3 | Insigni-ficant |
| | | | Free education and Mid day meal | 83.3 | 86.67 | |
| | | | Complete child development programme | 6.6 | 8.3 | |
| | 2. Why do they send children to AWC | | For food | 80 | 46.67 | Insigni-ficant |
| | | | For education | 91.6 | 93.3 | |
| | | | For health services | 66.67 | 30 | |
| Co-operation | | | Co-operation in AWC by mothers | 76.7 | 56.7 | 0,021* |

*Note:* * indicates that the Test statistics is significant at 5 per cent level of significance.

*Source:* Field Survey, February 2015.

Regarding the indicators taken under supply side indicators, out come indicators and demand and co-operation from community it is justified that similar indicators were taken to access the effectiveness of ICDS in two of the national level studies, i.e. the study "Three decades of ICDS" as well as the Planning Commission Report 2011. Although all the indicators taken in the national level studies were not included in this study due to lack of time and the resources were limited, but best efforts have been made to get a true picture and as per the objectives of the study.

The indicator taken on the supply side under man power was the profile of the AWW, under which AWW's education qualification and the trainings received was taken in this study. Similar indicators were used in most of the past studies at the national level. As per national study by NCEAR 2001 and NIPCCD 2006 study showed that the higher percentage of AWWs are in the education qualification of either being matriculate or passed higher secondary passed. And the findings of this study too show the same result, as higher percentage of AWW are under the group of matriculation and higher secondary passed. But there is difference when compared between rural and urban as there was higher percentage of AWW in the category of matriculation as compared to higher level in higher secondary passed in urban sector, but as per the Mann Whitney test this difference between rural and urban is not significant. The education qualification of the AWW is important because it affects to a great extent the effective function of the AWC and understanding the norms and effectively implementing them in the actual field. Similarly, the percentage AWW who received job training are important for the effective implementation of the ICDS programme and it was found in the study almost 100 per cent of the AWWs have received training. Similar findings regarding the trainings of AWW were also found in the various national level studies.

The next supply side indicator under materials received is infrastructure under which, where the AWC running in *pacca* or *kachcha* building. It is seen most of the AWC is running in *pacca* house except a few centres in both rural and urban and when compared with previous national studies which shows lower percentage running in *pacca* houses. Moreover, regarding the where the AWC is running it is the study that high percentage of AWC are running in own building both in rural and urban. A proper permanent all weathered building in needed for functioning and running of the ICDS services. Regarding the presence of sanitation 1531 AWC has been targeted in 2012-13 under Total Sanitation Camping under taken by Government of India in both Kamrup and Kamrup Metro districts, but this is not sufficient as lag still exist in coverage of AWC by sanitation both in urban and rural blocks. Past studies shows that the coverage of AWC by sanitation or toilet facility is dismantle, even the present study shows that out of the surveyed AWC 63.3 per cent had sanitation facility in rural and 50 per cent in urban and needs. The study also shows that there is no significant difference between rural and urban AWCs and the modal source of drinking water being nearby public tap in both rural and urban centres. Both sanitation and drinking water are two basic facilities for the people and also for sound health and it is important to avail the AWC with these basic facilities as ICDS aims at bringing nutrition and health security of the children. Regarding the presence of working weighting machine it was found from the past studies that there have been adequate presence of weighting machines in the AWC, but in the study it was found that only 63.3 per cent in rural and 50 per cent in urban had working weighting machines, which deviates from the existing literature and there is a need of weighting machines at AWC as one of the objective of ICDS growth monitoring of the children and is a very important point for the effectiveness of ICDS at AWC level.

As per the needs of ICDS there is a need for proper co-ordination among the community health workers and the AWC and the people of the community, as the different studies shows that ANM plays an important role in delivery of different health services at the AWC and there is regularity in their visits to AWC, similar findings were seen in the study as ANM being the most visited health personal to the AWC in both rural and urban. But there is irregularity of these visits in urban areas and this can be mainly due to the fact that in urban there is not much demand for health services at the AWC as alternatives are easily available. Moreover, it was seen and also reported by the AWW in the rural areas that they had a very good co-operation and co-ordination between the government health centres, community health workers and the people of the community. Moreover, the regular home visits by the AWWs and the community health workers helps to bring awareness among the people of the community that ICDS is not just a food programme, but a complete health, nutrition and child development programme.

Regarding the regularity of supplementary nutrition in the previous studies it is seen that the delivery of supplementary nutrition to the registered beneficiaries was above average of 65 per cent. In this study it was seen that there was regularity of supplementary nutrition to the children 3-6 years both in rural and urban areas as it is one of the main factor of attracting children to the AWC both for nutrition and PSE. Also the people are well aware of this and demand for this service both in rural and urban areas and this is one of the driving factors for regularity of supplementary nutrition to the children who attend AWC. But there is irregularity in the delivery of dry THR to the other beneficiaries in the urban area but on the other hand there is regularity in rural areas. This is mainly because in urban many of the registered beneficiaries are not aware of these services of ICDS and does not demand for the services to the AWW, moreover, they also do not have time to visit the AWC and demand for this services and also because easy availability from alternative sources. But the scenario is not same in rural areas.

Past studies suggest that about 60 per cent of the children are covered by PSE and there is regular delivery of PSE in AWCs. Again the recent study by Planning Commission in 2011 showed that in Assam 90 per cent of the AWCs were providing PSE and 93.4 per cent of AWC were trained for delivery of PSE in Assam. This study shows that there is regularity of PSE in both rural and urban AWCs, moreover greater emphasis is being given on PSE by the AWW as both in rural and urban areas as the stakeholders demand proper PSE for their children apart from supplementary nutrition. At the same time AWW are losing children from their centres both is rural and urban centres because of rapid privatisation of education services in both rural and urban areas and easy availability of these alternatives both is rural and urban areas. Also because there is some kind of peer-pressure in today's society and notion that private educational institutions are better than those of the government. Moreover, regarding the quality of PSE kit given to the children attending AWC, the AWWs complained that it was not of good quality and cannot be used properly by the children.

Regarding the money received by the AWW in the joint account to run the AWC there was delays in receiving the funds according to most of the AWW, this was mainly arising due to the gap in communications between the different functionaries (AWW, Supervisors, CDPO, DSWO and the Social Welfare Directorate office) and departments and office responsible for implementing and functioning of ICDS in Assam. Also at the time of survey many of the AWW reported that the money received last for running the AWC was not adequate for them and there was irregularity of delivery of supplementary nutrition both in rural and urban centres.

Regarding the outcome indicators like immunization, receiving of medicines and nutrition and health education as reported by the AWW the recent report by Planning Commission 2011 shows that 32.6 per cent of the children are immunised, 40.5 per cent children have received medicines and 23.9 per cent of adolescent and pregnant women have received and 52 per cent received nutrition and health education. This study shows that of the survey areas of the Kamrup and Kamrup Metro districts almost 100 per cent immunization have taken place and at the same time the mothers of the children and the AWW are well aware of the immunization of the children both in rural and urban areas.

The other main outcome indicators of ICDS are the presence of underweight children, malnourished, i.e. age for weight, IMR and MMR. As various literature suggest that children covered by ICDS services tend to be more healthy and also there has also been drop in severe malnutrition with the introduction of ICDS in India. Even papers by Shanti Ghosh (2006) suggest that ICDS must not be limited to only food programmes, but as a true health, nutrition and development programme. It also suggest that, underweight children in are more inclined towards child mortality and some of the reasons for this are poor living condition and lack of awareness of the young child's food requirements and also poor nutrition and young age of the mothers. This study shows that there higher number of underweight children were registered under urban slum AWC than rural AWC, this in because in the urban areas the AWC in the slum areas and also those areas resided by lower income groups showed greater presence of underweight children. Moreover, when we examine the mothers profile comparing rural and urban it is seen that the average age of the mothers in the urban areas were lower in the urban areas, i.e. below 25 years as compared to between (25-30) years in rural. Also equal cases of child mortality was found in both rural and urban centres as compared to 58 per 1000 live birth in rural and 34 per 1000 live birth in urban Assam as on 2011. So, it can be said that the ICDS services has not been able to achieve its targets and goals in Assam as this is clearly being indicated from the study as the outcome indicators are not good even in a small sample taken from the districts which includes the capital of Assam.

As the literature in various national level studies suggest that there is an average of 50 per cent to 60 per cent co-operation from the community and co-operation is more from the women's organisation or the members of the community and community leaders in solving problems of the AWC. This study shows that there is co-operation from the community both in rural and urban, but the involvement of the women of the community and the mothers of the children whose children attend AWC is higher in rural AWC, moreover, the involvement of the community in solving problems of AWC and engaging in the works of the AWC is high in rural areas as seen and experienced in the field, be it providing space for running the AWC or helping the AWW in transportation of the supplementary nutrition to the centre or the helping the AWW in distributing the dry THR. This is mainly because in rural areas the people are more aware of the different function and services to be received from the ICDS also there is co-operation and co-ordination among the people of the community in the rural areas, but this thing is missing in the urban areas. This is because in the rural areas in a particular locality there are limited number of families residing and are usually permanent resides of that area everyone is known to each other whereas in urban areas the case is just opposite. Again in rural areas there is lack of alternate sources in terms of access to health services or access of food from the market, but in urban areas there is availability of alternate sources. Since there is more awareness and active initiation and involvement of the community in the different functions of ICDS it is seen that the services of ICDS are more demand driven in rural areas by the stakeholders.

From AWW prospective, it is seen that rural is performing better compare to urban in most of the cases: infrastructure though not statistically significant, regularity of health persons visit, regularity of THR, co-operation from community and involvement of women, less presence of underweight children and also the services being demand driven.But some of the responses show same performance in rural and urban like: source of drinking water being public tap, visiting the AWC by ANM, regularity of cooked meals, presence of infant mortality cases and the services mostly demanded by stakeholders and PSE being the service which is mostly demanded. It can be said that since in the rural areas the services of ICDS are more demand driven, awareness about the services of ICDS, there is greater initiation and involvement of the community in ICDS programme and also at the same time there is lack of easy availability of alternatives than urban areas, there is greater effectiveness of the services of ICDS in rural areas of Kamrup. As the literature in the previous chapter suggest that ICDS is community based programme and requires active initiation and involvement of the community and the stakeholders for its effective implementation. Since to some extent there is initiation and involvement of the community and stakeholders in the rural blocks of Kamrup therefore ICDS have been functioning effectively in the rural blocks as compared to the urban blocks.

From the general profile of the mothers in both rural and urban, as reported by the mothers there are greater number of children in the urban who are underweight. One of the main reasons for this may be because of the significant difference in age gap of mothers interviewed in rural and urban areas. In urban areas a significant number of mothers were below 25 years of age or even below 18 years of age, but in rural areas this was not as such. On the other hand the income indicator show that most of them belong to low income groups with monthly income of the family being below Rs. 10000. Most of the mothers interviewed in urban areas were not permanent resident of the city whose husbands' work in the informal sector and lived in rented houses and a significant part of the income goes on rent of house. In urban areas the expenses on food, lodging and transportation is much higher than that of rural areas. This can be one of the reasons that there is lack of attention on the nutritional needs of the children and mothers. This also shows that some of the reasons of greater presence of underweight children in the urban areas are poor living conditions, lack proper nutritional food for the children, unable to bear the expenses of young child's food requirements and young age and poor nutrition of the mothers; which are also the same reasons discussed in Shanti Ghosh's papers. On the other hand in the rural though they have income below Rs. 10000, they did not have to spend on lodging as most of them resided on their own land and there were easily availability of seasonal fruits and vegetables from their own land, which added to the nutritional status of both mothers and children.

It is seen in the output indicators of this study that there is high registration of mothers in the AWC during pregnancy and the percentage of receiving services from AWC especially supplementary nutrition is higher in rural as compared to urban. Moreover in terms of referral services ASHA plays an active role in rural areas. This is mainly because, as seen in the field that there was greater co-ordination between the health centres, AWC and also the people of the community in the rural blocks. Everybody knows each other well and there is regularity of home visits by ASHA, whereas this scenario is missing in the urban areas. There are no regular home visits by the ASHA. This is because the population in the urban regions is densely settled and most of the low income groups are not permanent residents of the city and keeps moving from one place to place frequently so the AWW and the community health workers have a tough time to identify the target population. Again in urban areas there is easy availability of alternative sources and most of the time the people are unaware of the services of the community health workers and AWC in the urban areas.

Other output indicators taken in the study are regular weighting of the children at AWC, discussion of nutrition and growth charts, receiving of medicines and regularity of meetings with the mothers as responded by the mothers whose children attend AWC. Although urban is performing slightly better than rural in terms of regularity of weighting children and discussion of nutrition and growth charts, but the regularity of meetings at the AWC is better in rural. This is because in some of the AWC in the urban there is no adequate space at the AWC for holding meetings and also because the mothers themselves reported that they do not seek time to get involved in the works of the AWC and go for regular meetings in the urban areas.

Regarding the input indicator on the quality of supplementary nutrition, PSE and regularity of opening of the AWC, it is seen that there is not much difference in the responses of the respondents from rural and urban, most respondent has responded the quality of supplementary nutrition as good in urban and acceptable in rural; on the other hand the quality of PSE as somewhat good by most of the respondents of both rural and urban. The quality of food and PSE is maintained by the AWC for children who attend AWC and its regularity because, both these services are the most demanded services of ICDS and these services attract the people of the community to the AWC. Moreover, when officials come on supervision to the AWC, these two services are mainly seen when they visit the AWC, apart from immunization and health check up. On the other hand the people of the community also perceive AWC as a feeding centre and providing PSE, rather than a centre for complete child nutrition and health monitoring centre. It was also seen that the AWW also gives more emphasis on these two services.

Regarding what knowledge the respondents have about ICDS, it is already clear from the discussion in the previous paragraph that ICDS is mainly perceived by the respondents as a free education and mid-day meal programme and also they mainly send their children to AWC for education and food.

It was seen in this study that there is greater co-operation of the mothers in the work and meetings of the AWC in the rural areas. But regarding asking for the deficiency of the services equal percentage ask for the deficiency of the services in both rural and urban. The deficiency asked by the mothers is mainly regarding the regularity of the AWC opening, supply of supplementary nutrition and discussion about the PSE.

From the analysis of the responses of the mothers whose children attend AWC it can be concluded that, those services of ICDS has been available to them with quality and regularity of which they are aware of and the services which have been demanded by them. Therefore, it is seen that higher the people are aware of and demand the services along with co-operation higher is its effectiveness. This awareness and demand is different in rural and urban areas and may be a major cause of difference in effectiveness of the services of ICDS, as effectiveness of the community based programmes to a great extent depends on the awareness and demand for the services by the members of the community which has also been discussed in the literature of chapter one.

As far as the findings of this study is concerned, primary data was collected from AWW and mothers whose children attend

AWC. Data was collected from both categories of respondents about the supply side indicators, outcome indicators and level of demand for the services of ICDS and involvement of the community in the ICDS programme. The supply side indicators both from the prospective of AWW and mothers shows that gap exist in the overall functioning of ICDS both in rural and urban areas. But this gap is more in the urban areas as compared to rural and in many cases the difference is statistically significant. The areas where there is significant difference between rural and urban are fuel source, regularity of health personal visits, ASHA visits to the AWC, regularity of take home dry ration, receiving of medicines by children 3-6 years and amount of money received by the AWC from the AWW's prospective. Again the areas where there is significant difference from the prospective of the mothers are registration of mothers during pregnancy, receiving of services from AWC during pregnancy, referral service by ASHA and regularity of opening of AWC. It is interesting to see that from both the prospective rural AWC is performing better than urban AWC though service gap exist even in rural AWC. The findings also show that the outcome indicators especially in terms of presence of underweight children (weight for age) rural areas are better as compared to urban areas. Regarding the co-operation, awareness of ICDS programme and to what extend the services of ICDS are demand driven it can be concluded that there is greater awareness about the ICDS programme in rural areas along with greater co-operation of the community especially mothers and women's of the community in rural areas.

## Limitation of the Study

Since the study was conducted in a short period of time there was lack of resources and time. With the limited resource and time best efforts have been made to collect the random samples from both rural and urban areas. Sincere efforts were also made to choose the various variables under the different indicators with the given time and resources. The study could have been carried for a larger sample size, more numbers of indicators and samples collected from more interior rural areas given the time and resources which I plan to do in near future and make a better comparative study on the performance of ICDS in rural and urban areas of Assam.

## Conclusion

The findings shows that there is difference in performance of ICDS in rural and urban on one hand and community participation and involvement of women in the ICDS programme increases its effectiveness. Therefore, it can be concluded that since in the rural areas the services of ICDS are more demand driven, awareness about the services of ICDS, there is greater initiation and involvement of the community in ICDS programme and lack of easy availability of alternatives than urban, there is greater effectiveness of the services of ICDS in rural areas of Kamrup.

The study will contribute to the existing literature of studies on ICDS especially at the district level. Though in most of the national level studies on ICDS, Assam as a whole has been included but there has not been much research at district level comparing rural and urban AWCs. The study concludes that there is difference in effectiveness of ICDS in selected rural and urban areas of Assam and at the same time its effectiveness increase with greater initiation and involvement of the community is the ICDS programme as it is a community based programme.

## References

Banerjee, Sangita, Community Participation in ICDS: A Study on Community Participation in ICDS at North Kolkata. *Researches in ICDS upto 2008. NIPCCD, 3*(1): 284-289.

Chudasama, R.K., Kadri, A.M., Verma, P.B., Patel, U.V., Joshi, N., Zalavadiya, D. and Bhola, C. (2014.). Evaluation of Integrated Child Development Services Programme in Gujarat, India. *Indian Journal of Paediatrics,* 51(9): 707-711.

Dreze, Jean, and Sen, Amartya (2013). *An Uncertain Glory: India and its Contradictions.* Princeton University Press, Princeton.

Dreze, Jean, (August 26, 2006). Universalisation with Quality: ICDS in a Rights Perspective, *Economic and Political Weekly, 41*(34): 3706-3715.

Directorate of Economics and Statistics, Assam. *Statistical Handbook Assam, 2013.* Assam: Directorate of Economics and Statistics, Assam.

Dobies, Ann, K., Mroue, Martin, Mustafa, Thahira, S., and Roy, Aditi, (2012). "Adding Value To Integrated Child Development Services (ICDS): A Case Study of the ICDS Accreditation Process in Assam, India".

Dornan, Paul, and Kumar, Vijay, (June 2013). *Delivering the MDGs in India: Targeting Children's Nutrition and Education*. Retrieved from: www.younglives.india.org.

Ghosh, Shanti, (August 26, 2006). Food Dole or Health, Nutrition and Development Programme. *Economic and Political Weekly, 41*(34), 2305-2314.

Gupta, Arti., Gupta, Sanjeev K., and Nongkynrih, Baridalyne, ( March 2013). Integrated Child Development Services (ICDS) Scheme: A Journey of 37 years. *Indian Journal of Community Health. 25*(1): 77-81.

Gupta, Arun, (August 26, 2006). Infant and Young Child Feeding. *Economic and Political Weekly, 41*(34): 1472-1482.

International Institute for Population Science, Deonar Mumbai, (2008). *National Family Health Survey (NFHS 3) 2005-06*. Mumbai: International Institute for Population Science (http://www.rchiips.org/nfhs/assam_report_for_website.pdf).

Ministry of Women and Child Development (2013) *ICDS Mission—The Broad Framework For Implementation*. Delhi: Ministry of Women and Child Development.

Ministry of Women and Child Development. Government of India (2014) *Annual Report 2013-14*. Delhi: Ministry of Women and Child Development. Government of India.

National Institute of Public Cooperation and Child Development (NIPCCD), (2006).*Three Decades of ICDS—An Appraisal*. Delhi: Ministry of Women and Child Development. Government of India. (http://nipccd.nic.in/reports/icdsvol3.pdf.)

National Institute of Public Cooperation and Child Development (NIPCCD), (2008). *Research on ICDS: An Overview*. Ministry of Women and Child Development.

Patwari, A.K. (May 2013). Millennium Development Goals and Child Undernutrition. *(http://www.indianpediatrics.net/may2013/may-449-452.html)*

Programme Evaluation Organisation, New Delhi (2011), *Evaluation of ICDS*, Planning Commission, Government of India.

Rajivan, Anuradha, K. (August 26, 2006). Tamil Nadu: ICDS with a difference. *Economic and Political Weekly, 41*(34): 1445-1454.

Saiyed, F., and Seshadri, S., Impact of the Integrated Package of Nutrition and Health Services. *Indian Journal of Paediatrics, 67*(5): 322-328.

Sen, Amartya (2001). Development as Freedom. *Oxford India,* pp. 195 and 202.

Sinha, Dipa (August 26, 2006). Rethinking ICDS: A Rights Based Perspective. *Economic and Political Weekly, 41*(34), 2262- 2270.

Smith, Stephen C., and Todaro, Michel P. (2008). *Economic Development*. 10th edition.

Social Statistics Division (October 2013), Towards Achieving Millennium Development Goals, India 2013. *Ministry of Statistics and Programme*

*Implementation, Government of India.* (http://mospi.nic.in/mospi_new/upload/MDG_pamphlet29oct2013.pdf)

*Status of Implementation of Food Schemes in Assam,* (October 2010). Institute of Development Action, Office of Commission of Supreme Court (CWP196/2001) and Office of Advisor to Supreme Court Commission, Assam.

UNICEF, (May 2011). *The Situation of Children in India—A Profile*. Delhi: UNICEF (http://www.unicef.org/india/The_Situation_of_Children_in_India_A_profile_20110630_.pdf)

# PART 4
# Education, Nutrition and Health

# 13
# Survey on Knowledge and Attitude Regarding Tuberculosis among Rajshahi University Students in Bangladesh

*Md. Masud Rana, Md. Rafiqul Islam* and
*Md. Golam Hossain*

## Introduction

World Health Organization (WHO) declared that tuberculosis (TB) as a global emergency as because more than two billion people in the world is infected with mycobacterium tuberculosis. They have the chance of developing TB at any stages of life. Furthermore, the infection rate is higher in developing countries like Bangladesh. TB is the second leading cause of death after human immune deficiency virus (HIV), as the greatest killer worldwide due to a single infectious agent (DGHS, 2013). Every year, more than 1.3 million people die around the globe due to TB (WHO, 2013). Of them, over 82 deaths occur in 22 high burden countries (HBCs) and Bangladesh rank 6th among 22 HBCs. TB is a major cause of morbidity and mortality globally with an estimated 8.6 million incident cases. In 2012, among 1.3 million deaths, 0.32 million was associated with HIV. Though HIV is low, TB is a serious public health problem in Bangladesh due to other associated factors. Low awareness, education, income and high population density, smoking, diabetes, certain drugs and other associated diseases are the causal factors for TB.

The Ministry of Health and Family Welfare, Directorate General of Health Services (DGHS) in Bangladesh are providing free diagnostic and treatment support to every irrespective of age, race, sex, occupation, geography or education through its National Tuberculosis Control Programme (NTP, 2013). The Ministry of Health in Bangladesh is also conducting dissimilar sessions, seminars, workshops, meeting, conferences, and orientation on TB from using mass media and other media to aware the people at all level. Though most of the students have knowledge on common symptoms of TB and them apparent that TB is curable, we wait for that lack of knowledge still exists regarding treatment and various types of TB such as pulmonary and extra pulmonary or latent TB which is an important problem encountered while managing the disease. On the other hand, TB has been associated with stigma due to lack of knowledge and awareness about the disease. Though Bangladesh has adopted internationally recommended strategy for TB control directly observed treatment short course (DOTs) (WHO, 2013). In STOP TB strategy in 2006 for effective control of TB in Bangladesh and also achieved more than 92 treatment success rate through public private partnership and involvement of huge health care providers, still it requires more attention on knowledge and awareness of the community people concerning many areas; specially about diagnostic and treatment service opportunities, availability of services, mode of transmission, effect as well as impact of disease, DOTs, type of disease etc. Without proper diagnosis in early stage and irregularity of treatment can be a serious threat for the country as a whole due to chance of increasing spread and development of drug resistant (DR) TB. The DR-TB is a double burden for the society due tc more duration of sufferings, high treatment cost and more chance of deaths. So, people at all level need to be aware for early health seeking and regularity of treatment. Several studies have surveyed the knowledge about TB and they found that reported poor knowledge, attitudes and practices regarding TB among general population (Huang *et al.*, 2012; Diallo *et al.*, 2009) among pre-university students (Reddy *et al.*, 2014) high and secondary school students. Most of the survey took place among medical students, health care workers and other occupation (Behnaz *et al.*, 2014; Laurenti *et al.*, 2013).

However, some researchers have surveyed the knowledge about TB among non-medical university students in other countries (Smolovic *et al.*, 2012; Bertolozzi *et al.*, 2011). We assume that a significant portion of middle and higher educated people have poor knowledge on TB including Rajshahi University students in Bangladesh. On the other hand, there is no survey on level of knowledge and awareness about TB among Rajshahi University students in Bangladesh. Specifically with respect to Bangladeshi populations surveyed the knowledge about TB transmission among ever-married women in Bangladesh (Khandoker *et al.*, 2011). Another study surveyed knowledge about TB in two areas in northern Bangladesh to assess and compare the level of knowledge, attitude and practice towards leprosy and TB among two communities (Croft & Croft,1999). Special attention should be paid to Rajshahi University students considering their potential influence on the family and their contribution to the nation's workforce in near future in a particular nation. Due to their unique role in near future in the society, it is important to investigate the knowledge about communicable disease like TB. Considering the level of knowledge on common symptoms, disease agent, type of disease, latent infection, source of gaining knowledge, vaccination against TB, treatment system is fundamental information about TB which is necessary to analyse. Association between the knowledge and attitude about TB of Rajshahi University students and significant socio-economic factors such as gender, religion, residence, parents' education, occupation and income, type of family, in order to ensure corrective measures can be assumed.

Therefore, the objective of this study is to assess the knowledge about TB among Rajshahi University students in Bangladesh.

## Materials and Methods

In the present study, a total sample consisted of 839 (male 572 and female 267) selected from Rajshahi University students residing in student halls at the University of Rajshahi, Bangladesh. The University of Rajshahi is the second largest university in Bangladesh, with students coming from all over the country. The university has sixteen (11 for male and 5 for female) halls of residence accommodating a total of 25,000 students (20,000 male and 5,000 female) at any particular time. Students were interviewed from March to August 2013 using a semi-structured questionnaire containing pre-coded and open-ended questions. This study was approved by Northwestern University's Institutional Review Board and the CPS Research and Review Board.

### *Sample Size Determination and Sampling*

The following formula has been used for determining sample size:

$$n = \frac{N}{1 + Nd^2},$$

where $n$ = required sample size,
N = population size (in here 25000),
d = marginal error (we considered, $d = 0.033$).

We assumed 95 confidence level. The formula provided that the significant sample size was 839 for this study. Since our population was heterogeneous and population divided into different groups (male and female), within the group are homogeneous, stratified random sampling with a proportional allocation technique was used for selecting sample from University of Rajshahi.

### *Statistical Analysis*

After collecting data, responses were converted to English for data entry and analysis with Statistical Package for Social Sciences (SPSS) version 17.0. The two items 'editing and coding' were processed in computer. $\chi^2$-test was utilized in this study to find the association between knowledge about TB and some selected socio-economic and demographic factors. A value of $p<0.05$ was regarded as statistically significant in the analysis.

## Results and Discussion

The knowledge and attitude about TB of 839 Rajshahi University students, among them 572 (68.2%) and 267 (31.8%) were male and female, respectively. 70.4 per cent and 29.6 per cent students came from rural and urban, respectively. More than 94 students confirmed that they knew the term TB and 5.6 per cent were confused about the term. Among the subjects 43.7 per cent, 18.4 per cent, 23.7 per cent and 14.2 per cent were first time learned about the term TB from electronic media, print media, relatives and friends and other sources, correspondingly (Table 13.1).

TB is a communicable disease but for 33.7 per cent students it was apparent that TB is as non-communicable disease and 14.8 per cent students answered that they did not have idea about the expression communicable and non-communicable regarding TB.

**Table 13.1:** Frequency Allowance of Gender, Residence, Initial Knowledge about TB among University of Rajshahi Students

*(%)*

| *Variable* | *Group* | *Frequency n* |
|---|---|---|
| Gender | Male | 572 (68.2) |
| | Female | 267 (31.8) |
| Residence | Rural | 591 (70.4) |
| | Urban | 248 (29.6) |
| Did you know about TB? | Yes | 792 (94.4) |
| | No | 47 (5.6) |
| From where did you hear about TB? | Electronic Media | 367 (43.7) |
| | Print Media | 154 (18.4) |
| | Relative/Friend | 199 (23.7) |
| | Others | 119 (14.2) |

*Note:* Figures in the parentheses represent percentage.
*Source:* Data collected from University of Rajshahi, Bangladesh.

However, 51.5 per cent respondents answered properly that TB is a communicable disease. The knowledge of communicable disease regarding TB, male had higher percentage (53.7%) than female (46.8%) and $\chi^2$-test demonstrated that the alliance between the knowledge of type of TB disease (communicable or non-communicable or no idea) and gender was statistically significant ($p<0.05$). The respondents who came from rural environment had higher knowledge (53.1%) than urban (47.6%) and we noticed that the association between the type of TB disease and residence was significant ($p<0.05$). Students who came from single family had more knowledge (52.2%) about the communicable disease of TB than their counterparts (48.8%) and the association between the type of TB disease and type of family was significant ($p<0.05$). Father's education, occupation and income were not significantly associated with perception of communicable or non-communicable TB disease (Table 13.2).

Among the respondents, 42.8 per cent believed that TB is a bacterial disease, but outstanding respondents had incorrect or no perception about the disease agent those who answered viral (32.4%), others (2.1%) and don't know (22.6%) (Table 13.3). Among the students, female had higher knowledge (48.7%) about the agent of TB than male (40%) and we observed that the association between knowledge about the agent of TB and gender was

**Table 13.2:** Knowledge about Type of TB Disease and its Association with Socio-economic and Demographic Factors of University of Rajshahi Students

*(in %)*

| *Variables* | *Group* | *Is TB communicable disease?* | | | *$\chi^2$-Value* | *p-Value* |
|---|---|---|---|---|---|---|
| | | *Yes, 432 (51.5)* | *No, 283 (33.7)* | *No idea, 124 (14.8)* | | |
| Religion | Muslim | 383 (50.9) | 255 (33.9) | 114 (15.2) | 1.218 | 0.544 |
| | Hindu | 49 (56.32) | 28 (33.7) | 10 (12.0) | | |
| Gender | Male | 307 (53.7) | 178 (31.1) | 87 (15.2) | 5.52 | 0.043 |
| | Female | 125 (46.8) | 105 (39.3) | 37 (13.9) | | |
| Parents' Occupation | Labour | 5 (62.5) | 2 (25) | 1 (12.5) | 2.32 | 0.970 |
| | Farmer | 145 (53.1) | 90 (33.0) | 38 (13.9) | | |
| | Business | 105 (49.5) | 70 (33.0) | 37 (17.5) | | |
| | Serviceholder | 149 (51.2) | 102 (35.1) | 40 (13.7) | | |
| | Other | 28 (50.9) | 19 (34.5) | 8 (14.5) | | |
| Parents' Education | No Education | 71 (53.8) | 38 (28.8) | 23 (17.4) | 7.25 | 0.298 |
| | Primary | 69 (50.4) | 45 (32.8) | 23 (16.8) | | |
| | Secondary | 105 (52.5) | 61 (30.5) | 34 (17.0) | | |
| | Higher | 187 (50.5) | 139 (37.6) | 44 (11.9) | | |
| Residence | Rural | 314 (53.1) | 182 (30.8) | 95 (16.1) | 8.42 | 0.015 |
| | Urban | 118 (47.6) | 101 (40.7) | 29 (11.7) | | |
| Parents' Income | Poor | 180 (54.1) | 106 (31.8) | 47 (14.1) | 3.63 | 0.458 |
| | Middle | 227 (49.1) | 166 (35.9) | 69 (14.9) | | |
| | Rich | 25 (56.8) | 11 (25.0) | 8 (18.2) | | |
| Type of Family | Single Family | 349 (52.2) | 231 (34.5) | 89 (13.3) | 5.79 | 0.045 |
| | Joint Family | 83 (48.8) | 52 (30.6) | 35 (20.6) | | |
| Smoking Status | No | 391 (51.5) | 256 (33.7) | 112 (14.8) | 0.004 | 0.998 |
| | Yes | 41 (51.3) | 27 (33.8) | 12 (15.0) | | |

*Note:* Figures in the parentheses represent percentage.
*Source:* Data collected from University of Rajshahi, Bangladesh.

significant ($p<0.05$). Respondents who came from single family had more knowledge (44.8%) about the agent of TB than their counterparts (34.7%) and the association between these two factors was significant ($p<0.05$). Other independent variables, father's education, occupation, income, subjects' residence and smoking status were not statistically significant with students' knowledge about the agent of TB (Table 13.3).

A significant percentage (77.7%) of respondents were believed that TB is a major public health problem as it spread from man to man through coughing or sneezing while 22.3 per cent had no knowledge regarding public health problem (Table 13.4). Female

**Table 13.3:** Knowledge about Agent of TB and its Association with Socio-Economic and Demographic Factors of University of Rajshahi Students

*(in %)*

| *Variables* | *Group* | *Distribution of Opinion on which agent is responsible for this disease?* | | | | $\chi^2$-*value* | *p-value* |
|---|---|---|---|---|---|---|---|
| | | *Bacteria, 359 (42.8)* | *Virus, 272 (32.4)* | *Other, 18 (2.1)* | *Don't know, 190 (22.6)* | | |
| Religion | Muslim | 320 (42.6) | 239 (41.8) | 17 (2.3) | 176 (23.4) | 3.294 | 0.349 |
| | Hindu | 39 (44.9) | 33 (37.9) | 01 (1.2) | 14 (16.1) | | |
| Gender | Male | 229 (40.0) | 185 (32.3) | 14 (2.4) | 144 (25.2) | 9.030 | 0.029 |
| | Female | 130 (48.7) | 87 (32.6) | 4 (1.5) | 46 (17.2) | | |
| Parents' occupation | Labour | 4 (50.0) | 2 (25.0) | 0 (0.0) | 2 (25.0) | 18.390 | 0.104 |
| | Farmer | 114 (41.8) | 87 (31.9) | 7 (2.6) | 65 (23.8) | | |
| | Business | 88 (41.5) | 72 (34.0) | 2 (0.9) | 50 (23.6) | | |
| | Serviceholder | 141 (48.5) | 86 (29.6) | 6 (2.1) | 58 (19.9) | | |
| | Other | 12 (21.8) | 25 (45.5) | 3 (5.5) | 15 (27.3) | | |
| Parents' education | No Education | 48 (36.4) | 47 (35.6) | 2 (1.5) | 35 (26.5) | 11.992 | 0.214 |
| | Primary | 53 (38.7) | 42 (30.7) | 4 (2.9) | 38 (27.7) | | |
| | Secondary | 79 (39.5) | 68 (34.0) | 5 (2.5) | 48 (24.0) | | |
| | Higher | 179 (48.4) | 115 (31.1) | 7 (1.9) | 69 (18.6) | | |
| Residence | Rural | 238 (40.3)) | 201 (34.0) | 15 (2.5) | 137 (23.2) | 6.213 | 0.102 |
| | Urban | 121 (48.8) | 71 (28.6) | 3 (1.2) | 53 (21.4) | | |
| Parents' income | Poor | 126 (37.8) | 113 (33.9) | 9 (2.7) | 85 (25.5) | 7.107 | 0.303 |
| | Middle | 213 (46.1) | 144 (31.2) | 9 (1.9) | 96 (20.8) | | |
| | Rich | 20 (45.5) | 15 (34.1) | 0 (0.0) | 9 (20.5) | | |
| Type of family | Single Family | 300 (44.8) | 213 (31.8) | 13 (1.9) | 143 (21.4) | 6.583 | 0.046 |
| | Joint Family | 59 (34.7) | 59 (34.7) | 5 (2.9) | 47 (27.6) | | |
| Smoking Status | No | 327 (43.1) | 249 (32.8) | 16 (2.1) | 167 (22.0) | 2.035 | 0.565 |
| | Yes | 32 (40.0) | 23 (28.8 | 2 (2.5) | 23 (28.8) | | |

*Note:* Figures in the parentheses represent percentage.
*Source:* Data collected from University of Rajshahi, Bangladesh.

students (83.5%) had higher perception about TB as a public health problem than male (75.0%), and the association between the knowledge about TB major public health problems and gender was significant ($p<0.01$). Student his or her father was service holder had more knowledge (81.4%) than their counterparts and the association between the knowledge about TB public health problem and father occupations was significant ($p<0.01$).

**Table 13.4:** Knowledge about Public Health Concern regarding TB and its Association with Socio-economic and Demographic Factors of University of Rajshahi Students

*(in %)*

| Variables | Group | Number of Response who are or not whether aware TB a problem for public health? | | χ2-value | p-value |
|---|---|---|---|---|---|
| | | Yes 652 (77.7) | No 187 (22.3) | | |
| Religion | Muslim | 586 (77.9) | 166 (22.1) | 0.192 | 0.662 |
| | Hindu | 66 (75.9) | 21 (24.1) | | |
| Gender | Male | 429 (75.0) | 143 (25.0) | 7.630 | 0.006 |
| | Female | 223 (83.5) | 44 (16.5) | | |
| Parents' occupation | Labour | 5 (62.5) | 3 (37.5) | 13.747 | 0.008 |
| | Farmer | 215 (78.8) | 58 (21.2) | | |
| | Business | 162 (76.4) | 50 (23.6) | | |
| | Service holder | 237 (81.4) | 54 (18.6) | | |
| | Other | 33 (60.0) | 22 (40.0) | | |
| Parents' education | No Education | 104 (78.8) | 28 (21.2) | 5.789 | 0.122 |
| | Primary | 96 (70.1) | 41 (29.9) | | |
| | Secondary | 161 (80.5) | 39 (19.5) | | |
| | Higher | 291 (78.6) | 79 (21.4) | | |
| Residence | Rural | 455 (77.0) | 136 (23.0) | 0.604 | 0.437 |
| | Urban | 197 (79.4) | 51 (20.6) | | |
| Parents' income | 6000 and less | 101 (71.6) | 40 (28.4) | 8.331 | 0.040 |
| | 6001–10000 | 148 (77.1) | 44 (22.9) | | |
| | 10001–20000 | 270 (79.9) | 68 (20.1) | | |
| | 20001–35000 | 103 (83.1) | 21 (16.9) | | |
| | 35001 and above | 30 (68.2) | 14 (31.8) | | |
| Type of family | Single Family | 526 (78.6) | 143 (21.4) | 1.590 | 0.207 |
| | Joint Family | 126 (74.1) | 44 (25.9) | | |
| Smoking Status | Yes | 593 (78.1) | 166 (21.9) | 0.801 | 0.371 |
| | No | 59 (73.8) | 21 (26.2) | | |

*Note:* Figures in the parentheses represent percentage.
*Source:* Data collected from University of Rajshahi, Bangladesh.

Concerning BCG vaccine against TB in children, most respondents (93%) were aware (Table 13.4). Among the students, female (76.8%) were more aware about the vaccination of TB than male. We noticed that the association between the knowledge about the vaccination of TB and gender was statistically significant ($p<0.01$). $\chi^2$–test demonstrated that the others selected factors used in this study were not significantly associated with knowledge about vaccination of TB (Table 13.5).

**Table 13.5:** Knowledge about Vaccination (BCG) of TB and its Relationship the Socio-Economic and Demographic Factors of University of Rajshahi Students *(in %)*

| *Variables* | *Group* | *Response of Respondents on whether they have knowledge about Vaccination of TB?* | | *χ2-value* | *p-value* |
|---|---|---|---|---|---|
| | | *Yes* 780 (93) | *No* 59 (7) | | |
| Religion | Muslim | 509 (67.7) | 243 (32.3) | 0.880 | 0.348 |
| | Hindu | 61 (70.1) | 26 (29.9) | | |
| Gender | Male | 365 (63.8) | 207 (36.2) | 14.053 | 0.001 |
| | Female | 205 (76.8) | 62 (23.2) | | |
| Parents' occupation | Labour | 4 (50.0) | 4 (50.0) | 2.857 | 0.582 |
| | Farmer | 178 (65.2) | 95 (34.8) | | |
| | Business | 148 (69.8) | 64 (30.2) | | |
| | Serviceholder | 201 (69.1) | 90 (30.9) | | |
| | Other | 39970.9) | 16 (29.1) | | |
| Parents' education | No Education | 81 (61.4) | 51 (38.6) | 4.049 | 0.256 |
| | Primary | 90 (65.7) | 47 (34.3) | | |
| | Secondary | 140 (70.0) | 60 (30.0) | | |
| | Higher | 259 (70.0) | 111 (30.0) | | |
| Residence | Rural | 393 (66.5) | 198 (33.5) | 1.905 | 0.168 |
| | Urban | 177 (71.4) | 71 (28.6) | | |
| Parents' income | 6000 and less | 91 (64.5) | 50 (35.5) | 2.129 | 0.712 |
| | 6001-10000 | 126 (65.5) | 66 (34.5) | | |
| | 10001-20000 | 234 (69.2) | 104 (30.8) | | |
| | 20001-35000 | 88 (71.0) | 36 (29.0) | | |
| | 35001 and above | 31 (70.5) | 13 (29.5) | | |
| Type of family | Single Family | 463 (69.2) | 206 (30.8) | 2.444 | 0.118 |
| | Joint Family | 107 (62.9) | 63 (37.1) | | |
| Smoking Status | Yes | 56 (70.0) | 24 (30.0) | 0.257 | 0.879 |
| | No | 514 (67.7) | 245 (32.3) | | |

*Note:* Figures in the parentheses represent percentage.
*Source:* Data collected from University of Rajshahi, Bangladesh.

More than 97 respondents strongly believed that TB is a curable disease among them male and female were 96.7 per cent and 99.6 per cent respectively. The association between the knowledge about TB curable and gender was significant ($p<0.01$). Higher educated father's child had more knowledge (99.2%) than secondary (96.5%), primary (98.5%) and no educated father's child (93.9%), and the association between knowledge about curable disease of TB and father education was significant (p<0.01) (Table 13.6).

**Table 13.6:** Knowledge about the TB is curable its Relationship the Socio-Economic and Demographic Factors of University of Rajshahi Students *(in %)*

| *Variables* | *Group* | *Distribution of Opinion of the Respondents on whether TB is Curable* | | $\chi^2$*-value* | *p-value* |
|---|---|---|---|---|---|
| | | *Yes 819 (97.62)* | *No 20 (2.38)* | | |
| Religion | Muslim | 733 (97.5) | 19 (2.5) | 0.636 | 0.425 |
| | Hindu | 86 (98.9) | 01 (1.1) | | |
| Gender | Male | 553 (96.7) | 19 (3.3) | 6.795 | 0.009 |
| | Female | 266 (99.6) | 01 (.4) | | |
| Parents' occupation | Labour | 7 (87.5) | 1 (12.5) | 3.636 | 0.458 |
| | Farmer | 267 (97.8) | 6 (2.2) | | |
| | Business | 207 (97.6) | 05 (2.4) | | |
| | Serviceholder | 284 (97.6) | 7 (2.4) | | |
| | Other | 54 (98.2) | 01 (1.8) | | |
| Parents' education | No Education | 124 (93.9) | 08 (6.1) | 13.176 | 0.004 |
| | Primary | 135 (98.5) | 02 (1.5) | | |
| | Secondary | 193 (96.5) | 07 (3.5) | | |
| | Higher | 367 (99.2) | 03 (.8) | | |
| Residence | Rural | 578 (97.8) | 13 (2.2) | 0.291 | 0.589 |
| | Urban | 241 (97.2) | 07 (2.8) | | |
| Parents' income | 6000 and less | 136 (96.5) | 05 (3.5) | 5.305 | 0.257 |
| | 6001–10000 | 185 (96.4) | 07 (3.6) | | |
| | 10001–20000 | 331 (97.9) | 07 (2.1) | | |
| | 20001–35000 | 124 (100.0) | 0 (0.0) | | |
| | 35001 and above | 43 (97.7) | 01 (2.3) | | |
| Type of family | Single Family | 653 (97.6) | 16 (2.4) | 0.001 | 0.976 |
| | Joint Family | 166 (97.6) | 4 (2.4) | | |
| Smoking Status | Yes | 79 (98.8) | 01 (1.2) | 0.489 | 0.485 |
| | No | 740 (97.5) | 19 (2.5) | | |

*Note:* Figures in the parentheses represent percentage.
*Source:* Data collected from University of Rajshahi, Bangladesh.

This study demonstrated the knowledge and attitude about TB, particularly on common symptoms, disease agent, communicable or non-communicable, latent TB, vaccination against TB, treatment system etc. The study also examined the perception of respondents about TB as a public health problem, source of gaining knowledge, urban-rural and male-female ratio, father's education and income etc. 94.4 per cent of Rajshahi University students declared that they have heard the term tuberculosis or TB. Only 5.6 per cent were confused about the term. They have heard the term TB from various sources. Of them, electronic media were 43.7 per cent, print media 18.4 per cent, relatives and friends 23.7 per cent and other sources were 14.2 per cent. In other study, similar results were found among other people in Rajshahi city including students (Sayem & Islam, 2013). It indicate that electronic media is a strong media to communicate people at all level to aware, inform and guide them for receiving information and services of TB with free of cost from their nearest distance. Friends and relatives were also playing a vital role in disseminating information to others. Different sessions, meetings, workshops, drama, rally is influencing others as discussion matter. Print media, bill boards, leaflets; posters have also impact in disseminating information to the community people. Nearly half (51.5%) of the students properly knew that TB is a communicable disease and it spread from man to man. 14.8 per cent had no knowledge as communicable disease while 33.7 per cent had wrong believe that indicates less involvement of university students in TB related sessions, meetings or workshops. Though several partner NGOs are working for ACSM activities in Rajshahi district, they need to perform adequate sessions or meeting with university students. According to sex, male were more informed than female due to frequent movement, gathering or discussion. And surprisingly, students who come from rural area had more knowledge (53.10%) regarding communicable disease. This may due to frequent advertisement through Bangladesh television (BTV) which is largely observed by rural people. But urban people is usually enjoy other Television channels like dish television (TV) channels. Now-a-days, dish TV channels are expanding to rural areas of Bangladesh. So, it is necessary to widely utilize dish TV channels as electronic media for TB related advertisement. Poverty, illiteracy, higher fertility has higher chance of developing TB. Once TB developed in any family, all members of the family become experienced and gained knowledge about symptoms, services and management of TB. But our study shows that father's education and income had no significant association on knowledge of university students regarding TB. This may due to no direct experience of gaining knowledge. In our study, only 42.8 per cent believed that TB is a bacterial disease while other had no knowledge or wrong perception. It may indicate less inclusion of TB disease idea in general education curriculum. In developing countries like Bangladesh, more than half of whole populations are infected with TB as latent TB. Those latent TB have the chance of reactivation to active disease at any time when environment is favourable for reactivation. Our study revealed that only 13.7 per cent have knowledge on latent TB. Poor nutrition, diabetes or immunosuppressive drugs, smoking or certain diseases can reactivate TB. University of Rajshahi students should know more about latent TB and its environmental condition.

The respondents were asked for latent TB as more intricate question and only 13.7 per cent answered positively while 86.3 per cent respondents did not have idea about latent TB (Table 13.7). Those who had knowledge about latent TB, male had higher knowledge (15.4%) than female (10.1%). We observed that the association between the knowledge about latent TB and gender was significant ($p<0.05$). Smoker students had more knowledge (22.5%) than their counterparts (12.8%), and the association between the knowledge about latent TB and smoking status was significant ($p<0.05$). Other preferred factors were not statistically significant ($p>0.05$) with the knowledge about latent TB (Table 13.7%).

The knowledge on treatment system through DOT for each TB patient was surveyed among students. Solitary 91.4 per cent knew about DOT while 8.6 per cent did not have knowledge about treatment system through DOT (Table 13.8). Hindu students had higher knowledge (37.9%) about DOT than Muslim (27.4%), and we observed that the association between knowledge about DOT and religion was significant ($p<0.05$). Male students had more knowledge (30.9%) than female (23.2%), the association between the knowledge about DOT and gender was significant ($p<0.05$). Students who came from single family had more knowledge (30.2%) than their counterparts (21.8%). We noticed that the association between the knowledge about DOT and type of family was significant ($p<0.05$). We did not find significantly ($p>0.05$) associated between other variables and knowledge about DOT (Table 13.8).

**Table 13.7:** Knowledge about Latent TB and its Socio-Economic and Demographic Factors of University of Rajshahi Students

| *Variables* | *Group* | *Distribution of Respondents on whether they know about latent TB?* | | $\chi^2$-*value* | *p-value* |
|---|---|---|---|---|---|
| | | *Yes 115 (13.7)* | *No 724 (86.3)* | | |
| Religion | Muslim | 103 (13.7) | 649 (86.3) | 0.001 | 0.980 |
| | Hindu | 12 (13.79) | 75 (86.21) | | |
| Gender | Male | 88 (15.4) | 484 (84.6) | 4.28 | 0.039 |
| | Female | 27 (10.1) | 240 (89.9) | | |
| Parents' occupation | Labour | 1 (12.5) | 7 (87.5) | 1.29 | 0.863 |
| | Farmer | 33 (12.1) | 240 (87.9) | | |
| | Business | 32 (15.1) | 180 (84.9) | | |
| | Service holder | 40 (13.7) | 251 (86.3) | | |
| | Other | 9 (16.4) | 46 (83.6) | | |
| Parents' education | No Education | 15 (11.4) | 117 (88.6) | 2.41 | 0.492 |
| | Primary | 16 (11.7) | 121 (88.3) | | |
| | Secondary | 33 (16.5) | 167 (83.5) | | |
| | Higher | 51 (13.8) | 319 (86.2) | | |
| Residence | Rural | 83 (14.0) | 508 (86.0) | 1.92 | 0.661 |
| | Urban | 32 (12.9) | 216 (87.1) | | |
| Parents' income | 6000 and less | 19 (13.5) | 122 (86.5) | 4.72 | 0.317 |
| | 6001–10000 | 33 (17.2) | 159 (82.8) | | |
| | 10001–20000 | 39 (11.5) | 299 (88.5) | | |
| | 20001–35000 | 20 (16.1) | 104 (83.9) | | |
| | 35001 and above | 4 (9.1) | 40 (90.9) | | |
| Type of family | Single Family | 94 (14.1) | 575 (85.9) | 0.330 | 0.565 |
| | Joint Family | 21 (12.4) | 149 (87.6) | | |
| Smoking Status | No | 97 (12.8) | 662 (87.2) | 5.78 | 0.016 |
| | Yes | 18 (22.5) | 62 (77.5) | | |

*Note:* Figures in the parentheses represent percentage.
*Source:* Data collected from University of Rajshahi, Bangladesh.

Almost all Bangladeshi has adopted with expanded programme on immunization (EPI) programme and our study shows that with the success of EPI in Bangladesh, 93 per cent of the respondents believed that BCG vaccination is effective against childhood TB. Of them, female are more aware than male. This

**Table 13.8:** Knowledge about DOT Programme and its Association with Socio-Economic and Demographic Factors of University of Rajshahi Students

| *Variables* | *Group* | *Distribution of Response on whether they know about DOT Programme?* | | *χ2-value* | *p-value* |
|---|---|---|---|---|---|
| | | *Yes 767 (91.4)* | *No 72 (8.6)* | | |
| Religion | Muslim | 206 (27.4) | 546 (72.6) | 4.250 | 0.039 |
| | Hindu | 33 (37.9) | 54 (62.1) | | |
| Gender | Male | 177 (30.9) | 395 (69.1) | 5.330 | 0.021 |
| | Female | 62 (23.2) | 205 (76.8) | | |
| Parents' occupation | Labour | 03 (37.5) | 05 (62.5) | 1.307 | 0.860 |
| | Farmer | 82 (30.0) | 191 (70.0) | | |
| | Business | 56 (26.4) | 156 (73.6) | | |
| | Serviceholder | 81 (27.8) | 210 (72.2) | | |
| | Other | 17 (30.9) | 38 (69.1) | | |
| Parents' education | No Education | 40 (30.3) | 92 (69.7) | 0.354 | 0.950 |
| | Primary | 38 (27.7) | 99 (72.3) | | |
| | Secondary | 58 (29.0) | 142 (71.0) | | |
| | Higher | 103 (27.8) | 267 (72.2) | | |
| Residence | Rural | 177 (29.9) | 414 (70.1) | 2.101 | 0.147 |
| | Urban | 62 (25.0) | 186 (75.0) | | |
| Parents' income | 6000 and less | 39 (27.7) | 102 (72.3) | 1.470 | 0.832 |
| | 6001–10000 | 54 (28.1) | 138 (71.9) | | |
| | 10001–20000 | 96 (28.4) | 242 (71.6) | | |
| | 20001–35000 | 34 (27.4) | 90972.6) | | |
| | 35001 and above | 16 (36.4) | 28 (63.6) | | |
| Type of family | Single Family | 202 (30.2) | 467 (69.8) | 4.728 | 0.030 |
| | Joint Family | 37 (21.8) | 133 (78.2) | | |
| Smoking Status | Yes | 28 (35.0) | 52 (65.0) | 1.842 | 0.175 |
| | No | 211 (25.14) | 548 (65.32) | | |

*Note:* Figures in the parentheses represent percentage.
*Source:* Data collected from University of Rajshahi, Bangladesh.

may due to mothers are more caring than father. Previously, people in Bangladesh thought that TB is not curable. But now, almost all people of Bangladesh strongly believe that TB is a curable disease. Advocacy, communication and social mobilization (ACSM) activities of NTP have turned them into adoption of such believe and our study also shows that 97.6 per cent of the respondents strongly believed that TB is a curable disease. But treatment system was not properly imprinted in the mind of the university students. 91.4 per cent of the respondents knew about DOT system for TB treatment while 8.6 per cent had no knowledge about DOT system in our study. As public health concern, most of the respondents (77.7%) believed that TB is a major public health problem as it spread from man to man through coughing or sneezing. In our study, among the respondents, female had higher perception (83.5%) as public health problem than male (75.0%).

## Conclusion

In this study 839 students of University of Rajshahi were surveyed of their knowledge about TB and established the association between the knowledge about TB and some selected socio-demographic factors. This study revealed that more than 50 per cent of students believed that TB is communicable disease, 93 per cent of students correctly answered about TB vaccination. More than 77 per cent of students agreed that TB is major health problem in Bangladesh, 97 per cent of students believed that TB is curable disease, and 42.8 per cent of students knew that bacteria is the agent for TB. Only 13.7 per cent of students had idea about latent TB and 28.5 per cent of heard about DOT programme. Poor knowledge about TB was noted among male students and the students came from urban areas and single family, those who were smoker and his/her parent was service holder and higher educated.

## Acknowledgements

The authors gratefully acknowledge the authority of Students' Residence Hall, University of Rajshahi, Bangladesh for giving permission to take data from students.

## References

Akin, S., Gorak, G., Unsar, S., Mollaoglu, M., Ozdilli, K., and Durna, Z. (2011). Knowledge of and attitudes toward tuberculosis of Turkish nursing and midwifery students. *Nurse Education Today,* 31(8): 774-79.

Behnaz, F., Mohammadzade, G., Mousavi-e-Roknabadi, R.S., and Mohammadzadeh, M. (2014). Assessment of knowledge, attitudes and practices regarding tuberculosis among final year students in Yazd, Central Iran. *Journal of Epidemiology and Global Health*. 4(2): 81-85.

Croft, R.P., and Croft, R.A. (1999). Knowledge, attitude and practice regarding leprosy and uberculosis in Bangladesh. *Leprosy Review, 70*(1): 34-42.

Directorate General of Health Services (DGHS, 2013). National Tuberculosis Control Programme (NTP, 2013), National Guidelines and Operation Manual for Tuberculosis Control; 5th edition, Mohakhali, Dhaka, Bangladesh. Available at http://tbcare2.org/sites/default/files/National%20Guidelines%20for%20the%20Management%20of% 20Tuberculosis%20in%20Children_2.pdf

Diallo, S., Diarra, B., Diop, S., Toloba, Y., Berthé, F., Sissoko, B., Gomez, P., M'Baye, O., and Keita, B. (2009). Knowledge of the Bamako general population on tuberculosis. *Le Mali Medical,24*(1): 48-51.

Huang, Y., Zhong, J.M., Chen, S.H., Chen, B., and Wang, X.M. (2012). Investigation analysis on public awareness of tuberculosis knowledge in Zhejiang province. *Zhonghua Yu Fang Yi Xue Za Zhi, 46*(4): 352-54.

Khandoker, A., Khan, M.M., Krämer, A., and Mori, M. (2011). Knowledge about tuberculosis transmission among ever-married women in Bangladesh. *The International Journal of Tuberculosis and Lung Disease, 15*(3): 379-84.

Laurenti, P., Federico, B., Raponi, M., Furia, G., Ricciardi, W., and Damiani, G.(2013). Knowledge, experiences, and attitudes of medical students in Rome about tuberculosis. *Medical Science Monito*, 19: 865-874. doi: 10.12659/MSM.889515

Montagna, M.T., Napoli, C., Tafuri, S., Agodi, A., Auxilia, F., Casini, B., Coscia, M.F., D'Errico, M.M., Ferrante, M., Fortunato, A., Germinario, C., Martinelli, D., Masanotti, G.M., Massenti, M.F., Messina, G., Montuori, P., Mura, I., Orsi, G.B., Quarant a, A., Sotgiu, G., Stefanati, A., Tardivo, S., Torregrossa, M.V., Tortorano, A.M., Veronesi, L., Zarrilli, R., and Pasquarella, C. (2014). Knowledge about tuberculosis among undergraduate health care students in 15 Italian Universities: a cross-sectional study. *BioMed. Central Public Health, 14*: 970. doi: 10.1186/1471-2458-14-970.

Muñoz Sánchez, A.I., and Bertolozzi, M.R. (2011). Functioning of the concept of vulnerability to tuberculosis amongst university students. *Ciencia Saude Coletiva, 16* (2): 669-75.

Sayem, M. A. and Islam M. M. (2013). *Activities of NTP, Bangladesh: A Special Focus on Promotional Activities*. Internship report. Master of Business Administration, Institute of Business Administration, University of Rajshahi (p. 56).

Naidoo, S., and Taylor, M. (2013). Association between South African high-school learners' Knowledge about tuberculosis and their intention to seek healthcare. *Global Health Action,* 6: 21699. Avaialble at http://dx.doi.org/10.3402/gha.v6i0.21699.

Reddy, V., Bennadi, D., Gaduputi, S., Kshetrimayum, N., and Siluvai, S. (2014). Oral Health Related Knowledge, Attitude, and Practice among the pre-university students of Mysore city. *Journal of International Society Preventive and Community Dentistry,* 4(3): 154-58.

Smolovic, M., Pesut, D., Bulajic, M., and Simic, M. (2012). Knowledge and attitudes towards tuberculosis in non-medical students: University of Belgrade. *Pneumologia, 61*(2): 88-91.

Tanimowo, M.O. (1999). Knowledge, attitudes and practices regarding tuberculosis among senior secondary school students. *East Africa Medical Journal, 76*(1): 47-50.

World Health Organization (WHO, 2013). Global TB Repot, Geneva, Switzerland.

Zhao, Y., Ehiri, J., Li, D., Luo, X., and Li, Y. (2013). A survey of TB knowledge among medical students in Southwest China: is the information reaching the target. *BMJ Open,* 3(9): e003454. doi: 10.1136/bmjopen-2013-003454.

# 14
# The Influence of Education on Hygiene and Sanitation Practices among the Scheduled Caste Women of Silchar Town, Assam

*Rajiya Shahani* and *Kakoli Choudhury*

## Introduction

Health is a positive state of well-being, where every part of the body and mind is in harmony and in proper functioning balance with every other part. According to World Health Organization (WHO) "Health is the state of complete physical, mental, spiritual and social well-being and not merely absence of disease".[1] The greatest threat encountered by human health is the disease and illness that effects the normal functioning of a human body. To facilitate a fuller participation of its members, society adopts some unspoken and sometimes advised set of rules which can be summarized as health and hygiene behaviours to overcome diseases and illness. The health and hygiene of an individual is largely depends on the adequate availability of water for drinking and proper sanitation. According to World Health Organization, about two million people die every year due to diarrheal diseases.[2] Education plays an important role in the community hygiene. To prevent illness and have positive health attitude, correct and complete knowledge of health is necessary.

Education and awareness plays a pivotal role in realization, adaptation and formulation of hygiene and sanitation practices. Education brings out and develops the best in an individual. Education seeks to activate the best in man, thereby making for the all round development of his personality thereafter family, community and society. It is a very important flexible resource ; a resource that allows educated people to make good decisions about their health and health behaviour and benefit from the socio-economic resources (good jobs, high income etc.) that tend to come from achieving a adequate level of education which in regard of hygiene means, adopting healthy and useful behaviour, without which people remain unaware of various easily adoptable hygienic behaviour related to their good health and causes the consequences like practicing of poor hygienic behaviour, unhygienic living conditions causing prevailing of diseases. Educating school children on basic hygiene and sanitation is very importance because most children are eager to learn and therefore instill and promote positive behavioural change in other children as well as at home, in family and community level as they are and will be the future parents who will pass on good hygiene practices that they learn in school to their children. While the effect of educating adult on hygiene and sanitation is indeed most significant.

Nath *et al.*, (2010) in their research paper entitled *"Study on Perception and Practice of Hygiene and Impact on Health in India"* assess the level of health awareness and hygienic practices and their health impacts in urban *vis-à-vis* rural areas in five states of Eastern India—Assam, Bihar, Jharkhand, Odisha, and West Bengal. This study attempts to gauge the existing level of awareness of public health and hygiene issues and how it influences the hygiene practices in the community. The study demonstrates that basic socio-economic factors, such as religion, education and level of economic status, play a pivotal role in conditioning the perception and practice of hygiene.

Postma *et al.*, (2004) in their paper *"Life Skills-based Hygiene Education"* based on the outcomes of the first life skill-based hygiene education workshop organized in New York and experiences from a number of countries like Burkina Faso, Colombia, Nepal, Nicaragua, Vietnam and Zambia and three states in India, involved in a multi-year school sanitation and hygiene education programme prepared with financial support from UNICEF (United Nations International Children Emergency Fund), identifying actual relationship between education and hygienic behaviour in practical field, differ from traditional education, life skill-based hygiene education programme targets children and their formative childhood in school atmosphere to impart knowledge about hygiene education so that they can pass on in their families and communities. The study found that life-skill approach became the part of the overall review of the existing curriculum for primary education in Zambia and it identified the teaching of life-skills as an area of curriculum reform. In other places also children formulated the knowledge they acquired in school to their family and community level.

Sekhon *et al.*, (2013) in their article entitled *"A School based Survey on Hygiene in a Rural Area of Northern India"* reveals the good hygienic behaviour among the 350 children in a government school in a rural area of north India. The survey was conducted using the Global School-based Student Health Survey (GSHS) Core Questionnaire Modules. The study result shows that all the students adhere to the good habit of washing hands after using toilets or latrine which reveals a good standard of hygiene. However, steps are required to be taken so as to improve the status of personal hygiene of all the school children, who are found lacking in the aspect, various coordinated primordial as well as primary preventive measures like imparting health education.

WHO (World Health Organization) (2011), in the article, *"Water, Sanitation and Hygiene Interventions and the Preventions of Diarrhea"* discussed as diarrhea most often results from the pathogens from faeces that have not been disposed of properly, or from the lack of hygiene. Such lack of access to safe, clean drinking water and basic sanitation as well as poor hygiene cause nearly 90 per cent of all deaths from diarrhoea, mainly in children, while 87 per cent of the world's population now have access to improved water sources, 39 per cent still lack access to improved sanitation. The study found that there should be (a) the provision of an improved water supply; (b) water safety planning; (c) household water treatment and safe storage; (d) improved sanitation facilities; and (d) hygiene education for primary prevention of diarrhea.

The objective of the study is to examine the impact of education on hygiene and sanitation practices among scheduled caste people. It also explores the effect of other socio-economic indicators on health condition of the Scheduled Caste People.

## Methodology

The study has been conducted in Silchar town of Cachar District in Assam. A sample of 150 women has been taken. The study is exploratory in nature. The primary data has been collected through field study based on interview scheduled and group discussion. The secondary data has been collected from books, journals, newspapers, articles, reports etc. The analysis of the data has been done through SPSS and is presented in the form of tabulation. Silchar is located in the southern part of Assam.

## Socio-Economic Profiles of the Respondents

**Age-group of the Respondents:** Age-group of the respondents has been stratified as 15-24, 25-34 and 35-44 respectively. Twenty nine per cent of the respondents belong to the age-group of 15-24. Fifty four per cent of the respondents belong to the age-group of 25-34 and 17 per cent of the respondents belong to the age-group of 35-44.

**Education Qualification of the Respondents:** Almost 46 per cent of the respondents are educated up to graduate level. thirty per cent are found to be educated up to higher secondary level, 17 per cent are qualified to high school level. Only a few (5%) are educated to primary level and 2 per cent of the respondents are found to be illiterate.

**Education Qualification of the Respondent's Husbands:** Forty seven per cent of the respondent's husbands are found to be qualified up to graduate level. Thirty five per cent are educated up to higher secondary level. Fourteen per cent are found to be educated up to high school level. Only 3 per cent are educated up to primary level and rest 1 per cent are found to be illiterate.

**Occupation of the Respondents:** Thirty seven per cent of the respondents are being engaged in services among them 11 per cent are engaged in Government services while 26 per cent are engaged in private sector jobs. The rest 60 per cent of the respondents are housewives and rest 3 per cent are skilled workers.

**Occupation of the Respondent's Husband:** Eighty three per cent are found to be engaged in services among them 64 per cent are engaged in Government jobs and 19 per cent are engaged in private sector jobs. Fifteen per cent are engaged in business and rest 2 per cent are unemployed.

**Monthly Household Income of the Respondents:** Almost 70 per cent of the respondents have household income of more than 5,001. Twenty per cent of them have income within 4,001-5,000.

Seven per cent have household income within 3,001-4,000. Two per cent have household income within 2,001-3000 and a few (1%) have household income within 1,001-2,000.

**Other Socio-Economic Profiles:** One hundred per cent of the respondents belong to Scheduled Caste and belief Hinduism. One hundred per cent of the respondents live in the *pucca* house. In every house there is electricity facility available. The main source of drinking water is supply water. Most of the houses have their own supply water connection only a few do not have water facility available at their homes. So, they collect water from a common municipal connection.

## Pattern of Washing Hands among the Respondents

The habit of handwash refers to the simplest and easiest form of hygiene practices which little effort in actual meaning can prevent spread of the bacterial diseases without, which bacterial contaminants easily transfers through hand to inside the body mostly which become the main cause of diarrhea.

**Table 14.1:** Distribution of the Respondents on the basis of Handwash Habit

| Cleaning Agent | *Before Eating* | *After Using Toilet* |
|---|---|---|
| | *Frequency* | *Percentage* |
| Ash | 3 (2) | 5 (3.3) |
| Sand | 5 (3) | 2 (1.3) |
| Plain Water | 41 (27) | 1 (0.07) |
| Soap | 88 (59) | 141 (94) |
| None | 13 (9) | 1 (0.07) |
| **Total** | **150 (100)** | **150 (100)** |

*Note:* Figures in the parentheses represent percentage.
*Source:* Field survey.

Table 14.1 shows that most (88%) of the respondents have quite a good habit of washing hands with soap, but 27 per cent respondents wash with plain water before eating where 9 per cent do not wash hands before eating.

**Table 14.2:** Type of Latrines among the Respondents

| *Type of Latrine* | *Frequency* | *Percentage* |
|---|---|---|
| Pucca | 125 | 83 |
| Semi-Pucca | 19 | 13 |
| Kaccha | 6 | 4 |
| **Total** | **150** | **100** |

*Source:* Field survey.

Table 14.2 shows 94 of the respondents wash hands with soap after using toilet while only. 3.3 per cent of the respondents use ash. 1.3 per cent of them use sand and only. Seven per cent use plain water.

## Types of Latrine of the Respondents

Proper type of latrine and its maintenance can prevent many bacterial diseases. The distribution of type of latrines among the respondents in the study area is given in Table 14.3.

**Table 14.3:** Distribution of the Respondents according to Sources Drinking Water

| *Source of Drinking Water* | *Frequency* | *Percentage* |
|---|---|---|
| Supply water | 142 | 94.66 |
| Tube well | 6 | 4 |
| Well | 1 | 0.67 |
| Pond | 1 | 0.67 |
| **Total** | **150** | **100** |

*Source:* Field survey.

The data in Table 14.3 shows that 83 per cent of the respondents are using pucca latrines. Thirteen per cent are using semi-pucca latrines and only 04 per cent of the respondents are using kaccha latrines.

## Source of Drinking Water of the Respondents

Water has been crucial importance in the well being of health as well as the reason for illness. This difference comes from the source of the drinking water. It is water and its poor source which causes the different types of water related diseases like diarrhea, cholera etc. The distribution is shown in Table 14.4. 94.66 per cent of the respondents are depend upon supply water. Four per cent of the respondents are using tube well which also includes the bore well or private source of water. Only 67 per cent depends on well and pond or river water.

**Table 14.4:** Distribution of the Respondents according to Sources Drinking Water

| *Source of Drinking Water* | *Frequency* | *Percentage* |
|---|---|---|
| Supply water | 142 | 94.66 |
| Tube well | 6 | 4 |
| Well | 1 | 0.67 |
| Pond | 1 | 0.67 |
| **Total** | **150** | **100** |

*Source:* Field survey.

## Purification of Drinking Water

Water purification can also prevent the spreading of diseases. A quite good scenario of the purification habit is revealed. 61.4 per cent of the respondents use only filtration whereas 36 per cent of the respondents use the both method of filtration. 1.3 per cent use only boiling process and 1.3 per cent of the respondents does not use any purification method (Table 14.5).

**Table 14.5:** Distribution of the Respondents on the basis of Purification Method

| *Methods* | *Frequency* | *Percentage* |
|---|---|---|
| Filter | 92 | 61.4 |
| Boil | 2 | 1.3 |
| Filter + Boil | 54 | 36 |
| None | 2 | 1.3 |
| **Total** | **150** | **100** |

*Source:* Field survey.

## Disposal of Daily Waste/Garbage by the Respondents

Disposal of daily waste is very much important especially in urban area where the density of population is very high. Proper disposal of waste and garbage can help to keep the environment pollution free. It is shown in Table 14.6. 61.3 per cent of the respondents dispose the waste in common municipal pit whereas 32.7 per cent of the respondents simply throw the waste/garbage outside the fencing. And only 6 per cent of the respondents use to dispose the garbage in personal composite pit.

**Table 14.6:** Status of Garbage Disposal among the Respondents

| *Disposal Pattern* | *Frequency* | *Percentage* |
|---|---|---|
| Personal Composite Pit | 9 | 6 |
| Common Municipal Pit | 92 | 61.3 |
| Throw Outside the Fencing | 49 | 32.7 |
| **Total** | **150** | **100** |

*Source:* Field survey.

## Pattern of Sufferings of the Respondents from Diseases during Last 6 Months

Table 14.7 shows that 22 per cent of the respondents were suffering or suffered from diarrhea which is considered to be water, hand-wash and sanitation related disease. Where 18 per cent suffered from viral fever, 10 per cent Jaundice, 14 per cent Gastric/ Acidity, 4 per cent from Cholera and other disease sufferings constitutes 8 per cent. Twenty four per cent of the respondents did suffer from skin diseases during last 6 months from the date of survey.

**Table 14.7:** Pattern of Disease Suffering among the Respondents

| *Type of disease* | *Frequency (n = 50)* | *Percentage* |
|---|---|---|
| Diarrhea | 11 | 22 |
| Viral Fever | 9 | 18 |
| Jaundice | 5 | 10 |
| Gastric/Acidity | 7 | 14 |
| Cholera | 2 | 4 |
| Other | 4 | 8 |
| Skin diseases | 12 | 24 |

*Source:* Field survey.

### Pattern of Access to Mass Media among the Respondents about Sanitation and Hygiene Awareness

Mass media has a significant role in creation of awareness about health and hygienic behaviour among people now a day. Table 14.8 shows that 92 per cent of the respondents do have access to mass media. 1.3 per cent of respondents do not have access to mass media about hygienic behaviour, while 6.7 per cent of them occasionally accesses.

**Table 14.8:** Awareness Pattern of the Respondents about Sanitation and Hygiene

| *Remarks* | *Frequency* | *Percentage* |
|---|---|---|
| Yes | 138 | 92 |
| No | 2 | 1.3 |
| Occasionally | 10 | 6.7 |
| **Total** | **150** | **100** |

*Source:* Field survey.

### Sanitation Coverage and Perception Level

Overall, the study shows an increasing trend in health awareness among the higher educated respondents with improvement in sanitation coverage. Specifically, there was a low but positive correlation found between the sanitation coverage and level of awareness.

### Relation between Education and Perception Level

Awareness of hygiene tended to increase with the educational level of the respondents. Most of the respondents with an adequate level of education had a sufficient level of awareness or perception of hygiene. However, among the respondent with no formal education, have a lower level of hygiene perception.

### Perception Level Across Different Economic Level

Respondents at higher economic level were found to be more aware of hygiene and health issues. The higher economic group had the highest awareness of safe storage and handling of drinking water, safe disposal of human excreta etc.

### Practice of Hygiene Across Different Economic Level

Similar to awareness or perception, the reported hygienic practices also improved with increases in economic level. Higher levels of hygiene practice were recorded for higher economic group for instance, the monthly income category of 15,000 and above.

### Impact of Perception on Practice of Hygiene in the Community

In the study area, in which part of it, good perception of hygiene and practices were being made, that particular sub-area found to be clean and healthy, with systematic disposal of garbage in municipality pit and better level of drainage system.

### Impact of Hygiene Practice on Disease Burden in the Community

In the area of study were some of the poor economic background peoples were living, a negative correlation score found between the hygiene awareness and the incidence of the water borne diseases. Where in comparatively better socio-economic conditioned sub area, respondents were found comparatively less affected by water born diseases. Considering the brief analysis of the study, it has been clearly understood that, though the some of the respondents have a lower level of education such as primary, under metric including the illiterate, they have a adequate level of hygiene perception and practices like hand-wash, proper handling and filtering of drinking water at personal level which might be due to frequent access to mass media and the awareness programmes while these perception and practices found in a better format among the few higher educated respondents highlighting the significance of education. These three factors, carelessness of certain government authority, poverty and lack of education are interrelated in the study area and are the crucial reason that are affecting the area's environment, becoming the hindrance of development good hygienic atmosphere.

## Conclusion

Considering the analysis of this study, it has been clearly understood that, majority of the respondents have higher levels of education, which resulted in having an adequate level of hygiene perception and practices like hand-wash, proper handling and filtering of drinking water at personal level. But still some areas are found to be unhygienic, because of non-availability of common municipal pit. Rarely one or two pits are available the conditions of which are very pathetic due to lack of proper maintenance. Secondly, the study shows the existence of a significant difference of economic status of two groups of people. Poor people cannot think about proper sanitation though they have the little knowledge about the importance and value of it. This is the reason because of which most of the poor people of study area are using *kachcha* latrine and other worst type of sanitation facilities. Last but not the least, negligence and unawareness among the educated group are found to be one of the main reasons behind unhygienic condition. These three factors are crucial reasons that are affecting the study area's environment and becoming the hindrance for development of good hygienic atmosphere. While, though educating the people, making them aware and removal of poverty would be a time consuming process, but if proper steps and scheme are adopted by the government these problems may be solved.

## References

Theodore Hough, William Thompson Sedgwick (2008) "Elements of hygiene and sanitation", (pp. 1-288), United States, Biblio Bazar Publisher Nath, Kumar Jyoti; Chowdhury, Barenyo; Sengupta, (2010) "Study on Perception and Practice of Hygiene and Impact on Health In India", Dhaka, Bangladesh, February 2010, *South Asia Hygiene Practitioners' Workshop* (pp. 1-11) Retrieved from http://www.Ifh-Homehygiene.Org/Review/Study-Perception-And-Practice-Hygiene-And-Impact-Health-India (accessed on 15/09/2015)

Postma, Leonie; Getkate, Renate and van Wijk, Christine, (2004) "Life Skill-Based Hygiene Education: A guidance document on concepts, development and experiences with life" *Delft, the Netherlands, IRC International Water and Sanitation Centre.* No. 42 (pp. 1-144) Retrieved from http://www.wsp.org/Hygiene-Sanitation-Water Toolkit/

Resources/Readings/life%20skills%20Postma.pdf (accessed on17/09/2015)

Reddy, V. Ratna (2001) "Declining Social Composition in India", *E-journal of Economic and Political Weekly*, 36(29), (July 21-27, 2001): 2750-2751.

Sekhon, Harindar; Minhas, Sukhmeet, (2014) "A School based Survey on Hygiene in a Rural area of Northern India", *"International Journal of Pharma Research and Health Sciences"*, volume 2 (2), 2014: 179-184. Retrieved from http://www.pharmahealthsciences.net/pdfs/volume2/14_MS_1445.pdf (accessed on 15/09/2015).

World Health Organization (WHO), (2011), Report on Water, Sanitation and Hygiene Interventions and the Preventions of Diarrhea, Retrieved from http://www.who.int/elena/titles/bbc/wsh_diarrhoea/en/ (accessed on 17/09/2015).

World Health Organization, (WHO), Definition of Health, Retrieved from http://www.who.int/about/definition/en/print.html (accessed on 17/09/2015).

World Health Organization (WHO), on Diarrheal disease, Retrieved from http://www.who.int/mediacentre/factsheets/fs330/en/ (accessed on 17/09/2015)

Hygiene (n.d.) obtained from http://en.m.wkikipedia.org/wiki/hygiene Profile of North East India (n.d.) obtained from http://en.wikipedia.org/wiki/Northeast_India

Ministry of Women and Child Development (n.d.) Retrieved from http://wcd.nic.in/recommendations-rcmn2005-06.htm

General Information about North East India (n.d.) Retrieved from http://www.iitg.ernet.in/rcilts/phaseI/n_e.html

# 15
# Prevalence of Exclusive Breast-feeding Practices and Associated Factors among Mothers in North Eastern Region, India
## A Cross-Section Study

*Kh. Jitenkumar Singh*

## Introduction

Breast-feeding is a well established and recommended intervention for the improvement of child nutrition. Studies have shown that it reduces deaths in infants and young children (WHO, 2000; Black *et al.*, 2008; Jones *et al.*, 2003). The World Health Organization (WHO) recommends the practice of exclusive breast-feeding (EBF) of infants for the first six month of life after birth to achieve optimal growth, development and health (WHO, 2001; WHO, 2015; GoI, 2004). EBF means that the infant receives only breast milk upto six months of age. During this six-month period, no other liquids or semisolid or solids food or breast-feeding substitute should be given to the infants, not even water, with the exception of oral rehydration salt solution, or drops/syrups of vitamins, minerals or medicines (WHO, 2015). Previous studies have reported that EBF can protect the child from atopic ecyema (Ip *et al.*, 2009 and Kramer *et al.*, 2003), the risk of allergy, asthma, type II diabetes (Kramer *et al.*, 2001), leukaemia (Pettitt *et al.*, 1997) and obesity in later life (Jones *et al.*, 1998). Previous research established the benefits of EBF to health and well-being for both infants and mothers (Kramer, 2010). A child who is EBF for first six month of the life after birth is more likely to protected from gastrointestinal infections, respiratory illness, morbidity and death (Ip *et al.*, 2009 and Kramer *et al.*, 2003; Jones *et al.*, 2003), which has a great contribution in reducing under five mortality. Exclusive breast-feeding is a safe, economical and emotionally satisfying means of feeding babies, it provides babies the perfect nutrition and everything they need for healthy growth and brain development. Throughout the world, in developed and developing countries alike, inappropriate feeding of infants leading to their poor nutrition is a significant problem affecting socio-economic progress in general (Akri, 1989). EBF is estimated to prevent approximately 10 per cent of child deaths and could play an important role in meeting India's Millennium Development Goal 4 of reducing child mortality. The Indian Government developed the Infant and Young Child Feeding (IYCF) guideline in 2004 (MoHFW, 2004) and improving infant and young child feeding practices with a strong emphasis on promotion of exclusive breast-feeding upto six months, is a priority under the governments various programme's.

Understanding of factors (or predicators) that influence EBF for mothers is important to be able to breastfeed exclusively to the recommended six months. Various factors (or predicators) have been found to be associated with EBF: socio-demographic factors; biosocial factors; cultural factors and employment status. Previous studies have reported several factors (or predicators) of EBF. Several factors (or predicators) have been shown to be associated with EBF: variations between urban and rural areas, mother employment status, level of education, knowledge about breast-feeding practices, occupation, household income, mother's smoking status, socio-economic position, parity, positive attitude towards EBF, initiation of breast-feeding, mode of delivery, place of delivery infants birth weight, infant's age, discarding colostrum and community beliefs (Merten & Ackermann-Liebrich, 2004; Lande *et al.*, 2003; Aidam, Pe'rez-Escamilla and Lartey, 2005; Shirima, Greiner, Kylberg and Gebre-Medhin, 2000; Egata, Berhane and Worku, 2013; Setegn *et al.*, 2013; Tan, 2011). Although breast-feeding is universal in India, but exclusive breast-feeding and appropriate weaning practices rate are not satisfactory, diverse socio-cultural factors influence these practices, which vary from region to region (IIPS, 2007). In India, the prevalence of EBF is low, 43.1 per cent in 1992-93, and 46.5 per cent in 1998-99 and slightly less than half of children i.e., 46.4 per cent in 2005-06 (IIPS,

1994; IIPS, 2000, IIPS, 2007). This study attempts to assess the prevalence of EBF and associated factors among mother having infants aged less than six months in North Eastern region, India.

North Eastern region is comprised of eight small states, namely, Assam, Arunachal Pradesh, Manipur, Meghalaya, Mizoram, Nagaland, Sikkim and Tripura. Table 15.1 shows the socio-demographic profiles of the eight North Eastern states. Highest population density is in Assam (398) and lowest density is in Arunachal Pradesh (17). Arunachal Pradesh has the highest and Sikkim has the lowest 0-5 year population constituting respectively 29 per cent and 5 per cent of the state total population. Meghalaya reports the highest and Tripura the lowest natural growth rate of 16.6 and 9.9 per 1000 population respectively. Mizoram has highest percentage of urban population, 52.1 per cent and Arunachal Pradesh has the lowest urban population, 5.1 per cent. Majority of population in Mizoram are Scheduled Tribe, 94.4 per cent. There is no Schedule Caste population in Arunachal Pradesh and Nagaland states, but 17.8 per cent Schedule Caste in Tripura. The female literacy rate is highest in Mizoram, 89.3 per cent and others states are also higher than the national average female literacy except for Arunachal Pradesh. According to Sample Registration System 2013, infant mortality rates (IMR) were found to be lower than the country's average of 47 deaths per 1000 live birth in all the states except Assam (54). This study emphasizes that women characteristics and household environment in which a child is born and brought up, are important determining factors of child health, more so in the context of the isolated and inaccessible areas of North Eastern region. The region is not only physically isolated from the rest of the country due to mountains terrain and poor infrastructure, it has diverse socio-cultural practices bringing up children, given that the region is inhabited by numerous tribal and ethnic groups. These indigenous people live mostly in rural areas and mountainous terrain in traditional thatched roof huts without basic amenities. The lack of basic amenities and diverse socio-cultural practices of exclusive breast-feeding is directly or indirectly responsible for the prevalence of exclusive breast-feeding practices in this region. This chapter presents a study to enrich the understanding of the extent of exclusive breast-feeding in North Eastern region, India and its associated factors.

**Table 15.1:** Profiles and Demographic Characteristics of States in North-Eastern Region, India

| Variables | Arunachal Pradesh | Assam | Manipur | Meghalaya | Mizoram | Nagaland | Sikkim | Tripura |
|---|---|---|---|---|---|---|---|---|
| Land Area (sq. km.)[1] | 83743 | 78438 | 22327 | 22429 | 21081 | 16579 | 7096 | 10486 |
| Total population in million[1] | 1.38 | 31.21 | 2.57 | 2.97 | 1.10 | 1.98 | 0.61 | 3.67 |
| Population size—% of national population[1] | 0.1 | 2.6 | 0.2 | 0.2 | 0.1 | 0.2 | 0.1 | 0.3 |
| 0–5 (population in million)[1] | 0.18 | 3.94 | 0.32 | 0.49 | 0.15 | 0.24 | 0.05 | 0.39 |
| 0–5 (% of state population)[1] | 29.03 | 12.62 | 15.96 | 16.43 | 5.08 | 17.55 | 4.82 | 10.66 |
| Population density[1] | 17 | 398 | 115 | 132 | 52 | 119 | 86 | 350 |
| Urban percentage (%)[1] | 5.1 | 14.1 | 6.0 | 20.0 | 52.1 | 28.9 | 25.2 | 26.2 |
| Female literacy rate (%)[1] | 57.7 | 66.3 | 72.4 | 72.9 | 89.3 | 76.1 | 75.6 | 82.7 |
| Schedule Tribe percentage (%)[1] | 68.8 | 12.5 | 35.1 | 86.2 | 94.4 | 86.5 | 33.8 | 31.8 |
| Schedule Caste percentage (%)[1] | 0.0 | 7.2 | 3.8 | 0.6 | 0.1 | 0.0 | 4.6 | 17.8 |
| Sex ratio—Females per 1000 males[1] | 938 | 958 | 992 | 989 | 976 | 931 | 890 | 960 |
| 0–5 Sex ratio Females per 100 males[1] | 970 | 963 | 930 | 972 | 971 | 943 | 953 | 961 |
| Birth rate[2] | 19.3 | 22.4 | 14.7 | 23.9 | 16.1 | 15.4 | 17.1 | 13.7 |
| Death rate[2] | 5.8 | 7.8 | 4.0 | 7.6 | 4.3 | 3.1 | 5.2 | 4.7 |
| Natural growth rate[2] | 13.4 | 14.5 | 10.6 | 16.4 | 11.8 | 12.3 | 11.8 | 9.0 |
| Infant mortality rate[2] | 32 | 54 | 10 | 47 | 35 | 18 | 22 | 26 |

*Sources*: 1. Census of India, 2011, 2. *Sample Registration System*, Vol. 49, No. 1, 2014.

## Data and Methods

The present study was based on a publicly available datasets, the National Family Health Survey, NFHS-3 (2005-06). The International Institute for Population Sciences and Macro-International conducted the National Family Health Survey (NFHS-3) in India during 2005-06. The information provided NFHS-3 survey data is cross-sectional. The NFHS-3 was a useful and valid source of information on breast-feeding from a nationally representative sample households. The survey sample was selected using systematic, multi-stage stratified cluster sampling. A total of 20,470 households were selected for the sample, of which 21,843 were interviewed in North Eastern region, India (IIPS, 2007). NFHS-3 data use cluster-sampling to draw upon women respondents *via* multistage stratified sampling. The urban and rural samples within each state were drawn separately and the sample within each state was allocated proportionally to the size of the state's urban and rural populations. A uniform sample design was adopted in all states. In each state, the rural sample was selected in two stages, with the selection of Primary Sampling Units (PSUs), which are villages, with proportional to population size (PPS) at the first stage, followed by the random selection of households within each PSU in the second stage. In urban areas, a three-stage procedure was followed. In the first stage, wards were selected with PPS sampling. In the next stage, one census enumeration block (CEB) was randomly selected from each sample ward as a selected PSU. A list of households was obtained for each PSU. In the final stage, households were randomly selected within each selected PSU. All eligible ever-married women between the ages of 15 to 49 living in the sample households were interviewed. Details of clustering and sample selection are explained in the reports (IIPS, 2007). The women's questionnaire covered the topics: background characteristics (current age, education, religion, etc.), reproductive behaviour and intentions, marriage and cohabitation, knowledge and use of contraception, quality of care and contacts with health personnel, antenatal, delivery, and post-natal care, general health, child immunizations, breast-feeding, child health and child feeding practices, fertility, women's and children's nutrition, utilization of ICDS services, status of women and spousal violence, sexual life, HIV/AIDS and other sexually transmitted infections, respectively (IIPS, 2007). Information on duration of breast-feeding and breast-feeding practices was collected through a series of questions from eligible women who had live births during the five years preceding the survey (IIPS, 2007). The socio-demographic characteristic of breast-feeding mother (respondent) and median duration of breast-feeding analysis were based on alive children born to women during three years preceding the survey and the total weighted sample size was 5123. Median duration of breast-feeding were computed based on the current status data on breast-feeding 5123 weighted sample. Exclusive breast-feeding analysis was restricted to the last-born children age less than 6 months, living with the mother, alive and total weighted sample size was 954 which was extracted from weighted 5123 sample.

### Analysis

Univariate analysis was carried out for all variables to describe their characteristics using descriptive analytical methods (frequencies, proportion and 95% C.I.). Computation of median duration of EBF: children who received only mother's milk as the sole nutrition source, except for vitamin, mineral and/or medication drops or syrups, full breast-feeding: children who received either exclusive breastfed or received breast milk and plain water only, and any breast-feeding: children who received mother's milk as well as another fluid or food, including other milk or child formulae, were based on current status data. Information was first obtained on the proportion of children currently being breastfed according to the children's age in months. The distribution is smoothed by average of three groups, then percentage (or proportion) of children in each groups were calculated (Rutstein and Rojas, 2012). The prevalence of EBF was calculated based on the respective age of the infants. Proportion of EBF was also estimated further for the following categorization 0-1, 2-3 and 4-5 month of age. It should be noted that this indicator does not represent the proportion of infants who are exclusively breastfed until their sixth month of age. In bivariate analysis, differences in the proportion of EBF were assessed among the different level of each predictor. Crude Odds Ratio (OR) with 95 per cent confidence intervals (95% C.I.) and Pearson's chi-square ($\chi^2$) tests were performed to identify associations between categorical variables. Mann-Whitney test was used to test for a difference in exclusive breast-feeding tendencies between urban resident's mother and rural resident's mother and between Hindu mother and non-Hindu mother. Kruskal-Wallis test was also used to test for a difference in exclusive breast-feeding tendencies of mother with different age at birth and infant birth interval. Variance inflation factors (VIF) was used to identify collinearity among explanatory variables. The function calculates the VIF values for all explanatory variables, removes the variable with the highest value, and repeats until all VIF values are below the threshold. Independent variables, which falls below threshold are selected. In multivariate analysis, selected independent variables were considered for a multivariate logistic regression analysis to identify the association between the dichotomous outcomes variable: EBF (Yes/No) and explanatory factors among mothers having infants aged less than 6 month. Adjusted Odds Ratio (AOR) and 95 per cent confidence interval (95% C.I.) were reported for the model. To account for the complex sampling design, Bootstrap method was performed to estimate 95 per cent CIs around prevalence estimates. All analyses were performed using R software (R-CRAN, version 3.2.1) and Rstudio with packages epicalc, survey and lme4. All estimates were adjusted for study design and sampling weight to address the complex survey design. All tests were two-sided and $p < 0.05$ was considered statistically significant. The Hosmer and Lemshow goodness-of-fit test was used to assess whether the necessary assumption for the application of logistic regression were fulfilled and p value > 0.05 was considered a good fit.

## Definition of Variables

### Outcome Variable

The outcome variable, exclusive breast-feeding (EBF) was defined based on the WHO key infant feeding indicators and guide to DHS statistics (IIPS, 2007). EBF was defined as giving the infant who were currently breast-feeding and no other liquids or drink or solids – not even water except for oral rehydration salt (ORS), drops and syrup (vitamins, minerals and medicines). With the present study, the outcome variable, EBF was categorized as a dichotomous variable EBF: coded as 1; and Non-EBF: coded as 0. The missing data (0.3%) on breast-feeding was treated as Non-EBF.

### Explanatory Variables

Place of residence was classified into two categories: urban and rural areas. Mother age at birth from 15 to 49 years old were coded as: 15-19, 20-24, 25-29 and 30-49. Level of education of mother was also grouped into three categories: illiterate i.e., no education, literate, less than middle school and middle school complete and higher. Religion variable was categorized into Hindu and non-Hindu. Social status was classified into two categories: SC/ST (relatively disadvantaged group includes Schedule Caste and Scheduled Tribe who are socially and economically marginalised) and others (relatively advantaged). Occupation of mother was defined as the working status of the mother and categorised into two categories: working and not working. The wealth index is an international composite indicator of more than 40 household assets variables (IIPS,

2007). It is categorised into poorest, poor, middle, rich and richest. Mother having antenatal care (ANC) visits are more likely to promote exclusive breast-feeding practices during the first six months. Antenatal visit by a mother were reorganised into three groups (No visit, 1-3, 4 or more visits). In relation to place of delivery, option were categorised into two categories namely institutional and non-institutional. The generic mode of delivery: normal or caesarean section were also considered. Birth order was also categorized into three categories: one, two and three or more birth order. Birth interval was categorised into three categories: No previous birth, less than 24 month and birth interval greater than or equal 24 months. An infant's size at birth was categorised based on mother's perception into very small, small, average, large and very large. This was later re-categorised into two group: small and or average and large. In infant's sex was grouped as reported in the survey – male or female. Infant's age was computed in month (in CMC) and further grouped into four categories: <2 month, 2-3 month, 4-5 month and 6 and above. In terms of region, all the eight states in the North Eastern region, India, were considered. All explanatory variables used in the analysis are from NFHS-3.

**Ethics Statement**

The study is based on data available in the public domain, therefore, no ethical issue is involved.

**Results**

Socio-demographic characteristics of the respondents are presented in Table 15.2. Majority (77.4%) of the mothers residing in rural area. Mother's age at birth ranged from 15 to 49 years. The distribution also showed that 38.9 per cent had middle school complete or higher education, and 31 per cent were literate, but less than middle school. Majority of mothers (65.3%) were belongs to Non-Hindu by religion, 57.6 per cent were schedule caste or schedule tribe, and 59.2 per cent of the respondent were not working, 25.4 per cent and 28.4 per cent of mothers were from poorer and middle wealth quintile. About 72 per cent of mothers have received any antenatal care. With regards to the place of delivery, 1837 (35.9%) delivered their youngest child at health

**Table 15.2:** Socio-Demographic Characteristics of Breast-feeding Mother-Based on Children Born to Women During Three Years Preceding the Survey in North Eastern Region, India, NFHS 3, 2005-06.

| *Characteristics (N=5123)* | *Nominal Categories* | *Weighted sample* | *Weighted proportion* | *95% C.I.* |
|---|---|---|---|---|
| Place of residence | Urban | 1158 | 22.6 | [21.1-24.2] |
| | Rural | 3965 | 77.4 | [75.8-78.9] |
| Mother age at birth (Years) | 15 – 19 | 686 | 13.4 | [12.3-14.6] |
| | 20 – 24 | 1600 | 31.2 | [29.9-32.6] |
| | 25 – 29 | 1491 | 29.1 | [27.8-30.4] |
| | 30 – 49 | 1346 | 26.3 | [24.9-27.7] |
| Educational status of mother | Illiterate | 1567 | 30.6 | [28.4-32.9] |
| | Literate,<middle school | 1585 | 30.9 | [29.2-32.8] |
| | Middle school complete and higher | 1970 | 38.5 | [36.2-40.8] |
| Religion | Hindu | 1779 | 34.7 | [31.4-38.2] |
| | Non-Hindu | 3344 | 65.3 | [61.8-68.6] |
| Social status | SC/ST | 2948 | 57.6 | [53.8-61.2] |
| | Others | 2175 | 42.4 | [38.8-46.2] |
| Occupation of mother | Not working | 3032 | 59.2 | [56.5-61.8] |
| | Working | 2091 | 40.8 | [38.2-43.5] |
| Wealth quintile | Poorest | 622 | 12.2 | [10.4-14.1] |
| | Poorer | 1301 | 25.4 | [23.5-27.4] |
| | Middle | 1457 | 28.4 | [26.6-30.4] |
| | Richer | 1097 | 21.4 | [19.7-23.3] |
| | Richest | 646 | 12.6 | [11.3-14.1] |
| Antenatal visits | No visit | 1427 | 27.9 | [25.6-30.3] |
| | 1 – 3 | 1854 | 36.2 | [34.3-38.2] |
| | ? 4 | 1842 | 35.9 | [33.5-38.5] |
| Place of delivery | Non institutional | 3286 | 64.1 | [61.5-66.7] |
| | Institutional | 1837 | 35.9 | [33.3-38.5] |
| Mode of delivery | Vaginal delivery | 4754 | 92.8 | [91.9-93.6] |
| | Caesarean section delivery | 369 | 7.2 | [6.4-8.1] |
| Birth order | One | 1485 | 29.0 | [27.5-30.5] |
| | Two | 1294 | 25.3 | [23.9-26.7] |
| | Three and above | 2344 | 45.7 | [43.9-47.7] |

*(Contd.)*

| *Characteristics (N=5123)* | *Nominal Categories* | *Weighted sample* | *Weighted proportion* | *95% C.I.* |
|---|---|---|---|---|
| Birth Interval | No previous birth | 1492 | 29.1 | [27.6-30.7] |
| | < 24 months | 825 | 16.1 | [15.0-17.3] |
| | ? 24 months | 2806 | 54.8 | [53.2-56.3] |
| Size of baby | Large and average | 3967 | 77.4 | [75.8-79.0] |
| | Small | 1156 | 22.6 | [21.0-24.2] |
| Gender of infant | Male | 2598 | 50.7 | [49.2-52.2] |
| | female | 2525 | 49.3 | [47.8-50.8] |
| Age of infant (month) | < 2 | 235 | 4.6 | [3.9-5.2] |
| | 2 – 3 | 361 | 7.0 | [6.2-7.8] |
| | 4 – 5 | 358 | 7.0 | [6.2-7.7] |
| | 6 and above | 4169 | 81.4 | [80.2-82.5] |
| States | Arunachal Pradesh | 401 | 7.8 | [6.0-10.2] |
| | Assam | 829 | 16.2 | [12.8-20.3] |
| | Manipur | 1069 | 20.8 | [17.7-24.4] |
| | Meghalaya | 586 | 11.4 | [8.8-14.7] |
| | Mizoram | 423 | 8.3 | [6.3-10.7] |
| | Nagaland | 1098 | 21.4 | [18.3-25.0] |
| | Sikkim | 372 | 7.3 | [5.4-9.8] |
| | Tripura | 345 | 6.8 | [5.0-9.0] |

*Note:* C.I.: Confidence interval. 4874-unweighted cases; 5123-weighted cases.

*Source*: Based on author's computation from NFHS-3 (2005-06).

institutions. The mode of delivery distribution indicated that most 4754 mothers (92.8%) had a normal vaginal delivery. A significant proportion (45.7%) of the respondents were mother who had given birth to three or more children. Majority of participants (54.8%) were had birth interval greater than equal to 24 months, 29.1 per cent were no previous birth. According to the mothers' perceptions, 77.4 per cent of infant were of average size at birth, male and female were almost equal proportion.

Median duration of exclusive breast-feeding, full breast-feeding and any breast-feeding were computed based on 5123 (weighted sample) among last-born children born in the three years preceding the survey living with mothers. Table 15.3 shows the median duration of EBF, full breast-feeding and any (total) breast-feeding were 2.1 months, 4.0 months and 33.2 months respectively. Median duration of EBF in rural areas was 2.2 months, 2.3 months

**Table 15.3:** Median Duration of Exclusive Breast-feeding, Full Breastfeeding and Any Breast-feeding Among Last-Born Children Born in the Three Years Preceding the Survey Living with Mother by Background Characteristics, North Eastern Region, India, NFHS-3, 2005-06.

| *Characteristics (N=5123)* | *Nominal Categories* | *Median duration# (months) of breastfeeding among last-born children born in the last three years* | | |
|---|---|---|---|---|
| | | *Exclusive breast-feeding* | *Full breast-feeding* | *Any Breast-feeding* |
| Place of residence | Urban | 2.0 | 3.6 | 33.7 |
| | Rural | 2.2 | 4.2 | 35.2 |
| Educational status of mother | Illiterate | 2.3 | 4.3 | 35.2 |
| | Literate, < middle school | 2.0 | 4.1 | 31.4 |
| | Middle school complete and higher | 2.2 | 3.8 | 32.7 |
| Religion | Hindu | 1.2 | 4.2 | 36.0 |
| | Non-Hindu | 1.7 | 3.9 | 26.0 |
| Social status | SC/ST | 1.2 | 3.9 | 25.7 |
| | Others | 3.0 | 4.2 | 34.5 |
| Occupation of mother | Not working | 2.2 | 4.1 | 31.7 |
| | Working | 2.1 | 3,8 | 34.4 |
| Wealth quintile | Poorest | 3.1 | 5.1 | 36.0 |
| | Poorer | 3.3 | 5.1 | 34.2 |
| | Middle | 1.8 | 3.9 | 36.0 |
| | Richer | 1.4 | 3.7 | 29.1 |
| | Richest | 1.0 | 3.4 | 31.3 |
| Gender of infant | Male | 1.9 | 4.2 | 35.2 |
| | Female | 2.4 | 3.9 | 31.1 |
| Birth Interval | No previous birth | 2.1 | 4.2 | 35.3 |
| | < 24 months | 1.8 | 3.5 | 34.0 |
| | ? 24 months | 2.4 | 4.5 | 32.7 |
| Antenatal visits | No visit | 2.6 | 4.3 | 34.2 |
| | 1–3 visit | 2.2 | 4.2 | 31.0 |
| | ? 4 visit | 1.7 | 3.7 | 33.8 |
| Place of delivery | Non-institutional | 2.2 | 4.2 | 32.1 |
| | Institutional | 2.0 | 3.8 | 34.2 |
| Birth order | One | 1.8 | 3.6 | 34.1 |
| | Two | 2.4 | 4.3 | 34.0 |
| | Three or more | 2.2 | 4.2 | 33.0 |
| **Total** | | **2.1** | **4.0** | **33.2** |

Note: # represents the median duration after adjusting for study design and sample weight.

*Source*: Based on author's computation from NFHS-3 (2005-06).

for illiterate mothers, 1.7 months for Non-Hindu, 3.0 months for non-Schedule Caste and non-Schedule Tribe social status. Median duration of EBF was higher 3.1 months and 3.3 months for poorest and poorer wealth quintile, 2.4 month each for female infant, infant birth interval = 24 months, and birth order 2 infants, respectively. Median duration of full breast-feeding were 4.2 month and 4.3 month for mothers who are residing in rural areas and respondents who are illiterate in education. Median duration of full breast-feeding were higher among mothers belonging to poorest and poorer wealth quintile, 5.1 months each and 4.5 months for infant having birth interval =24 months.

Median duration of any (total) breast-feeding were higher among Hindu mothers by religion, belonging to poorest and poorer wealth quintile, 36 month each. Median duration of any breast-feeding was 35.3 months for infants having no previous birth. Median duration of any breast-feeding was 35.2 months each for mothers residing in rural areas, illiterate's mothers and male by sex of infants. But, lowest median duration were found 26.0 months for Non-Hindu mothers and 25.7 months for mother belonging to Schedule Caste or Schedule Tribe.

From this study, the prevalence of exclusive breast-feeding among mothers with infants age less than six month 46.2 per cent (95% CI=42.1-50.2) whereas 51.2 per cent (95% CI=46.7-55.7) and 56.6 per cent (95% CI=51.8-61.5) were exclusively breastfed upto five month and four month. The prevalence of exclusive when stratified by infant age from one to five months ranged between 26.4 per cent (95% CI=20.0-33.7) and 75.9 per cent (95% CI=65.0-83.9) with the highest among less than one month old infants and lowest among five month old infants. There is observed prominent decline as the age of infant progresses, the prevalence of EBF were 64.3 per cent (95% CI=57.7-70.5) for infants less than 2 months, 51.8 per cent (95% CI=45.4-58.1) between 2-3 month and 28.5 per cent (95% CI=23.8-34.1) between 4-5 months. As a child grows in months, exclusive breast-feeding decreases (Table 15.4).

In the first month of life, 63 per cent and 65 per cent of infants in urban areas and rural areas received EBF which declined to 51 per cent and 52 per cent in 2-3 months and 29 per cent each by the age of 4-5 months (Fig. 15.1). 67 per cent, 64 per cent and 61 per cent of infants age <2 month received EBF among different mother's age at birth 15-19, 20-34 and 35-49 years, and decline as the age of infant

**Table 15.4:** Infant Age Distribution and Prevalence (95% CI) of Exclusive Breast-feeding (weighted) Among Last-Born Children Living with Mother Who Were Less Than Six Month, North Eastern Region, India, NFHS-3, 2005-06.

| *Characteristics (N=954)* | *Weighted sample* | *Weighted proportion of exclusive breast-feeding* | |
|---|---|---|---|
| | | Sample (%)# | 95% C.I. |
| Infant age (months) | | | |
| < One | 87 | 66 (75.9) | [65.0-83.9] |
| One | 148 | 85 (57.4) | [48.9-65.9] |
| Two | 186 | 106 (57.0) | [48.6-64.7] |
| Three | 175 | 81 (46.3) | [37.9-54.9] |
| Four | 165 | 51 (30.9) | [23.8-39.6] |
| Five | 193 | 51 (26.4) | [20.0-33.7] |
| Infant age group (months) | | | |
| < 2 | 235 | 151 (64.3) | [57.7-70.5] |
| 2 – 3 | 361 | 187 (51.8) | [45.4-58.1] |
| 4 – 5 | 358 | 102 (28.5) | [23.5-34.1] |
| Infant age less than four month | 596 | 338 (56.7) | [51.8-61.5] |
| Infant age less than five month | 760 | 389 (51.2) | [46.7-55.7] |
| Infant age less than six month | 954 | 440 (46.2) | [42.1-50.2] |

*Note:* # the proportion represents the percentage (in the parenthesis) after adjusting for study design and sample weight.

*Source*: Based on author's computation from NFHS-3 (2005-06).

progresses, 47 per cent, 53 per cent and 51 per cent in 2-3 month and 23 per cent, 31 per cent and 15 per cent by age of 4-5 months (Fig. 15.2). Among mother who are belongs to Hindu and Non-Hindu by religion, 73 per cent and 59 per cent were provided EBF in infant <2 month, and which shows decline to 62 per cent and 46 per cent in 2-3 months, 33 per cent and 27 per cent in 4-5 months (Fig. 15.3). Prevalence of EBF for no previous birth infants were 60 per cent in infants <2 month, 48 per cent in 2-3 months and 27 per cent in 4-5 months. 68 per cent, 55 per cent and 32 per cent were provided EBF in infants <2, 2-3 month and 4-5 month and showing decline as age progresses. Tendency of EBF between urban and rural areas, mothers with different age group at birth, Hindu and Non-Hindu, and different birth interval were shows similar trends. From the Mann-Whitney test, W=18022, p-value=0.9079, hence no evidence to reject the null-hypothesis. That mother residing in urban areas and mother residing in rural areas have the same EBF tendency at the 5 per cent level. And for Hindu and non-Hindu mother, W=21428, p-value=0.6463, hence no evidence to reject the null

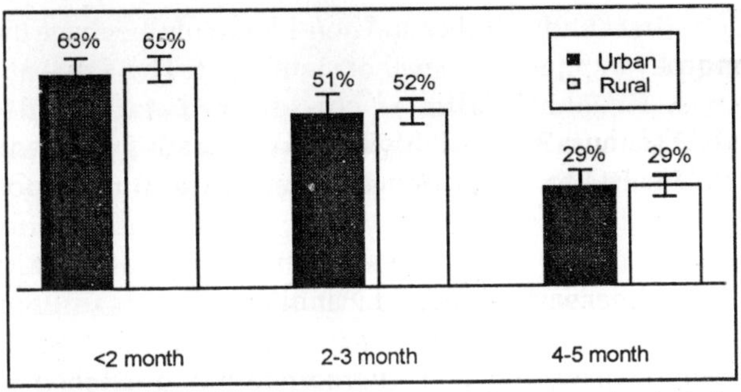


**Fig. 15.1:** Prevalence of exclusive breast-feeding practice in infants less than six months of age by place of residence.

*Source:* Author's Study.

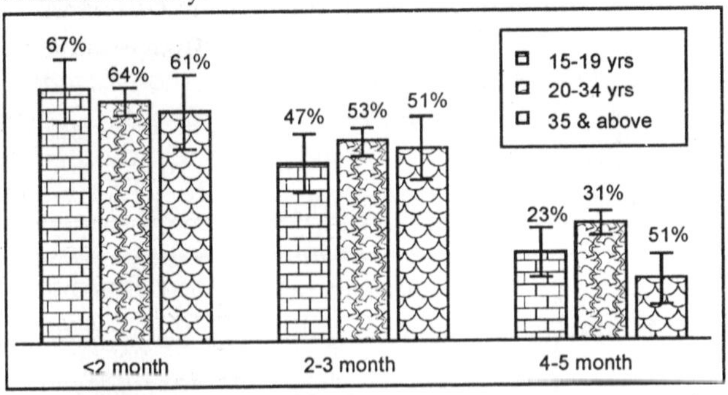


**Fig. 15.2:** Prevalence of exclusive breast-feeding practice in infants less than six months of age by maternal age.

*Source:* Author's Study.

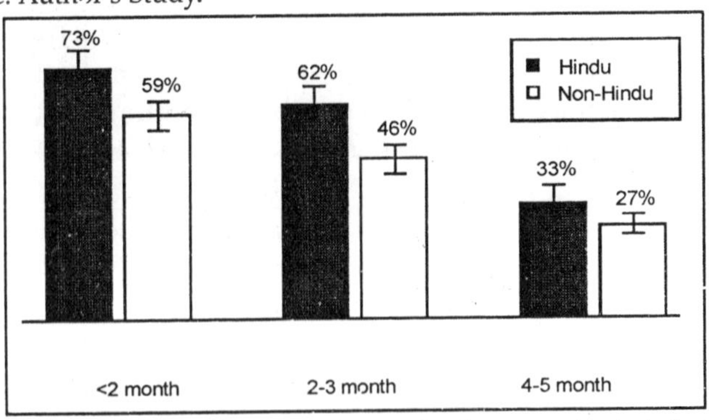


**Fig. 15.3:** Prevalence of exclusive breast-feeding practice in infants less than six months of age by religion.

*Source:* Author's Study.

hypothesis that Hindu mother and non-Hindu mother have the same EBF tendency at 5 per cent level of significant. The Kruskal-Wallis test gives, Kruskal-Wallis $\chi^2$ chi-squared=4.2092, df=3, p-value=0.2397, and Kruskal-Wallis chi-squared=2.5821, df=2, p-value=0.275, hence no evidence to reject the null-hypothesis, respectively. Therefore, likely to believe that there is no differences in EBF tendency between mothers with different age at birth and between mothers with different birth interval.

In bivariate analysis, the factors religion, social status, wealth index, birth order and age of infant were found association with EBF at 0.05 level of alpha (Tables 15.5 and 15.6). Evidence of an association was observed with religion of household (Crude OR=1.68, 95% CI=1.27-2.21). Mothers who are Hindu by religion had higher odds of EBF than those Non-Hindu mothers. Odds of EBF were found higher, for social status: others (non-Schedule Caste or non-Schedule Tribe) (Crude OR=1.74, 95% CI=1.33-2.27), poorest (Crude OR=1.79, 95% CI=1.07-2.99) and poorer (Crude OR=2.18, 95% CI=1.41-3.38), birth order one (Crude OR=1.26, 95% CI=0.89-1.78) and birth order three or more (Crude OR=1.75, 95% CI=1.16-2.64).

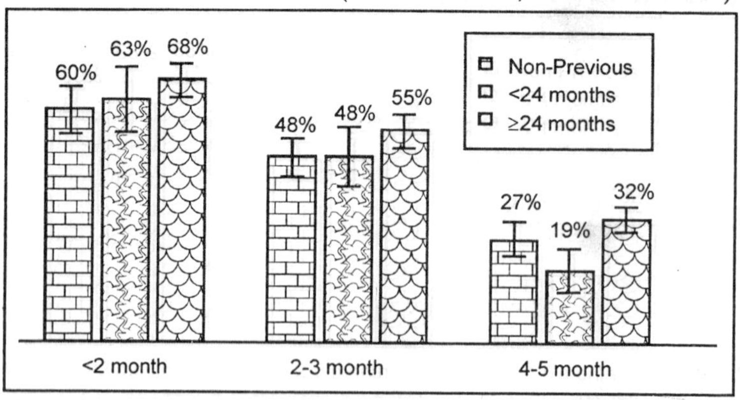


**Fig. 15.4:** Prevalence of exclusive breast-feeding practice in infants less than six months of age by birth interval.

*Source:* Author's Study.

In multivariate analysis no all factors showed significant association at 0.05 level of alpha, but again there was some evidence of association with religion: Hindu (p=0.024), social status: others (p=0.016) and wealth quintile: poorest (p=0.042) and poorer (p=0.007) and mother's age at birth (Table 15.7). Mother's age at birth between 20-24 years (AOR=1.25, 95% CI=0.93-2.01) were more likely to

**Table 15.5:** Bivariate Analysis of Socio-Demographic Variables (factors) Associated with the Interruption of Exclusive Breast-feeding Based on Last-Born Children Living with Mother Who Were Less Than Six Month in North-Eastern Region, India, NFHS-3, 2005-06

| *Characteristics (N=954)* | *Nominal Categories* | *EBF (n=440), n (%)#* | *Non-EBF (n=514), n (%)#* | $\chi^2$ | *p-value* | *Crude OR (95% C.I.)* |
|---|---|---|---|---|---|---|
| Place of residence | Urban | 93 (44.7) | 115 (55.3) | 0.1736 | 0.677 | 1.00 [reference] |
| | Rural | 347 (46.5) | 399 (53.5) | | | 1.20 [0.91-1.59] |
| Mother age at birth (Years) | 15 – 19 | 56 (44.1) | 71 (55.9) | 0.6925 | 0.875 | 1.00 [reference] |
| | 20 – 24 | 147 (48.0) | 159 (52.0) | | | 1.21 [0.79-1.86] |
| | 25 – 29 | 127 (45.2) | 154 (54.8) | | | 1.11 [0.72-1.72] |
| | 30 – 49 | 111 (46.0) | 130 (54.0) | | | 1.11 [0.72-1.74] |
| Educational status of mother | Illiterate | 146 (48.7) | 154 (51.3) | 1.7372 | 0.420 | 1.00 [reference] |
| | Literate,<middle school | 134 (42.9) | 178 (57.1) | | | 0.79 [0.57-1.11] |
| | Middle school complete and higher | 160 (47.1) | 181 (52.9) | | | 0.84 [0.61-1.16] |
| Religion | Hindu | 179 (55.2) | 145 (44.8) | 11.9236 | 0.006 | 1.68 [1.27-2.21] |
| | Non-Hindu | 261 (41.4) | 369 (58.6) | | | 1.00 [reference] |
| Social status | SC/ST | 220 (39.9) | 332 (60.1) | 14.1886 | 0.002 | 1.00 [reference] |
| | Others | 220 (54.7) | 182 (45.3) | | | 1.74 [1.33-2.27] |
| Occupation of mother | Not Working | 308 (46.8) | 350 (53.2) | 0.2838 | 0.594 | 1.00 [reference] |
| | Working | 132 (44.6) | 164 (55.4) | | | 0.98 [0.74-1.31] |
| Wealth quintile | Poorest | 66 (51.6) | 62 (48.4) | 15.6999 | 0.004 | 1.79 [1.07-2.99] |
| | Poorer | 151 (55.5) | 121 (44.5) | | | 2.18 [1.41-3.38] |
| | Middle | 96 (38.2) | 155 (61.8) | | | 1.11 [0.72-1.73] |
| | Richer | 83 (43.7) | 107 (56.3) | | | 1.33 [0.85-2.09] |
| | Richest | 44 (39.3) | 68 (60.7) | | | 1.00 [reference] |

*Notes:* # the proportion represents the percentage in the parentheses after adjusting for study design and sample weight.
EBF: Exclusive breast-feeding; Non-EBF: Non-Exclusive breast-feeding; n (%): Proportion per category.
C.I.: Confidence interval ; Crude OR: Crude Odds ratio.

*Sources:* Based on author's computation from NFHS-3 (2005-06).

provide EBF compared to mothers age at birth between 15-19 years. Keeping all factors constant mothers who are Hindu by religion had 1.6 times higher odds of EBF compared to those belonging to non-Hindu (AOR=1.55, 95% CI=1.06-2.28). The infants whose

**Table 15.6:** Bivariate Analysis of Variables (factors) Related to Antenatal Care (ANC) and Postnatal Care (PNC) Associated with the Interruption of Exclusive Breast-feeding Based on Last-Born Children Living with Mother Who Were Less Than Six Month in North Eastern Region, India, NFHS-3, 2005-06

| *Characteristics (N=954)* | *Nominal Categories* | *EBF (n=440) n (%)#* | *Non-EBF (n=514) n (%)#* | $\chi^2$ | *p-value* | *Crude OR (95% C.I.)* |
|---|---|---|---|---|---|---|
| Antenatal visits | No visit | 137 (51.5) | 130 (48.5) | 5.4698 | 0.066 | 1.58 [1.13-2.21] |
| | 1 – 3 | 162 (47.5) | 179 (52.5) | | | 1.33 [0.98-1.80] |
| | ? 4 | 141 (40.8) | 205 (59.2) | | | 1.00 [reference] |
| Place of delivery | Non- institutional | 285 (47.5) | 315 (52.5) | 0.8642 | 0.353 | 1.21 [0.92-1.58] |
| | Institutional | 156 (43.9) | 199 (56.1) | | | 1.00 [reference] |
| Mode of delivery | Vaginal delivery | 410 (46.1) | 480 (53.9) | 0.0298 | 0.863 | 1.00 [reference] |
| | Caesarean section | 30 (46.9) | 34 (53.1) | | | 1.03 [0.64-1.66] |
| Birth order | One | 125 (42.8) | 167 (57.2) | 8.5424 | 0.038 | 1.00 [reference] |
| | Two | 117 (49.4) | 120 (50.6) | | | 1.26 [0.89-1.78] |
| | Three and above | 181 (46.7) | 202 (53.3) | | | 1.75 [1.16-2.64] |
| Birth Interval | No previous birth | 127 (43.1) | 168 (56.9) | 4.1252 | 0.129 | 0.78 [0.58-1.05] |
| | < 24 months | 57 (41.0) | 82 (59.0) | | | 0.71 [0.47-1.08] |
| | ? 24 months | 256 (49.3) | 264 (50.7) | | | 1.00 [reference] |
| Size of baby | Large and average | 329 (45.4) | 395 (54.6) | 0.5769 | 0.448 | 1.00 [reference] |
| | Small | 112 (48.7) | 118 (51.3) | | | 1.14 [0.83-1.54] |
| Gender of infant | Male | 207 (43.7) | 267 (56.3) | 2.2384 | 0.135 | 1.00 [reference] |
| | female | 233 (48.5) | 247 (51.5) | | | 1.15 [0.89-1.50] |
| Age of infant (month) | < 2 | 151 (64.3) | 84 (35.7) | 40.5198 | 0.000 | 4.67 [3.26-6.71] |
| | 2–3 | 187 (51.8) | 174 (48.2) | | | 2.72 [1.98-3.74] |
| | 4–5 | 102 (28.5) | 256 (71.5) | | | 1.00 [reference] |

*Note:* # the proportion represents the percentage in the parentheses after adjusting for study design and sample weight. EBF: Exclusive breast-feeding; Non-EBF: Non-Exclusive breast-feeding; n (%): Proportion per category.

*Sources:* Based on author's computation from NFHS-3 (2005-06).

**Table 15.7:** Multivariate Analysis of Socio-Demographic Variables (factors) Associated with the Interruption of Exclusive Breast-feeding Based on Last-Born Children Living with Mother Who were Less Than Six Month in North Eastern Region, India, NFHS-3, 2005-06

| *Variables (N=954)* | *Categories* | *Crude OR (95% CI)* | *Adjusted OR (95% CI)* | *p-value* |
|---|---|---|---|---|
| Place of residence | Urban | 0.930 [0.660-1.310] | 1.305 [0.87-1.958] | 0.205 |
| | Rural (Ref.) | 1.00 | 1.00 | |
| Mother age at birth (Years) | 15 – 19 (Ref.) | 1.00 | 1.00 | |
| | 20 – 24 | 1.128 [0.756-1.684] | 1.253 [0.927-2.010] | 0.044 |
| | 35 – 49 | 0.899 [0.499-1.619] | 0.978 [0.458-2.083] | 0.583 |
| Educational status of mother | Illiterate (Ref.) | 1.00 | 1.00 | |
| | Literate,<middle school | 0.798 [0.561-1.134] | 0.927 [0.612-1.402] | 0.720 |
| | Middle school complete and higher | 0.937 [0.667-1.319] | 1.252 [0.814-1.924] | 0.284 |
| Religion | Hindu | 1.750 [1.273-2.406] | 1.554 [1.061-2.276] | 0.024 |
| | Non-Hindu (Ref.) | 1.00 | 1.00 | |
| Social status | SC/ST (Ref.) | 1.00 | 1.00 | |
| | Others | 1.829 [1.333-2.510] | 1.587 [1.093-2.303] | 0.016 |
| Occupation of mother | Not working (Ref.) | 1.00 | 1.00 | |
| | Working | 0.920 [0.675-1.254] | 0.943 [0.657-1.353] | 0.751 |
| Wealth quintile | Poorest | 1.639 [0.954-2.816] | 1.942 [0.976-4.114] | 0.042 |
| | Poorer | 1.927 [1.207-3.076] | 2.340 [1.257-4.358] | 0.007 |
| | Middle | 0.953 [0.589-1.541] | 1.213 [0.672-2.189] | 0.509 |
| | Richer | 1.190 [0.743-1.909] | 1.277 [0.760-2.145] | 0.356 |
| | Richest (Ref.) | 1.00 | 1.00 | |

*(Contd.)*

| *Variables (N=954)* | *Categories* | *Crude OR (95% CI)* | *Adjusted OR (95% CI)* | *p-value* |
|---|---|---|---|---|
| Place of residence | Urban | 0.930 [0.660-1.310] | 1.305 [0.87-1.958] | 0.205 |
| | Rural (Ref.) | 1.00 | 1.00 | |
| Mother age at birth (Years) | 15 – 19 (Ref.) | 1.00 | 1.00 | |
| | 20 – 24 | 1.128 [0.756-1.684] | 1.253 [0.927-2.010] | 0.044 |
| | 35 – 49 | 0.899 [0.499-1.619] | 0.978 [0.458-2.083] | 0.583 |
| Educational status of mother | Illiterate (Ref.) | 1.00 | 1.00 | |
| | Literate,<middle school | 0.798 [0.561-1.134] | 0.927 [0.612-1.402] | 0.720 |
| | Middle school complete and higher | 0.937 [0.667-1.319] | 1.252 [0.814-1.924] | 0.284 |
| Religion | Hindu | 1.750 [1.273-2.406] | 1.554 [1.061-2.276] | 0.024 |
| | Non-Hindu (Ref.) | 1.00 | 1.00 | |
| Social status | SC/ST (Ref.) | 1.00 | 1.00 | |
| | Others | 1.829 [1.333-2.510] | 1.587 [1.093-2.303] | 0.016 |
| Occupation of mother | Not working (Ref.) | 1.00 | 1.00 | |
| | Working | 0.920 [0.675-1.254] | 0.943 [0.657-1.353] | 0.751 |
| Wealth quintile | Poorest | 1.639 [0.954-2.816] | 1.942 [0.976-4.114] | 0.042 |
| | Poorer | 1.927 [1.207-3.076] | 2.340 [1.257-4.358] | 0.007 |
| | Middle | 0.953 [0.589-1.541] | 1.213 [0.672-2.189] | 0.509 |
| | Richer | 1.190 [0.743-1.909] | 1.277 [0.760-2.145] | 0.356 |
| | Richest (Ref.) | 1.00 | 1.00 | |

*Sources*: Based on author's computation from NFHS-3 (2005-06).

mothers were from non-Schedule Caste or non-Schedule Tribe by social status (AOR=1.59, 95% CI=1.09-2.30) were more likely to be EBF. On the other hand, the infants with wealthier mothers were less likely to be provided with EBF. The odds ratio for exclusive breast-feeding was about twice as higher for poorest mothers (AOR=1.94, 95% CI=0.98-4.14) and 2.8 times higher for poorer mothers (AOR=2.34, 95% CI=1.26-4.36) with compared to wealthier mothers. Infants below 2 (AOR=4.56, 95% CI=3.16-6.58) and infants between 2-3 months (AOR=2.73, 95% CI=1.94-3.86) were more likely to be exclusive breast-feeding than the infants in higher age.

## Discussions

The present study was based on the exclusive breast-feeding definition recommended by World Health Organization calculated (Rutstein and Rojas, 2012) to an infant in the last 24 hours recall preceding the survey. The NFHS surveys used the '24 hour recall' methodology to collect data on exclusive breast-feeding and its validity has been questioned by several authors (Dibley *et al.*, 2010, Chudasama, Patel and Kavishwar, 2009; Aarts, 2000). Its major denigration is that it misclassifies too many mothers as exclusively breast-feeding (Dibley *et al.*, 2010). It was reported as wide discrepancy on the prevalence of exclusive breast-feeding between current status based on a 24-hour recording and exclusive breast-feeding since birth (Dibley *et al.*, 2010). Studies also indicate that there is a significant tendency to under report small quantity items administered in addition to breast milk overestimating exclusive breast-feeding rates from current status data (Chudasama, Patel and Kavishwar, 2009; Aarts, 2000). Based on this definition, identified four factors: religion, social-status, wealth index and infant age were significantly associated with exclusive breast-feeding. In the present study, the overall prevalence or exclusive breast-feeding among mothers with infants less than six months of age was 46.2 per cent. This result was almost similar to the national figure 46.4 per cent (IIPS, 2007).

The median duration of exclusive breast-feeding was 2.1 months which was also reported as 2.0 month by NFHS-3, and any breast-feeding was 33.2 month which is higher than national level (24.4 months) as reported by NFHS-3 (IIPS, 2007). The median duration of exclusive breast-feeding, full breast-feeding, and any breast-feeding were relatively high for children form non-Schedule Caste or non-Schedule Tribes. It also observed that median duration 36 month for Hindu was higher than non-Hindu (26 month). The median duration of exclusive breast-feeding, full breast-feeding and any breast-feeding was also shorter in urban areas, and it decreases steadily with mother's education and wealth index. In the present study, mothers who are Hindu (55.2%), non-Schedule Caste or non-Schedule Tribe (54.7%) were more likely to practice exclusive breast-feeding as compared to mothers in non-Hindu (41.4%), Schedule Caste or Schedule Tribe (39.9%). The low practice of exclusive breast-feeding in non-Hindu and Schedule Caste or Schedule Tribe can be attributed to cultural beliefs. Cultural practices may be practical less in Hindu and non-Schedule Caste or non-Schedule Tribe, and hence, mothers in Hindu or non-Schedule Caste or non-Schedule Tribe tends to be more likely to practice exclusive breast-feeding. Results found that the mothers from households belonging to wealthier quintile had lower odds of exclusive breast-feeding than those belonging to poorest wealth quintile, and similar results to other studies (ORC Macro, 2005; Blas and Kurup, 2010) have reported prevalence of exclusive breast-feeding to be higher among children belonging to poorest wealth quintile.

The proportion of exclusive breast-feeding decreased considerably as infant age progresses. In North Eastern region, majority (64.3%) of infants less than 2 months were breastfed exclusively, dropping to 28.5 per cent when infants were 4-5 months of age. Infants age <2 month, 2-3 months and 4-5 months, proportion of EBF were 64.3 per cent, 51.8 per cent and 28.5 per cent as compared to 69.0 per cent, 50.9 per cent and 27.6 per cent reported in 2005-06 NFHS-3 (IIPS, 2007). This slightly different would be attributed to the sample size used, notwithstanding the finding of this study can be validated. The multivariable logistic regression analysis showed that age of infant was a predictor of exclusive breast-feeding practice, infants in the age group <2 months were 5 times more likely to be exclusively breastfed when compared to infants in the age group 4-5 months. Infants in the age group 2-3 months were about 3 times more likely to breastfed exclusively when compared to those infants in the age group 4-5 months. As the age of children approaches higher month, the rate of exclusive breast-feeding decreased significantly, which is similar to studies conducted in Iran, Uganda, Sudan and Ethiopia

(Alemayehu, Haidar and Habte, 2009; Bautista, 1997; Koosha, Hashemifesharaki and Mousavinasab, 2008; Engebretsen, 2007). This might be due to the fact that postpartum care is traditionally given in the first few months after birth where mothers remain at home, creating a chance to exclusively breastfeed their infant.

The present study encountered a number of limitations: the sample size used was small and limits its study ability to draw inferential causalities from the predictor variables and the practice of exclusive breast-feeding as based on cross-sectional data. The limitations include the recall bias inherent in 24 hour recall data, which could lead to a potential for exposure misclassification thus resulting in biased measures of association.

## Conclusion

The prevalence of exclusive breast-feeding was 46.4 per cent of infant age 0-5 months. The current study suggests the need for further intervention to promote exclusive breast-feeding. Being a Hindu by religion, non-Schedule Caste or non-Schedule Tribe, a young infant age and belonging to wealthier household were significantly associated with exclusive breast-feeding. Strengthening promotion of exclusive breast-feeding during the first six months of life, infant feeding advice/counselling both at household and community levels, focus on the factors associated with exclusive breast-feeding need to be addressed and implement the most appropriate and culturally acceptable ones were recommended in order to increase the proportion of women practicing exclusive breast-feeding.

## References

Aarts, C., Kylberg, E., Hornell, A., Hofvander, Y., Gebre-Medhin, M., Greiner, T. (2000). How exclusive is exclusive breast-feeding? A comparison of data since birth with current status data. *Int. J. Epidemiol.*, 29: 1041-1046.

Aidam, B.A., Pe'rez-Escamilla, R. and Lartey, A. (2005). Lactation counselling increases exclusive breast-feeding rates in Ghana. *J. Nutr.*, 135: 1691–1695.

Akri, J., Infant feeding (1989). The psychological basis. *Bull. World Health Organ*, 67: 8–9.

Alemayehu, T., Haidar, J., Habte, D. (2009). Determinants of exclusive breast-feeding practices in Ethiopia. *Ethiop. J. Health Dev*, 23: 12–18.

Bautista, L.E. (1997). Factors associated with initiation of breast-feeding in the Dominican Republic. *Rev. Panam. Salud. Publica.* 1: 200–207.

Black R.E., Allen L.H., Bhutta Z.A., Caulfield L.E., de Onis M, Ezzati M., Mathers C., Rivera J. (2008). Maternal and child undernutrition: global and regional exposures and health consequences. *Lancet*, 371: 243 260.

Blas E., Kurup A.S. (2010). Equity, social determinants and public health programme. Geneva: World Health Organization.

Chudasama R.K., Patel P.C., Kavishwar A.B. (2009). Determinants of exclusive breast-feeding in south Gujarat region of India. *J. Clinic Medic. Res.* 1(2): 102–108.

Dibley M.J., Roy S.K., Senarath U., Patel A., Tiwari K., Agho K.E., Mihrshahi S. (2010). South Asia Infant Feeding Research Network. Across-country comparisons of selected infant and young child feeding indicators and associated factors in four South Asian countries. *Food Nutr. Bull.* Jun, 31(2): 366-75. PMID:20707239

Egata, G., Berhane, Y. and Worku A. (2013). Predictors of non-exclusive breast-feeding at 6 months among rural mothers in east Ethiopia: a community-based analytical cross-sectional study. *Int. Breastfeed J.*, 8: 8.

Engebretsen I.M., Wamani H., Karamagi C., Semiyaga N., Tumwine J., Tylleskär T. (2007). Low adherence to exclusive breast-feeding in eastern Uganda: a community-based cross-sectional study comparing dietary recall since birth with 24-hour recall. *BMC Pediatr.*, 7: 10.

GOI (2004). Ministry of Human Resource Development, Department of Women and Child Development (Food and Nutrition Board), Government of India. Retrieved from http://wcd.nic.in/nationalguidelines.pdf.

International Institute of Population Sciences (IIPS) and Macro International (1994). National Family health Survey (NFHS 1), 1992-93, India. Mumbai: IIPS.

International Institute of Population Sciences (IIPS) and Macro International (2000). National Family health Survey (NFHS 2), 1998-99, India. Mumbai: IIPS.

International Institute of Population Sciences (IIPS) and Macro International (2007). National Family health Survey (NFHS 3), 2005-06, India: Volume I. Mumbai: IIPS.

Ip S, Chung M., Raman G., Trikalinos T.A., Lau J. (2009). A summary of the agency for health care research and quality's evidence report on breast-feeding in developed countries. *Breastfeed Med.*, 4(Suppl. 1): S17 S30.

Jones G., Steketee R.W., Black R.E., Bhutta Z.A., Morris S.S., Bellagio Child Survival Study Group (2003). How many child deaths can we prevent this year? *Lancet*, 362: 65–71.

Jones M.E., Swerdlow A.J., Gill L.E., Goldacre M.J. (1998). Pre-natal and early life risk factors for childhood onset diabetes mellitus: a record linkage study. *Int. J. Epidemiol.*, 27(3): 444–449.

Koosha A., Hashemifesharaki R., Mousavinasab N. (2008). Breast-feeding patterns and factors determining exclusive breast-feeding. *Singapore Med. J.*, 49:1002–1006.

Kramer, M.S. (2010). Breast is best: the evidence. *Early Hum. Dev.*, 86(11): 729–732.

Kramer M.S., Chalmers B., Hodnett E.D., Sevkovskaya Z., Dzikovich I., Shapiro S., Collet J.P., Vanilovich I., Mezen I., Ducruet T., *et al.*,(2001). Promotion of breast-feeding intervention trial (PROBIT): a randomized trial in the republic of belarus. *JAMA*, 285(4): 413–420.

Kramer M.S., Guo T., Platt R.W., Sevkovskaya Z., Dzikovich I., Collet J.P., Shapiro S., Chalmers B., Hodnett E., Vanilovich I., *et al.*,(2003). Infant growth and healthoutcomes associated with 3 compared with 6 mo of exclusive breast-feeding. *Am. J. Clin. Nutr.*, 78(2): 291–295.

Lande B., Andersen L.F., Baerug A., Trygg K.U., Lund-Larsen K., Veierod M.B., Bjorneboe G.E. (2003). Infant feeding practices and associated factors in the first six months of life: the Norwegian infant nutrition survey. *Acta Paediatr.*, 92: 152–161.

Merten S. and Ackermann-Liebrich U. (2004). Exclusive breast-feeding rates and associated factors in Swiss baby-friendly hospitals. *J. Hum. Lact.*, 20: 9–17.

MoHFW (2004). Ministry of women and child development-Government of India. National guidelines on IYCF. Retrieved from URL: http// wcd.nic.in/national guidelines.pdf, accessed on April 19, 2015.

ORC Macro, (2005). National Institute of Population Research and Training (NIPORT), Mitra and Associates: Bangladesh Demographic and Health Survey 2004. Dhaka, Bangladesh and Calverton, USA: NIPORT, Mitra and Associates, and ORC Macro.

Pettitt D.J., Forman M.R., Hanson R.L., Knowler W.C., Bennett P.H. (1997). Breast-feeding and incidence of non-insulin-dependent diabetes mellitus in pima Indians. *Lancet*, 350(9072): 166–168.

Rutstein S., Rojas G. (2012). Guide to DHS statistics. ORC Macro. Calverton, Maryland. September 2006. Retrieved from http:// www.dhsprogram.com/pubs/pdf/DHSG1/Guide_to_DHS_Statistics 29 Oct. DHSG1.pdf. accessed on 25/03/2015.

Setegn T., Belachew T., Gerbaba M., Deribe K., Deribew A., Biadgilign S. (2012). Factors associated with exclusive breast-feeding practices among mothers in Goba district, south east Ethiopia: a cross-sectional study. *Int. Breastfeed J.*, 7: 17.

Shirima R., Greiner T., Kylberg E., Gebre-Medhin M. (2000). Exclusive breast-feeding is rarely practised in rural and urban Morogoro, Tanzania. *Public Health Nutr.*, 4: 147–154.

Tan, K.L. (2011). Factors associated with exclusive breast-feeding among infants under six months of age in peninsular Malaysia. *Int. Breastfeed J.*, 6: 2.

WHO (2000). WHO Collaborative Study Team on the Role of Breast-feeding on the Prevention of Infant Mortality: Effect of breast-feeding on infant and child mortality due to infectious diseases in less developed countries: a pooled analysis. *Lancet*, 355(9202): 451 455.

WHO (2001). The optimal duration of exclusive breast-feeding: report of an expert consultation. Geneva: World Health Organization, Department of nutrition for health and development and department of child and adolescent health and development.

WHO (July, 2015). e-Library of Evidence of Nutrition Actions (eLENA). Breast-feeding-exclusive breast-feeding. http://www.who.int/elena/titles/ exclusive _breast-feeding /en.

WHO (July, 2015). Up to what age can a baby stay well nourished by just being breastfed? Retrieved from http:// www.who.int/features/qa/21/en/.

# 16
# Non-Communicable Conditions and the Poor

## A State level Analysis with Special Reference to North East India

*Mauli Sanyal*

## Introduction

Morbidity and mortality due to non-communicable diseases (NCDs) have been rising at a rapid pace in the last few decades. As per the World Health Organization (WHO, 2012). NCD related death rates in the world have gone up from 63 per cent in 2008 to about 68 per cent in 2012. Moreover, about three-quarters of NCD deaths, that is, nearly 28 million of deaths occurred in low and middle income countries. NCD related morbidity and mortality is projected to increase by 15 per cent by 2020. According to the WHO projections the increase will be more prominent in the WHO regions of Africa, South-East Asia and the Eastern Mediterranean regions. About 82 per cent of the deaths are caused by leading NCDs like cardiovascular diseases, cancers, diabetes and chronic lung diseases.

The situation is no different for India which is going through a period of epidemiological transition. NCD is capturing the upwardly mobile middle class people who are fast adopting the lifestyle of the West. Studies in India have shown a greater proportion of deaths caused by chronic diseases and NCDs like diseases of the circulatory system (Joshi *et al.*, 2006; Gajalakshmi & Peto, 2004). India has been declared as the diabetic capital of the world by the WHO (projected to reach a record high of 8 crores by 2030).

An associated issue for concern is that the burden of NCDs has severe economic consequences like high health care costs, impoverishment of families and the weakening of country economies. In fact the treatment cost for NCD is almost double the cost for that of other conditions and illness. According to Mahal *et al.*, (2010), the share of NCD related out-of-pocket health care expenditure rose from 31.6 per cent in 1995-96 to 47.3 per cent in 2004 in India. The chances of catastrophic hospitalization expenditures are higher for non- communicable diseases like Cancer than when hospitalization is due to any communicable disease and disabilities.

## Research Objective

This chapter tries to analyse the spread of NCD in India and the major states and impoverishment caused due to it. The spread of NCD and its effects across socio-economic classes is studied as a whole but the exercise is essentially targeted towards capturing the condition of the individuals in the lower income group or the "poor". Since NCD has always been viewed as the disease of the affluent, this chapter tries to verify the sanctity of this belief. The exercise will be repeated for the North East states in India to understand the scenario in this part of the country as well.

## Database and Methodology

### *Processing of the Raw Data*

The study is based on the unit level National Sample Survey 60th round data ("Morbidity and Health Care") during the period January to June 2004. In NSSO 60th round there are information both at the individual and household levels. The work is based on incidence of ailment of the individuals in the sample. We have considered only those incidences that have resulted in hospitalization via referral system (hospitalization in the last 365 days).

## Disease Classification

In order to study the disease pattern in the sample we need to classify the diseases into certain categories. There are various ways in which health services researchers classify diseases—some based on general information yet others following specific schemes. Diseases may be classified by their cause (e.g., bacteria, viral), whether they are communicable or non-communicable, and whether they are infectious or chronic in nature. Infectious diseases may be further classified by their specific mode of transmission, incubation period, and portal of entry into the body. In our study of the diseases, we have followed the WHO guidelines but with slight modifications as adopted in Mahal *et al.*, (2010) and grouped diseases into *Communicable, Non-Communicable and Other Conditions/Disabilities.* The details are available in the Appendix-1 to this chapter.

### Diseases and Socio-economic Status

Apart from biological factors and inheritable characteristics, poverty, inequality and socio-economic backgrounds play a role in determining who acquires what diseases. Socio-economic status (SES) is broadly defined as individuals or group's access to the basic resources required to achieve and maintain good health. The most commonly used indicators of SES are education, occupation and income or wealth. Depending on the nature of the disease each social dimension (education, income and occupation) assumes prominence in their effect on the countries health outcome. In our study we have conceptualized SES through income.

*The 60th Round does not explicitly give any income data and so the household expenditure per thousand of the population have been used as a proxy. The sample is then divided into five quintile groups as* Poorest, Poor, Middle, Rich and Richest.

### Hospitalization and Loss of Income

As a person acquires a disease and is hospitalized, he sacrifices a lot of things the most important being household income. Expenses incurred for treatment under various heads, of fooding and lodging of relatives and friends in need, and earning opportunity foregone during the stay in hospital, amounts to a significant loss in income. The situation is critical when the patient is the household head or a care giver. Literature shows that treatment seeking and cost burdens vary by the type of diseases (Russell, 2004; McIntyre *et al.*, 2006). In this study we try to find out the loss of household income due to ailment among various expenditure classes.

From the 60th Round data we chose the entry loss of household income due to hospitalization during the last 365 days as the proxy for the financial burden due to diseases and hospitalization. It is captured by the variable *"rlosshhi"* and has eight categories according to the loss amount. While doing a state level analysis we find that income loss in excess of rupees twenty thousand due to hospitalization in the last 365 days, is negligible for the sample and hence have been omitted.

## Health Care Financing

The impact of health systems payments are examined in terms of burden on households (Murray *et al.*, 2003; Xu *et al.*, 2003). The household's financial burden due to health system payments is generally represented by household financial contribution (HFC). Here expenditure on health includes contributions through general taxes, social health insurance contributions, private health insurance premiums, and out-of-pocket payments. In this chapter, we define HFC as the ratio of annual household expenditure on in-patient services *"ipexp"* to annual household expenditure *"ahhe"*.

The analysis begins with the study of the pattern of ailment across expenditure/income class using descriptive statistics. The next task has been to find out the loss of household income due to ailment related hospitalization. At the end the burden of illness is projected through HFC contributions. At each stage the analysis is repeated with the state level data. The study includes a multinomial logit analysis to understand the association between ailment and income category at the disaggregated level.

## Empirical Analysis

### *Distribution of Ailment (India and the Major States)*

An overview of the epidemiological situation in India (see Fig. 16.1) reveals that CDs (37%) and NCDs (39%) are more or less equal in their spread across the society with other diseases and disabilities just trailing behind.

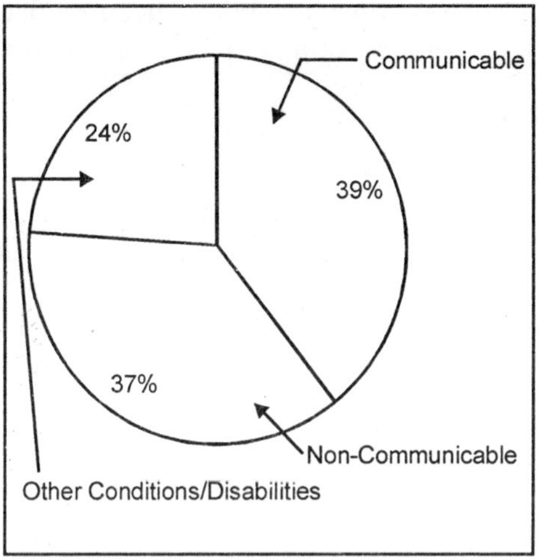


**Fig. 16.1:** Sample Profile by Ailment Category (in %).
*Source:* Author's calculations and NSSO, 2004, Report No. 507.

The incidence of NCDs is quite notable among most of the Indian states (as high as 47.3 per cent in Uttarakhand). As noted at the all India level, the difference between the incidence of CD and NCD is small. In many of the states like Andhra Pradesh, Haryana, Kerala, Maharashtra, Punjab, Tamil Nadu and Uttarakhand, the incidences of NCDs (incidence of more than 40%) have surpassed that of CDs. The details of the NCD incidences have been reported in Table 16.2. There are apprehensions regarding India heading towards an NCD epidemic. Incidentally, these are quite affluent states. Globalization and urbanization might be acting as the catalyst in changing the lifestyle and dietary habits of the Indians thus landing them in serious health hazards like raised BP, diabetes, distorted lipid profile and obesity. In fact four stimulants like tobacco smoking, alcohol abuse, physical inactivity and high intake of sodium are said to have triggered this NCD epidemic.

## SES and Disease

Since we are interested in the incidence of diseases of the poor, our next step is to link nature of diseases with the SES of the persons hospitalized. Literature claims that about 80 per cent of variability in morbidity and pre-matured mortality can be explained through differences in socio-economic status (Adler and Newman, 2002). In this study we have concentrated on the income component only.

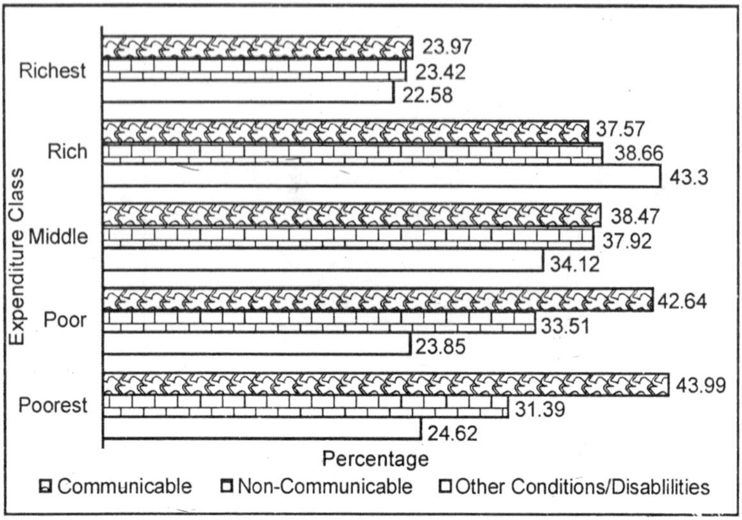


**Fig. 16.2:** Sample Profile by Expenditure Class (annual household expenditure, in %).

*Source:* Author's calculations and NSSO, 2004, Report No. 507.

As mentioned earlier we have tried to approximate income categories through expenditure classes. Initially we find that CDs dominate people in all expenditure classes except the 'Rich' where we find instances of NCDs (38.66%) higher (CD-37.57%). Moreover, this class has a very high rate of the diseases of 'Other Categories/ Disabilities' or OCD (43.33%). On a closer inspection (Fig. 16.2) we find that although CDs dominate the economically weaker sections, the percentage of people affected by any NCD in this class is also quite high (33.51%) and in cases more than the richest section (23.42%). So NCD is not limited only in the upper stratum of the society. Pollution, adulteration in food, unlimited use of pesticides and other environmental hazards might have played a role in this and have obviously affected the rich and poor alike.

To further understand the link between ailment category and expenditure class, we estimated a multinomial logit model (Table 16.1) with the variable "ailment" as the dependent variable and "expclass" as the explanatory variable. The variable ailment

**Table 16.1:** Ailment and Income Class-Regression Summary in terms of Relative Risk Ratios

| *Variable (ailment type)* | *RRR* | *Std. Err.* | *Z* | *P> Z* | *[95% Confidence Interval]* | |
|---|---|---|---|---|---|---|
| Communicable Disease (base outcome) | | | | | | |
| Non-communicable Disease expenditure class | | | | | | |
| Poor | 1.101526 | .044763 | 2.38 | 0.017 | 1.017195 | 1.192848 |
| Middle | 1.369019 | .0554185 | 7.76 | 0.000 | 1.264597 | 1.482062 |
| Rich | 1.429055 | .0578908 | 8.81 | 0.000 | 1.319979 | 1.547145 |
| Richest | 1.779083 | .0722451 | 14.19 | 0.000 | 1.642973 | 1.926468 |
| Constant | 0.7133891 | .0206444 | −11.67 | 0.000 | .674053 | .7550208 |
| Other Conditions and Disabilities expenditure class | | | | | | |
| Poor | 0.997001 | .0443725 | −0.01 | 0.995 | .9164071 | 1.090564 |
| Middle | 1.113462 | .0498321 | 2.40 | 0.016 | 1.019954 | 1.215543 |
| Rich | 1.103321 | .049765 | 2.18 | 0.029 | 1.00997 | 1.2053 |
| Richest | 1.182625 | .0543432 | 3.65 | 0.000 | 1.08077 | 1.29408 |
| Constant | 0.5596234 | .0174449 | −18.62 | 0.000 | .5264556 | .5948809 |

*Note:* Dependent variable is ailment type with Communicable Disease as the baseline comparison group and expenditure class is the independent variable. *Poorest* is the reference category used for expenditure class.

*Source:* Author's own calculations and NSSO, 2004, Report No. 502.

has three values depending upon whether it is CD, NCD or Other respectively. The explanatory variable as we know is categorical in nature (categories have been mentioned before in data base and methodology section).

The model has utilized 32,591 observations. The relative risk ratio as reported in the mlogit model suggests a positive significant (at 1%) relationship between ailment type and income category in India. Also belonging to the richest income class versus the poorest class increases the relative risk of contaminating a NCD as compared to CD by 1.78. The corresponding risk figure is less as we go down the income class. The relation however is not significant for the poor class. The findings reported are in line with the already established notion of NCD as the disease of the rich. However, one might get a different result if further divisions are made in the ailment category to include the chronic and non-chronic varieties and the data on hospitalization as out-patients are incorporated in the study. For the time being we have abstained from it. For the Other ailment category, a high positive significant probability of being affected by a disability increases relatively for the richest class as compared to the poorest class.

The state-level break-up gives a different picture. Among the various income classes we find an equally interesting fact that even in the lower income classes (Poor and Poorest), number of incidences of NCDs has outweighed that of CDs. The pattern gets distorted a little only among the middle income category.

As expected, incidence of NCD is high among the upper strata of the society (Table 16.2). But what is striking is that the states (Andhra Pradesh, Kerala, Punjab, Maharashtra and Uttarakhand) where NCD incidences are quite high among the poor (in the range 36%- 40% and above) are the ones where the overall cases of NCD related hospitalization is also high and there majority of them live in the urban areas. So acquiring NCDs might just be an effect of the living environment in such cases.

**Table 16.2:** Distribution of Ailments among Persons Hospitalized Across Major States in India

*(in %)*

| States | Persons Hospitalized | Communicable | Non-communicable | Others |
|---|---|---|---|---|
| Andhra Pradesh | 2351 | 33.52 | 42 38 | 24.11 |
| Assam | 906 | 58.76 | 24.83 | 16.41 |
| Bihar | 1548 | 41.68 | 32.62 | 25.70 |
| Gujarat | 1361 | 42.69 | 37.91 | 19.40 |
| Haryana | 697 | 34.10 | 44.32 | 21.58 |
| Himachal Pradesh | 677 | 32.59 | 38.67 | 28.74 |
| Karnataka | 1499 | 38.89 | 37.56 | 23.55 |
| Kerala | 1869 | 33.35 | 46.20 | 20.45 |
| Madhya Pradesh | 1564 | 43.97 | 34.74 | 21.28 |
| Maharashtra | 2707 | 35.74 | 38.32 | 25.94 |
| Odisha | 1142 | 47.01 | 25.57 | 27.42 |
| Punjab | 683 | 30.78 | 45.36 | 23.86 |
| Rajasthan | 1519 | 37.59 | 36.80 | 25.61 |
| Tamil Nadu | 2468 | 33.47 | 42.42 | 24.11 |
| Uttar Pradesh | 3997 | 36.87 | 35.09 | 28.04 |
| West Bengal | 2347 | 36.55 | 34.63 | 28.83 |
| Chhattisgarh | 556 | 52.36 | 27.72 | 19.93 |
| Jharkhand | 625 | 40.10 | 36.23 | 23.67 |
| Uttarakhand | 223 | 27.48 | 47.30 | 25.23 |

*Source:* Author's calculations and NSSO, 2004, Report No. 507.

## Ailment, Hospitalization and Loss of Income

An all-India level study reveals that loss of household income due to NCD related hospitalization in many cases are double the amount to that caused by CDs. In 50 per cent or more cases (Fig. 16.3) we find that loss of household income due to NCD related hospitalization is more than ten thousand rupees. This is nothing extraordinary as treatment of most NCDs requires longer stays at the hospital and hence greater abstains from regular life and loss of income both at the individual and household levels.

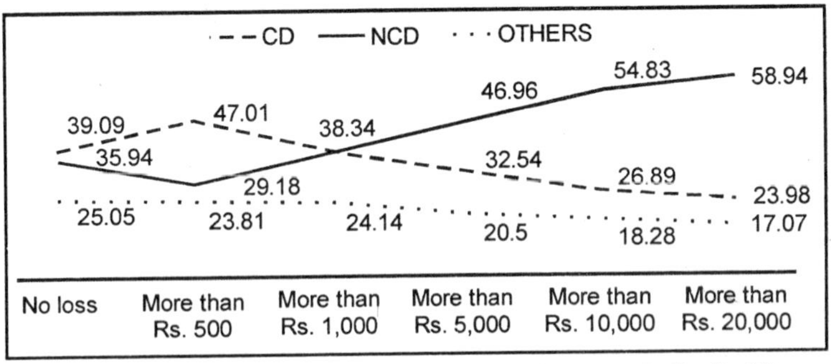


**Fig. 16.3:** Loss of Household Income Due to Ailment in India (in %).
*Source:* Author's Calculations and NSSO, 2004, Report No. 507.

Evidences from NSS data show that instances exist where the loss due to hospital stay amounts to a couple of thousands. In fact as most NCDs are chronic in nature and often involve a resurgence history, instances of consecutive hospitalization can deplete the income base of any household to the extent of impoverishment. In fact, in the last ten years the treatment cost for NCDs have increased by five times in the rural areas and almost three times in the urban localities. So, one can well conceive the plight of an already poor household under such circumstances.

For the state-level analysis we compared loss of income due to NCD and CD only. From the data we find that losses in household income due to NCD in the range of Rs. 2,000 to Rs. 20,000 is quite high for most of the states. For states like Andhra Pradesh (65.52%), Bihar (73.68%), Gujarat (85.71%) and Kerala (70%) of the NCD related hospitalization amounted to more than Rs. 20,000 as loss of income (Table 16.4).

**Table 16.3:** Distribution of Ailments across Income Class among Major States in India (%)

*(in %)*

| States | Poorest | | Poor | | Middle | | Rich | | Richest | |
|---|---|---|---|---|---|---|---|---|---|---|
| | CD | NCD | CD | NCD | CD | NCD | CD | NCD | CD | NCD |
| Andhra Pradesh | 34.40 | 38.89 | 38.31 | 36.98 | 34.64 | 42.92 | 26.85 | 49.38 | 27.60 | 51.95 |
| Assam | 62.67 | 23.33 | 68.95 | 16.84 | 55.02 | 28.92 | 54.55 | 25.45 | 48.74 | 31.93 |
| Bihar | 33.23 | 25.79 | 26.71 | 21.23 | 20.91 | 19.25 | 12.11 | 21.43 | 7.76 | 12.30 |
| Gujarat | 16.35 | 11.43 | 17.21 | 16.28 | 19.10 | 19.38 | 26.16 | 23.64 | 27.17 | 29.26 |
| Delhi | 57.14 | 28.57 | 38.89 | 38.89 | 19.35 | 58.06 | 54.55 | 34.09 | 32.00 | 48.00 |
| Haryana | 6.33 | 3.90 | 13.50 | 10.06 | 19.41 | 18.83 | 24.47 | 23.38 | 36.29 | 43.83 |
| Himachal Pradesh | 14.09 | 8.05 | 25.00 | 26.82 | 22.73 | 24.90 | 22.27 | 26.05 | 15.91 | 14.18 |
| Karnataka | 47.70 | 30.89 | 41.36 | 34.88 | 39.39 | 37.66 | 32.79 | 37.66 | 30.34 | 49.81 |
| Kerala | 28.89 | 48.89 | 36.24 | 44.96 | 31.92 | 47.57 | 35.47 | 43.84 | 32.75 | 46.60 |
| Madhya Pradesh | 44.95 | 30.56 | 47.62 | 29.69 | 43.71 | 35.69 | 43.17 | 38.01 | 38.08 | 44.35 |
| Maharashtra | 38.95 | 32.3 | 41.45 | 53.46 | 31.8 | 40.20 | 34.48 | 41.70 | 33.19 | 41.70 |
| Odisha | 49.73 | 20.87 | 40.18 | 27.68 | 47.06 | 28.02 | 52.04 | 27.55 | 42.11 | 40.10 |
| Punjab | 46.67 | 30.00 | 36.23 | 47.83 | 24.03 | 57.36 | 30.77 | 43.59 | 30.86 | 41.80 |
| Rajasthan | 41.08 | 27.57 | 34.51 | 39.79 | 36.75 | 38.55 | 40.28 | 35.21 | 36.36 | 39.21 |
| Tamil Nadu | 37.45 | 39.41 | 41.9 | 36.19 | 28.6 | 43.42 | 29.18 | 46.88 | 24.29 | 51.43 |
| Uttar Pradesh | 35.54 | 34.35 | 39.3 | 31.65 | 36.58 | 32.53 | 37.06 | 36.72 | 35.67 | 39.90 |
| West Bengal | 44.46 | 27.85 | 40.65 | 32.11 | 32.85 | 35.49 | 32.13 | 36.96 | 27.18 | 45.38 |
| Chhattisgarh | 55.79 | 23.61 | 53.54 | 22.05 | 55.71 | 30 | 40.81 | 37.88 | 44.64 | 42.86 |
| Jharkhand | 49.24 | 28.79 | 42.86 | 36.65 | 37.93 | 35.34 | 35.16 | 34.07 | 32.23 | 46.28 |
| Uttarakhand | 37.95 | 44.83 | 33.3 | 37.04 | 25.93 | 51.85 | 30.00 | 42.00 | 8.57 | 65.71 |

*Source*: Author's calculations and NSSO, 2004, Report No. 507.

**Table 16.4:** Loss of Household Income due to Ailment among Major States in India

*(in %)*

| States | No loss | | Rs. 500 or Less | | Rs. 1,000 or Less | | Rs. 2,000 or Less | | Rs. 5,000 or Less | | Rs. 10,000 or Less | | Rs. 20,000 or Less | |
|---|---|---|---|---|---|---|---|---|---|---|---|---|---|---|
| | CD | NC | CD | NC | CD | NC | CD | NC | CD | NC | CD | NC | CD | NC |
| Andhra Pradesh | 33.00 | 42.15 | 38.48 | 35.62 | 31.85 | 44.18 | 30.94 | 48.62 | 24.32 | 56.76 | 26.67 | 56.67 | 20.61 | 65.52 |
| Assam | 55.30 | 25.06 | 68.78 | 17.30 | 59.52 | 23.81 | 58.44 | 32.47 | 50.00 | 32.15 | 43.48 | 34.78 | 66.67 | 33.33 |
| Bihar | 43.67 | 26.97 | 47.75 | 27.42 | 39.82 | 27.88 | 35.15 | 43.14 | 32.20 | 51.69 | 26.83 | 65.85 | 21.05 | 73.68 |
| Delhi | 39.87 | 39.24 | 30.00 | 55.00 | 41.18 | 47.06 | 21.05 | 63.16 | 0 | 83.33 | 50.00 | 50.00 | – | – |
| Gujarat | 43.87 | 37.14 | 51.71 | 28.54 | 38.71 | 40.00 | 18.87 | 55.66 | 36.51 | 52.38 | 17.39 | 73.91 | 0 | 85.71 |
| Haryana | 50.00 | 44.74 | 18.8 | 15.13 | 15.81 | 9.87 | 6.84 | 10.20 | 7.26 | 11.18 | 1.28 | 6.91 | 0 | 1.32 |
| Himachal Pradesh | 29.55 | 27.59 | 33.18 | 17.24 | 12.27 | 17.62 | 12.73 | 14.94 | 7.73 | 13.79 | 1.82 | 4.60 | 1.36 | 2.30 |
| Karnataka | 41.99 | 36.50 | 48.37 | 26.98 | 26.14 | 43.18 | 24.14 | 55.17 | 16.18 | 61.76 | 31.58 | 47.37 | – | 33.33 |
| Kerala | 34.73 | 44.05 | 37.31 | 45.90 | 38.46 | 39.49 | 27.61 | 52.24 | 11.96 | 69.57 | 20.59 | 61.76 | 10.00 | 70.00 |
| Madhya Pradesh | 43.95 | 33.5 | 52.14 | 23.23 | 43.92 | 36.87 | 39.24 | 45.57 | 35.48 | 45.16 | 6.67 | 83.33 | 29.41 | 47.06 |
| Maharashtra | 34.80 | 38.11 | 45.45 | 29.86 | 31.87 | 38.75 | 25.12 | 50.72 | 33.10 | 50.34 | 18.18 | 56.82 | 40.00 | 40.00 |
| Odisha | 38.54 | 29.62 | 56.42 | 17.84 | 49.72 | 24.86 | 45.10 | 31.37 | 31.43 | 35.71 | 33.33 | 100 | 0 | 0 |
| Punjab | 34.46 | 41.51 | 32.98 | 44.68 | 27.42 | 45.16 | 26.39 | 54.17 | 12.82 | 64.10 | 8.33 | 25.00 | 57.14 | 28.57 |
| Rajasthan | 38.28 | 34.53 | 40.27 | 31.23 | 41.23 | 33.47 | 35.00 | 45.00 | 31.5 | 46.46 | 18.18 | 59.09 | 16.67 | 66.67 |
| Tamil Nadu | 30.93 | 43.17 | 42.94 | 32.69 | 27.18 | 52.26 | 30.99 | 45.77 | 21.81 | 62.50 | 21.05 | 68.42 | 0 | 100 |
| Uttar Pradesh | 36.00 | 32.65 | 42.72 | 29.02 | 38.64 | 35.78 | 32.98 | 41.44 | 26.04 | 49.65 | 32.98 | 50.00 | 28.95 | 60.00 |
| West Bengal | 37.19 | 32.26 | 44.77 | 29.65 | 26.20 | 42.79 | 30.43 | 37.27 | 16.83 | 62.38 | 20.00 | 44.00 | 30.00 | 30.00 |
| Chhattisgarh | 52.43 | 27.18 | 55.26 | 22.11 | 58.62 | 34.48 | 43.94 | 31.82 | 50.00 | 41.67 | 0 | 50.00 | 50.00 | 50.00 |
| Jharkhand | 38.61 | 34.65 | 47.98 | 30.06 | 37.14 | 32.86 | 41.67 | 35.00 | 38.33 | 46.67 | 30.43 | 60.87 | 0 | 76.92 |
| Uttarakhand | 17.80 | 54.24 | 40.43 | 31.91 | 42.31 | 38.46 | 22.22 | 77.78 | 46.15 | 38.46 | 25.00 | 37.15 | 0 | 0 |

*Note:* Percentage of persons with loss of household income in excess of Rs. 20,000 is insignificant for most of the states and is not reported.

*Source:* Author's calculations and NSSO, 2004, Report No. 507.

## Ailment and Out-of-pocket Payments

Two other important things associated with demand for hospital care are access and structure. Out-of-pocket cost for medical care to the patient, length of the queue and waiting time for various kinds of treatment, the proportion of medical care expenditures paid for by the government, voluntary health insurance, or other third-party payers, for medical care, the range of conditions accepted for treatment are the factors that decide the access part. Structure on the other hand deals with the characteristics of the system that deals with what happens to the patient after his/her entry to the system. The study regarding NCD related inpatient hospitalization shows that the hospitalization rate is increasing as we move up the income class. This however does not always imply that NCD is the disease of the affluent. In fact it may be a matter of concern for the poor because of the sublime factors acting on it. It might be so that the poor just cannot afford to avail hospital care as inpatients and not that they are least affected by NCDs. It points to some inherent problems in the economy.

The first one obviously relates to access problems that arise mainly due to the lack of adequate resources and financial protection mechanisms. It deters the poor from demanding in-patient health care even if needed. This in turn exposes the second fact that majority of health care spending is out-of-pocket in nature. Considering the formidable cost of treatment for most NCDs, the rich can only afford it and poor has no other option than to stay out of it.

Incidentally, catastrophic health expenditure is defined as expenditure in excess of 10 per cent and 20 per cent of total household consumption and in excess of 40 per cent of household capacity to pay (Xu *et al.*). It leads to impoverishment of the household. Health care expenditures become catastrophic in the absence of adequate protection and coverage by Government and third party payers. Literature also identifies that HFC is normally high for better off households (can avail private health care facilities) and also those that have a member having chronic illness and disability (Somkorta & Lagrada, 2009). In this chapter, we verified the results as reported in literature with NSS 2004 data for India.

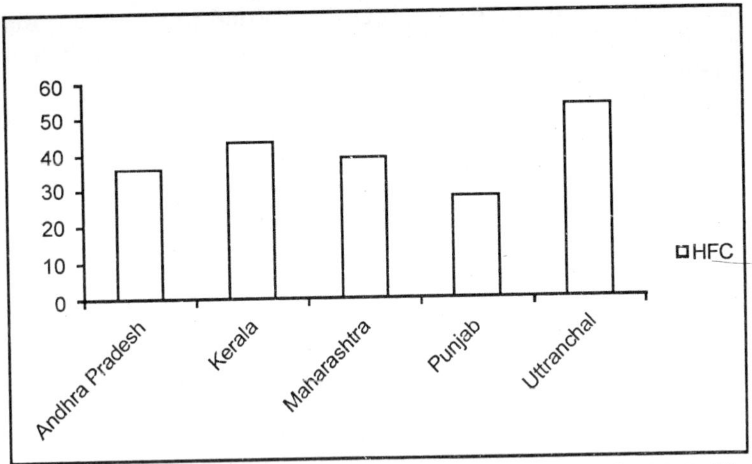


**Fig. 16.4:** Household Financial Contribution for Treatment of NCD (in %).
*Source:* Author's calculations and NSSO, 2004, Report No. 507.

In the study of the NSS data on NCD related hospitalization among the poor we find that at the all India level, for 25 per cent of the instances, HFC is more than 40 per cent. Again for the states where NCD rates are high, HFC rates in many cases crosses the 40 per cent threshold as in Kerala and Uttaranchal (Fig. 16.4). This is indeed alarming keeping in view the fact that many non-poor households can also fall into the poverty trap due to increase in HFC.

## The North East Scenario

Epidemiological study in North East India, however, shows that in general there is predominance of communicable disease over NCD in majority of the states. However, few states like Sikkim, Manipur and Mizoram show high level of NCD related hospitalization records (44.08%). The distribution for other North East states is shown in Fig. 16.5. However, one thing should be remembered that since we are dealing with only hospitalization data, unless the individual or household seek institutional care, their demand or need will not get reflected in the data set. So, it may be so that access, structure or affordability might have prevented the people of this region from getting hospitalized even after getting affected by an NCD. The second probability is that the lifestyle and environmental qualities (or living environment) of this region may be conducive to a good health status in general.

As for distribution of ailments across income class, we find incidence of NCD among the poor is negligible except for Sikkim, Manipur and Mizoram (Table 16.5). For these states, considering the fact that more than 80 per cent of the poor live in rural areas, the results are indeed thought provoking. In fact the huge amount of disparity is noted in the NCD related hospitalization rates across socio-economic groups among the seven states. But if the poor are hospitalized more in Sikkim compared to the other North Eastern states, it can indicate many other factors acting towards it (like development level and state level policies) and not just a higher NCD incidence. In fact higher rates of reduction in the poverty level in Sikkim may have been instrumental in empowering the poor to seek institutional medical care compared to the other states.

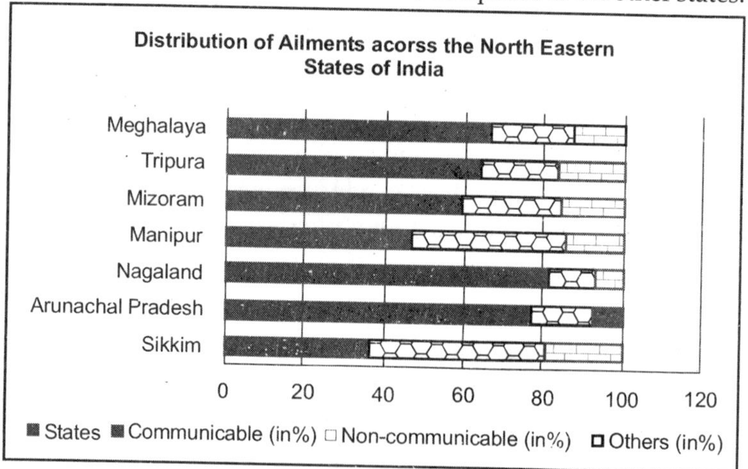


**Fig. 16.5:** Distribution of Ailments among Persons Hospitalized North East India.

*Source:* Author's calculations and NSSO, 2004, Report No. 507.

For Sikkim NCD related hospitalization rate among the lower income group is indeed very high (43.24% for the Poorest and 46.03% for the Poor). The corresponding figures for the households in the high income bracket are comparatively lower (43.59% for the Rich and 33.33% among the Richest). The low rate of

**Table 16.5:** Distribution of ailments across income class among North Eastern states of India

*(in %)*

| States | Poorest | | Poor | | Middle | | Rich | | Richest | |
|---|---|---|---|---|---|---|---|---|---|---|
| | CD | NCD | CD | NCD | CD | NCD | CD | NCD | CD | NCD |
| Sikkim | 40.54 | 43.24 | 34.92 | 46.03 | 33.33 | 46.3 | 41.03 | 43.59 | 33.33 | 33.33 |
| Arunachal Pradesh | 80.56 | 8.33 | 68.18 | 18.18 | 77.94 | 19.12 | 80.00 | 16.00 | 77.00 | 16.67 |
| Nagaland | 60.00 | 20.00 | 85.71 | 7.14 | 84.21 | 15.79 | 86.49 | 8.11 | 78.57 | 12.86 |
| Manipur | 54.05 | 27.10 | 43.82 | 41.57 | 53.69 | 36.95 | 42.49 | 39.9 | 36.23 | 46.38 |
| Mizoram | 38.89 | 55.56 | 65.00 | 25.00 | 69.64 | 12.50 | 64.8 | 18.4 | 53.14 | 30.86 |
| Tripura | 68.68 | 17.58 | 71.54 | 8.13 | 56.38 | 23.40 | 55.36 | 28.57 | 31.82 | 63.64 |
| Meghalaya | 95.00 | 5.00 | 77.78 | 14.81 | 82.61 | 13.64 | 57.38 | 26.23 | 51.35 | 28.38 |

*Source:* Author's calculations and NSSO, 2004, Report No. 507.

hospitalization due to NCDs in other North Eastern states might just be the result of access problems in those regions for the poor people. As mentioned earlier when people do not seek institutional health care, it might be the structural and accessibility hindrances that are acting strong.

Not much detail is available in the NSS 2004 data regarding the loss of household income due to in-patient hospitalization for NCD treatment. Anyhow we find that in case of Sikkim, NCD related loss of income is as high as Rs. 2000 in 60 per cent of the cases (Table 16.6). In Meghalaya on the other hand NCD related loss of this amount is higher (46.43%) compared to CD (35.71%).

As far as health care financing burden is concerned, HFC is not that alarming for the states where NCD related hospitalization rates are high (like Sikkim, Manipur and Mizoram). Instead in Tripura it is comparatively high among the other states in the North East (Fig. 16.6).

The picture obtained is a contradiction to the previous explanations given in terms of accessibility and affordability. Such anomalies cannot be sorted out based on secondary data and calls for detail primary level survey of these states.

## Conclusion

NCD epidemic is in full vogue in the world. The situation in India also hints that NCD related morbidity and mortality is steadily increasing. In this chapter, we focused on hospitalization as in-patients due to NCDs to analyse the situation in terms of effective

**Table 16.6:** Loss of Household Income due to Ailment among North Eastern States of India

(*in %*)

| State | Sikkim | | Arunachal Pradesh | | Nagaland | | Manipur | | Mizoram | | Tripura | | Meghalaya | |
|---|---|---|---|---|---|---|---|---|---|---|---|---|---|---|
| | CD | NC | CD | NC | CD | NC | CD | NC | CD | NC | CD | NC | CD | NC |
| No loss | 46.99 | 37.35 | 74.05 | 15.27 | 80.95 | 9.52 | 65.87 | 23.02 | 56.96 | 26.52 | 61.50 | 20.50 | 67.67 | 18.80 |
| Rs. 500 or Less | 40.35 | 38.60 | 77.42 | 16.13 | 87.50 | 12.50 | 45.45 | 31.82 | 70.83 | 20.83 | 73.96 | 14.69 | 78.05 | 12.20 |
| Rs. 1,000 or less | 25.00 | 45.83 | 79.17 | 12.5 | 89.66 | 6.90 | 34.86 | 51.38 | 64.71 | 11.76 | 45.45 | 21.21 | 72.00 | 20.00 |
| Rs. 2,000 or less | 19.51 | 60.98 | 81.11 | 14.44 | 78.85 | 11.54 | 28.57 | 55.10 | 63.04 | 25.00 | 39.29 | 42.86 | 35.71 | 46.43 |
| Rs. 5,000 or less | | | 71.43 | 23.81 | 80.00 | 16.67 | 32.30 | 54.72 | 62.50 | 25.00 | | | | |
| Rs. 10,000 or less | | | 50.00 | 50.00 | 75.00 | 25.00 | 22.73 | 45.45 | | 50.00 | | | | |

*Note*: "." Denote missing figures.

*Source*: Author's calculations and NSSO, 2004, Report No. 507.

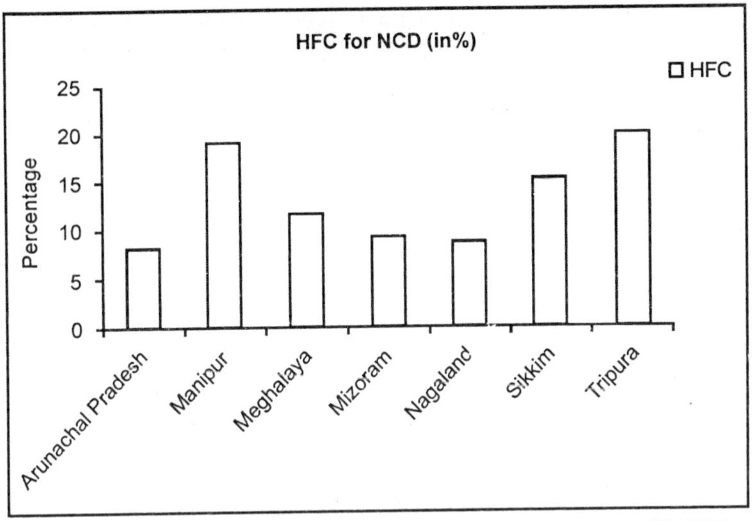


**Fig. 16.6:** Financial Contribution of Household for treatment of NCD in North East India (in %)

*Source:* Author's calculations and NSSO, 2004, Report No. 507.

demand. This is to say that disease for which no treatment is sought for can in turn intensify the menace caused by it. NSS 2004 data reveals that NCD related hospitalization is as high as 37 per cent. Its spread across socio-economic classes show that difference in the rates for the high and the low income groups is not much (38.66% for the Rich and 33.51% for the Poor). So even if CDs are the main causes of hospitalization for the poor in India (42.64%), NCD related hospitalization is slowly picking up. In fact recent figures show that NCDs (39% excluding injuries) have taken over CDs (24%).

The situation prevailing in the North East is very different from that in the rest of India. Even though the 2004 data reveals that CDs dominate in this part of India, the latest figures indicate that NCD has emerged as the killer disease here (incidence of about 60%). In fact Cancer of the oesophagus, lungs, nasopharynx, stomach and gall bladder is very common in these states. In many cases behavioural factors are responsible for this (in Mizoram about 42 per cent of the population has been identified as daily smokers, in the year 2010-11).

Hospitalization is however a derived demand for medical care. As mentioned earlier it depends upon access and structure. In countries like India with its vast social and economic disparities, affordable healthcare is beyond the reach of large sections of society. Health care infrastructure and funding is insufficient in our country and out-of-pocket expenditures are high as evidenced by the NSSO data. So, even if the poor seek medical care, they tend to over spend and adopt risky coping up strategies compared to the rich households. Thus, ill health due to NCD can disproportionately affect the poor. The issue has been under soft focus till date.

Ailment and hospitalization affects individuals directly through the costs of treatment and indirectly due to the loss of man days during the hospital stay and after. In the absence of proper third party insurance payments (about 0.43% of the population are insured as par NSSO 60th round data, 2004), out-of-pocket expenditures emerge as the chief mode of health care financing. In India in 16 per cent cases HFC for NCD related hospitalization as in-patients has crossed the 40 per cent threshold to be deemed as catastrophic expenditure. Thus, the role of SES as the principal deciding factor in determining hospitalization demand does not decrease as in other countries where third party insurance coverage is prominent and active at all levels.

Most of the health care programmes introduced by the government are curative in nature and covers immunization, maternity care and communicable diseases. The range and coverage provided under public insurance schemes are very limited and can hardly buffer the enormous cost for NCD treatment. About 86 per cent of rural population and 82 per cent of urban population are not covered under any scheme of health expenditure support (NSSO Report, 2012). As already shown loss of household income due to NCD is quite high. So, it is quite likely that the chances of impoverishment will increase for the people in the lower income bracket with increased incidences of NCD among them.

NCD deteriorates the quality of life of the patients both economically and socially. It leads to a significant loss of productivity and income. Loss in income leads to a consequent loss in investments in human capital especially education of the children which in turn reduces future income earning possibilities.

The poor family thus gets caught in a vicious cycle of disease and subsequent loss in household income.

It is known that low income countries like India have lower capacity to prevent and control such NCD epidemic. So, the study undertaken is crucial in reorienting the health system to address the needs of the individuals affected by NCDs on a case specific basis. Since the condition of the poor is really bad in this era of escalating health care cost and meagre social security infrastructure, the need lies in the estimation of the extent of push required to help them escape the disease-poverty trap. This however calls for a detailed micro-level analysis of the situation with latest data and primary level survey as and where necessary to get to the roots of the problems. This is so because in the presence of any anomaly between the policy decisions, development programmes and the target group, the victim will be none other than the economically weak and the deprived.

## References

Adler, N.E. and Newman, K.(2002). Socio-economic disparities in health: pathways and policies, *Health Affairs, 21*(2): 60-76.

Gajalakshmi, V. and Peto, R. (2004). Verbal autopsy of 80,000 adult deaths in Tamil Nadu, South India, *BMC Public Health*, 4: 47.

Government of India.(2004). *Morbidity, Health Care and the Condition of the Aged,* Report No. 507, National Sample Survey Organization, Socio-economic Survey, Sixtieth Round.

Government of India.(2012). *Key Indicators of Social Consumption in India: Health,* Report No. KI 71/25, National Sample Survey Organization, Socio-economic Survey, Seventy- first Round.

Joshi, R., Cardona, M., Iyengar, S., Sukumar, A., Ravi Raju C., Rama Raju, K., Raju, K., Srinath, K., Reddy, Lopez, A. and Neal, B. (2006). Chronic diseases now a leading cause of death in rural India – mortality data from the Andhra Pradesh rural health initiative, *International Journal of Epidemiology,* 35(6): 1522-1529.

Mahal, A., Karan, A. and Engelgau, M. (2010). The Economic Implications of Non-Communicable Disease for India, *HNP Discussion Paper,* 2009.

McIntyre, D., Thiede, M., Dahlgren, G. and Whitehead, M. (2006). What are the economic consequences for households illness and of paying for health care in low-and middle-income country contexts? *Social Science and Medicine,* 62: 858–865.

Murray, C.J., Xu, K., Klavus, J., Kawabata, K., Hanvoravongchai, P.,

Zeramdini, R., Mylena, A., Aguilar-Rivera, Evans, D.B. (2003). Assessing the distribution of household financial contributions to the health system: concepts and empirical application, In: Murray CJL, Evans DB, eds. *Health systems performance assessment: debates, methods and empiricism, Chapter 38,* World Health Organization, Geneva.

Russell, S. (2004). The economic burden of illness for households in developing countries: a review of studies focusing on malaria, tuberculosis and human immunodeficiency virus/acquired immunodeficiency syndrome, *American Journal of Tropical 15 Medicine and Hygiene, 7(2)*: 147–155.

Somkotra, T. and Lagrada, P. (2009). Which households are at risk of catastrophic health spending: experience in Thailand after Universal Coverage exploring the reasons why some households still incur high levels of spending—even under universal coverage—can help policymakers devise solutions, *Health Affairs,* 28(3): w467–w478 (published online March 2009;10.1377/hlthaff.28.3.w467)]

World Health Organization.(2012). *Deaths from NCDs,* http://www.who.int/gho/ncd/mortality_ _morbidity/ncd_total/en/index.html [Last accessed on 2012 July 31]

Xu, K., Klavus J., Kawabata, K., Evans D. B., Hanvoravongchai, P., Ortiz, J.P., Zeramdini, R., Murray, C. J.L. (2003). Household health system contributions and capacity to pay: definitional, empirical, and technical challenges. In: Murray CJL, Evans DB, eds. *Health systems performance assessment: debates, methods and empiricism, Chapter 39,* World Health Organization, Geneva.

**Appendix-1**

***Classifying the 2004 Household Survey Response Categories into Communicable, Non-Communicable and Other Categories***

## I. Communicable Conditions/Childhood Diseases

- Diarrhoea/Dysentery, Gastritis/peptic ulcer, worm infestation, Amoeboisis,
- Hepatitis/Jaundice
- Malaria, Mumps, Diphtheria, Whooping Cough, Fever of Unknown Origin
- Tetanus
- Filariasis
- Diseases of the skin,
- Gynaecological disorders
- Under-nutrition, anaemia
- Sexually transmitted diseases
- Respiratory (including ear/nose/throat) ailments
- Tuberculosis

## II. Non-Communicable Conditions

- Heart disease, hypertension
- Bronchial asthma
- Respiratory (including ear/nose/throat) ailments
- Disorders of joints and bones
- Diseases of the kidney/Urinary system
- Prostatic disorders
- Neurological disorders
- Psychiatric disorders
- Diabetes
- Cancers and other tumours
- Accidents/injuries/burns/fractures/poisoning

**III. Other Conditions/Disabilities**

- Goitre
- Eye ailments (cataract, glaucoma, conjunctivitis)
- Diseases of the mouth, teeth and gum
- Disabilities: locomotor, visual, speech hearing
- Other diagnosed ailments
- Other undiagnosed ailments

# Index